# The Biopolitics of
# Breast Cancer

# The Biopolitics of Breast Cancer

*Changing Cultures of Disease and Activism*

MAREN KLAWITER

UNIVERSITY OF MINNESOTA PRESS

MINNEAPOLIS • LONDON

All royalties earned from the sale of this book will be donated to the
Women's Cancer Resource Center in Berkeley, California, http://www.wcrc.org, and to
Breast Cancer Action in San Francisco, http://www.bcaction.org.

Excerpts from chapters 5, 6, and 7 were originally published as "Racing for the Cure,
Walking Women, and Toxic Touring: Mapping Cultures of Action within the Bay Area Terrain of
Breast Cancer," *Social Problems* 46, no. 1 (February 1999): 104–26; copyright 1999 by The Society
for the Study of Social Problems. An earlier version of chapter 8 was published as "Breast Cancer
in Two Regimes: The Impact of Social Movements on Illness Experience," *Sociology of Health
and Illness* 26, no. 6 (September 2004): 845–74; copyright Blackwell Publishers Ltd. and the
Foundation for the Sociology of Health and Illness.

The poem quoted in the Conclusion, "Alive/To Testify," by Wanna G. Wright, is reprinted
courtesy of the author. Wanna Wright is a twenty-seven-year breast cancer survivor and
women's health advocate.

Published by the University of Minnesota Press
111 Third Avenue South, Suite 290
Minneapolis, MN 55401-2520
http://www.upress.umn.edu

Library of Congress Cataloging-in-Publication Data

Klawiter, Maren.
The biopolitics of breast cancer : changing cultures of disease and activism / Maren Klawiter.
p. ; cm.
Includes bibliographical references and index.
ISBN 978-0-8166-5107-8 (hc : alk. paper) — ISBN 978-0-8166-5108-5 (pb : alk. paper)
1. Breast—Cancer—Political aspects—United States. 2. Biopolitics—United States. I. Title.
[DNLM: 1. Breast Neoplasms. 2. Cultural Characteristics. 3. Feminism.
4. Politics. WP 870 K63b 2008]
RC280.B8K568 2008
362.196'99449—dc22
2007050521

Printed in the United States of America on acid-free paper

The University of Minnesota is an equal-opportunity educator and employer.

15 14 13 12 11 10 09 08        10 9 8 7 6 5 4 3 2 1

IN HONOR OF MY PARENTS

*Marilyn and Fred Klawiter*

AND

IN MEMORY OF

*Jennifer Mendoza*

(1964–1996)

# CONTENTS

# ACKNOWLEDGMENTS

First and foremost, I want to thank the remarkable activists, educators, volunteers, staff members, and support group leaders whom I met, interviewed, and came to know during the course of this research, as well as the thousands of unknown, unnamed women and men who attended the numerous meetings, conferences, rallies, protests, readings, teach-ins, and other public events that make up a social movement. They are the subjects, sources, and inspiration for this book. I thank the following individuals in particular (some of whom are no longer alive): Bradley Angel, Kishi Animashaun, Davis Baltz, Linda Davis, Nancy Evans, Ann Fonfa, Mary Gould, Ann Hunter, Mary Jackson, Nancy Johnson, Yvette Leung, Susan Lewis, Allie Light, Andrea Martin, Chris Mason, Marilyn McGregor, Jacqueline Miranda, Josepha Moseley, Pamela Priest Naeve, Sara O'Donnell, Lu Pearson, RavenLight, Joan Reiss, Margo Rivera-Weiss, Irving Saraf, Beth Sauerhaft, Ginger Souders-Mason, Sherry Spargo, Karen Susag, Wendy Tanowitz, Gale Uchiyama, Helen Vozenilek, Jocelyn Whidden, Abby Zimberg.

I also extend a very special thank you to the following women, each of whom played an integral role in the development of the women's cancer community and generously contributed time, energy, and intellect to teach me about the biopolitics of breast cancer: Merijane Block, Judy Brady, Barbara Brenner, the late Susan Claymon, Carla Dalton, Diane Estrin, Wendy Favila, the late Francine Levien, the late Shannon McGowan, Roni Peskin-Mentzer, and Wanna Wright.

Second, and closely related, I express my deepest gratitude and appreciation to the dozens of women living with breast cancer who allowed me to interview them in confidence, usually in the privacy of their homes, and whose names do not appear in this book. The stories they shared and the forms of engagement, exchange, and expression that I witnessed in the support groups they attended taught me to pay attention to the deeply gendered and embodied dimensions of this disease. I am eternally grateful for their openness and generosity of spirit and for the abundant insights they offered. Here, I extend my warmest thanks and appreciation to Constance Cole, who not only provided the spark that started this project but was my friend, informant, and teacher throughout the academy.

Moving from the field to the academy, there are an equally large number of people to whom I am indebted. I thank Michael Burawoy, who supervised the dissertation on which this book is based. I cannot imagine what my years at the University of California, Berkeley, would have been like without him, nor would I want to. I am grateful for Michael's tremendous generosity, his contagious enthusiasm, and his always stimulating, always provocative, always demanding, and always inspiring blend of teaching and advising. I do not know how he manages to accumulate more students every year without abandoning the old ones, but I have learned that his support and generosity extend from the academic cradle to the grave. I am eternally grateful for Michael's steadfast support throughout the years and for the privilege of working with him.

Barrie Thorne also made a tremendous contribution to this project and to my development as a sociologist. I am enormously grateful to her for agreeing to serve on my dissertation committee so soon after joining the Berkeley faculty. Barrie provided insightful, incisive comments, excellent advice, and flawless editorial suggestions. She extended herself way beyond the call of duty, even feminist mentoring duty. She shared her enthusiasm, encouraged me, pointed me in promising directions, opened doors for me, and served as an excellent role model and mentor. She represents what is best about feminist faculty, and I am, also, forever in her debt.

Raka Ray's seminar on social movements first set me off on the careening course that ultimately resulted in this book. In that seminar I began to explore the issues, develop the fixations and irritations, and wrestle with the questions that I later returned to over and over again. I am grateful to Raka not only for her intellect and insights but also for her energy, warmth, and compassion.

Adele Clarke, from the University of California, San Francisco (UCSF), generously provided what the Berkeley Department of Sociology could not: depth, breadth, and theoretical sophistication in the sociological study of medicine, health, and illness. Adele opened her home to me and provided entrée to a wonderful community of graduate students that included Jennifer Fishman, Jennifer Fosket, Laura Mamo, and Janet Shim. Over the years I have learned a great deal from the UCSF gang (as I think of them), and for this I am immensely grateful.

I also thank Phil Brown, of Brown University, for his many acts of kindness over the years. I do not know how or why Phil became my personal patron after I left Berkeley, but I am thankful that he did, and I am grateful, as well, for the shining example that Phil sets of blending activism and academics: he is both a consummate professional and a public intellectual. We need more people like him.

For their thoughtful comments on this book manuscript, I thank Monica Casper, Verta Taylor, Steve Vallas, and, especially, Steven Epstein. For stimulating conversations, comments, and a willingness to share their own work in progress, I thank Susan Bell, Kim Clum, Peter Conrad, Nick Crossley, Joe Dumit, Scott Frickel, David Hess, Nadine Hubbs, Samantha King, Kyra Landzelius, Paula Lantz, Barron Lerner, Ruth Linden, Marie Menorét, Theresa Montini, Kelly Moore, Jackie Orr, Michael Orsini, Jennifer Pierce, Laura Potts, Volo Rabeharisoa, Regina Stolzenberg, Stephen Zavestoski, and the Berkeley Global Ethnographies Group (Joseph Blum, Sheba George, Zsuzsa Gille, Teresa Gowan, Lynne Haney, Steve Lopez, Seán Ó Riain, and Millie Thayer).

Shifting from individuals to institutions, I thank the Berkeley Department of Sociology, the Townsend Center for the Humanities, and the University of California, Berkeley, for their generous financial support during my graduate student years. I also thank the Robert Wood Johnson Foundation and the University of Michigan for the privilege of spending two years as a postdoctoral fellow in the Scholars in Health Policy Research Program. Although I did not work directly on this book during that period, it gave me a chance to rethink some things and move in new directions. At the University of Michigan and the Robert Wood Johnson Foundation, I am grateful to Renée Anspach, Michael Chernew, Alan

Cohen, Eileen Connor, Rodney Hayward, Catherine McLaughlin, and, especially, Paula Lantz for their guidance and generosity. A warm thank-you goes also to the University of Minnesota Press and my editor, Jason Weidemann, for professionalism, follow-through, advice, and enthusiasm at every stage of this project.

Finally, I thank Michael Allen for his risks and sacrifices, and my family and friends for their unwavering support and encouragement. In particular, I would like to thank my mother, Marilyn Klawiter, my father, Fred Klawiter, and my brother, Richard Klawiter. Without you, none of this would have been possible, and I know that you are almost as happy as I am that this book is finally finished! Cheers to us all!

# ACRONYMS

| | |
|---|---|
| ACS | American Cancer Society |
| ACT UP | AIDS Coalition to Unleash Power |
| AIs | aromatase inhibitors |
| AMA | American Medical Association |
| ASCC | American Society for the Control of Cancer |
| BAYS | Bay Area Young Survivors |
| BCA | Breast Cancer Action |
| BCCCP | Breast and Cervical Cancer Control Program |
| BCCPTA | Breast and Cervical Cancer Prevention and Treatment Act |
| BCDA | Breast Cancer Detection Awareness project |
| BCDDP | Breast Cancer Detection Demonstration Project |
| BCEDP | Breast Cancer Early Detection Program |
| BCERC | Breast Cancer and the Environment Research Centers |
| BCF | Breast Cancer Fund |
| BCPT | Breast Cancer Prevention Trial |
| BCRP | California Breast Cancer Research Program |
| BSE | breast self-examination |
| BVHP | Bayview–Hunters Point |

| | |
|---|---|
| CAM | complementary and alternative medicines |
| CDC | Centers for Disease Control and Prevention |
| CDHS | California Department of Health Services |
| CMCC | Charlotte Maxwell Complementary Clinic |
| COA | culture of action |
| COTC | Community Outreach and Translational Core |
| DCIS | ductal carcinoma in situ |
| DDMAC | Division of Drug Marketing, Advertising, and Communications |
| DES | diethylstilbestrol |
| DMAG | Data Management Advisory Group |
| DPH | Department of Public Health |
| FDA | Food and Drug Administration |
| FY | fiscal year |
| GM | General Motors |
| HIP | Health Insurance Plan of Greater New York |
| HRT | hormone-replacement therapy |
| IBIS-I | International Breast Cancer Intervention Study–I |
| ICI | Imperial Chemical Industries |
| LCIS | lobular carcinoma in situ |
| MBCW | Marin Breast Cancer Watch |
| NABCO | National Association of Breast Cancer Organizations |
| NBCAM | National Breast Cancer Awareness Month |
| NBCC | National Breast Cancer Coalition |
| NCAB | National Cancer Advisory Board |
| NCCC | Northern California Cancer Center |
| NCI | National Cancer Institute |
| NHLBI | National Heart, Lung, and Blood Institute |
| NIEHS | National Institute of Environmental Health Sciences |
| NIH | National Institutes of Health |

| | |
|---|---|
| NSMT | new social movements theory |
| ODAC | Oncology Drugs Advisory Committee |
| OWL | Older Women's League |
| PHN | post herpetic neuralgia |
| PPT | political process theory |
| Project LEAD | Leadership, Education, and Advocacy Development |
| RMT | resource mobilization theory |
| SAEJ | Southeast Alliance for Environmental Justice |
| SEER Program | Surveillance, Epidemiology, and End Results Program |
| SERMS | selective estrogen receptor modulators |
| STAR | Study of Tamoxifen and Raloxifene |
| TLC | Toxic Links Coalition |
| UCSF | University of California, San Francisco |
| UOA | United Ostomy Association |
| WCRC | Women's Cancer Resource Center |
| WEDO | Women's Environment and Development Organization |
| WFA | Women's Field Army |
| WHI | Women's Health Initiative |

# Mapping the Contours
# of Breast Cancer

On an unusually clear, hot summer day in downtown San Francisco, I stationed myself along Market Street to watch the 1993 Lesbian-Gay-Bisexual-Transgender Pride Parade. Although partitions separated the crowd from the parade participants, the event itself was highly interactive. Hundreds of thousands of onlookers lined the route, yelling, cheering, and applauding as parade participants wended their way down the street: waving, walking, marching, dancing, strutting, stomping, sashaying, floating, biking, and cruising through the Castro district in this, the official "Year of the Queer." Dykes on Bikes, the crowd-pleasing favorite, kicked off the parade. They were followed by an assortment of queer archetypes and gender benders, including drag queens, drag kings, Doc Marten butches, high-heeled femmes, bare-breasted women, and bare-bottomed men in leather and chains. It was a festive and carnivalesque event, a celebration of queer identities, cultures, politics, and communities.

AIDS was deeply woven into the fabric of this community and occupied a prominent position in the parade. It was represented in the form of numerous political, educational, direct-service, and health care organizations and by various contingents of HIV-positive people and people with AIDS. The crowd was enthusiastic in its support not only of people living with AIDS and HIV but of the panoply of organizations that had sprung up to address the AIDS epidemic. A giant rainbow flag that stretched the width of the street and extended well over a hundred feet was carried by marchers who threw rainbow-colored condoms into the crowd. The crowd, in turn, snatched the condoms from the air and threw coins onto the flag, which grew heavier and heavier, weighted down with the manna that would later be divided among local AIDS organizations.

About an hour into the parade, I watched as another marcher approached leading a small contingent of women. She wore a black leather miniskirt, leather straps, and a narrow black leather band that stretched across her back, curled around her sides, and left her breasts exposed. There was nothing particularly unusual about seeing a bare-breasted woman at the parade, but as she drew nearer, I realized that something was not normal. A moment later I was electrified by the sight of her—riveted by the vision of one large breast next to a smooth, flat surface. What registered for me, in the short space of a glance, was the image of a sexy, leather-clad woman unabashedly displaying her one-breastedness, visually broadcasting her encounter with what was supposed to be a shameful, mutilating, desexualizing, and deadly disease. The sight of this marcher's provocative display was oddly exhilarating, and my reaction was visceral and immediate. Tears welling from my eyes, I yelled my encouragement and applauded wildly.

Meanwhile, the man standing next to me, with whom I'd exchanged pleasantries earlier in the day and who had enthusiastically expressed his appreciation of other provocateurs, was busy having his own, equally powerful experience of this scene and responding in his own, equally visceral manner. "That's disgusting!" he yelled in outrage, as the one-breasted marcher turned and walked in his direction. "Cover it up! Cover it up!" he screamed again and again, as she drew near.

His outburst was a lightning rod for my anger, which grew in intensity as it siphoned the energy from my own, now dissipating, feelings of elation. As we faced each other in mutual distaste and incomprehension, I found myself tongue-tied and confused. I could not explain my rage at his reaction, and I did not understand why the sight of this proud, one-breasted woman had moved me to tears. He, in turn, seemed equally tongue-tied and confused. And so, after a heated but mutually unenlightening exchange of sputtered insults, we moved away from each other and merged again with the crowd.

RavenLight, I later learned, was the name of the performer whose body politics unexpectedly revealed the architecture of the closet that protected women with breast cancer from encountering the stigmatizing gaze of the

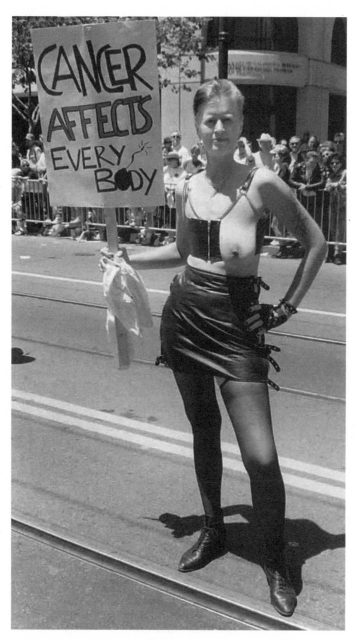

RavenLight marching in the 1993 San Francisco Lesbian-Gay-Bisexual-Transgender Pride Parade. Photograph copyright Cathy Cade.

public and protected the public from knowingly encountering the inhab-itants of this hidden "kingdom of the ill."[1] Without question, RavenLight's display derived its political power from the symbolically overloaded mean-ing of women's breasts in U.S. society. Signifying sexual pleasure and desire, as well as motherhood and nurturing, breasts had also, and with growing intensity, come to signify danger and risk: risk of disease, risk of defemini-zation, risk of deformity, risk of death. What was so startling about Raven-Light's display was that she mingled the "life-affirming" and "life-destroying" meanings of women's breasts in the space of one moment and one body. For me, and I think for the thousands of parade-goers who cheered for RavenLight that day, as well as for the handful of those who jeered at her, RavenLight's embodied politics touched a common nerve, a high-voltage cultural current. Eroticism, motherhood, and death—breasts embody and inspire a heady brew of emotions.

## BELTWAY ACTIVISM AND THE NATIONAL BREAST CANCER COALITION

A few weeks after RavenLight marched through the streets of downtown San Francisco, the breast cancer movement, or at least one slice of it, arrived on the cover of the *New York Times Magazine*. The now-famous cover photo of the August 15, 1993, issue featured a striking self-portrait of the artist and activist Matuschka with one half of the bodice of her elegant white dress cut away to expose a mastectomy scar where her right breast had been. Within days the *New York Times* received four times the usual volume of letters to the editor, and Matuschka reported being "besieged by television networks, radio stations, newspapers . . . and magazines all over the world."[2] Like the body politics of RavenLight, this image of Matuschka struck a powerful chord.

The lead article of the magazine, entitled "'You Can't Look Away Any-more': The Anguished Politics of Breast Cancer," focused on the rapid rise and remarkable success of the National Breast Cancer Coalition (NBCC), the Washington, D.C.–based breast cancer advocacy organization that had recently taken Congress and the White House by storm.[3] Founded in 1991 by a handful of women's cancer organizations scattered across the country, the NBCC was created to address the inadequacy of scientific research on breast cancer; the lack of medical progress in treating, diagnosing, and preventing it; and the absence of the voices of breast cancer survivors in breast cancer policy making.

As part of their campaign, the NBCC organized public marches, candle-light vigils, a demonstration on the front lawn of the White House, and rallies where "breast cancer survivors"—a new collective identity and political actor—demanded more scientific research, medical progress, and public awareness of the disease. Activists argued that breast cancer had been ne-glected by the federal government because it was a women's disease. This history of neglect, they argued, meant that they faced the same repertoire of ineffective medical treatments—"slash, burn, and poison"—as had their mother's generation. Drawing attention to the marked increase in breast cancer incidence rates that occurred during the 1980s, they argued that breast cancer had become "a silent epidemic" and that it deserved the same investment in research as diseases, like AIDS, that primarily affected men (AIDS was commonly viewed, in the early 1990s, as a disease of gay men).

In its first year of lobbying, the NBCC secured a $43 million increase in federal funding for breast cancer research—an increase of almost 50 per-cent over the previous year's allocation. The following year NBCC activists presented President Bill Clinton and the first lady, Hillary Rodham Clinton, with a truckload of hand-signed, hand-circulated, hand-delivered petitions representing the voices of 2.6 million Americans who supported the NBCC's demands for a comprehensive national strategy to end "the breast cancer epidemic." That year NBCC activists and their congressional allies secured an additional $300 million increase in federal funding earmarked for breast cancer research, bringing the total budget to $400 million. Almost overnight, it seemed, an astonishingly powerful breast cancer movement had converged on Washington: storming the gates, forcing open the coffers, and elbowing its way to a seat at the table.

The momentum of the NBCC grew throughout the 1990s. By 1997 federal funding earmarked for research on breast cancer had reached $500 million, and activists trained by the NBCC's innovative Project LEAD (Leadership, Education, and Advocacy Development) were serving on a broad range of scientific advisory panels. By 2003 the NBCC counted more than six hundred organizations as dues-paying members, and federal fund-ing for breast cancer research had climbed to more than $800 million. A decade after it was founded, the NBCC was voted one of the twenty-five most influential organizations in health policy in the United States by congressional staffers.[4]

And that, in a nutshell, is the well-known and widely accepted story of the U.S. breast cancer movement. It is a popular story; it is a true story; it is a compelling story; and it is easy to understand. Like all stories, however, it is also partial and incomplete—partial in that it is shaped by particular ways of seeing and asking questions; incomplete in that it privileges one site of activity and one organization. In this book I tell a different story about breast cancer activism. My account is also, and necessarily, partial and incomplete. The difference—and I believe it is an important one—is that I recognize that my account is partial and incomplete, and I incorporate that recognition into my understanding of social movements in general and my conceptualization of the breast cancer movement in particular.

The problem with the standard account of the breast cancer movement is not that it is partial or incomplete. The problem is that its partiality and incompleteness have been occluded. The same is true of the mainstream models that have guided research on social movements in the United States for the past twenty or thirty years. They have failed to adequately account for their partiality and limitations. As a result, the standard accounts and mainstream models have drowned out the voices of both activists and academics who raise different questions, tell different stories, and offer different perspectives. This book represents an intervention in, and an alternative to, the standard account of the breast cancer movement and the standard models of social movements. I hope that other scholars will interpret this intervention as an invitation to ask new questions about social movements and diversify the stories we tell about them.

But I am getting ahead of myself. Let me return to the San Francisco Bay Area, where the stories that I want to tell begin.

## MAPPING THE LOCAL CONTOURS OF BREAST CANCER

About a year after RavenLight marched through the streets of downtown San Francisco and the NBCC marched on Washington, I decided to take a closer look at the breast cancer movement. First, I wanted to understand why, in the early 1990s, women with breast cancer had emerged en masse from the architecture of the closet and reconstituted themselves as political actors. Why, after decades (indeed, centuries) of silence, isolation, and invisibility, had the experience of being diagnosed with breast cancer become a collectively shared, publicly declared, political identity? What made that transformation possible? Second, I wanted to know why the breast cancer movement was so popular with the cancer-free masses. Why did hundreds of thousands of women, in particular, sign petitions, write checks, buy T-shirts, attend rallies, and participate in breast cancer fashion shows and fitness fund-raisers? Why did this movement resonate so powerfully with so many women who had never faced a diagnosis of breast cancer and probably never would? Third, I wanted to know what the movement looked like "on the ground" in the San Francisco Bay Area. I'd been involved with social movements for long enough to know that the political culture of lobbying organizations in Washington, D.C., and the political culture of organizing outside the Beltway were often as different as night and day. I also knew that there were strong regional differences in the AIDS movement, and I wondered if the same were true for breast cancer.[5] Had the Bay Area's history as an incubator of social movements and its legacy of radical politics resulted in different configurations of activism? If so, what were they? Where did they come from? How did they develop? And where did the body politics of RavenLight fit in?

In 1994 I entered a volunteer training program at the Women's Cancer Resource Center (WCRC) in Berkeley, California, the first feminist cancer organization of its kind in the country (it was established in 1986). Through the center I became involved in a wide range of activities. For the next four years I conducted roving, multisited ethnographic research in a variety of settings: community cancer centers, advocacy organizations, public health departments, research study groups, fund-raising events, educational forums, political protests, street theater, public hearings, town hall meetings, early detection campaigns, political coalitions, breast cancer summits, and international conferences. I supplemented this ethnographic research with approximately two dozen taped interviews and oral histories of cancer activists, educators, cultural workers, and community-builders.[6]

At approximately the same time that I entered WCRC's training program, I began observing women's cancer support groups. Over the course of the next four years I observed support groups in four different institutional settings for periods of time ranging from two months to more than two years. The first group was held in a private for-profit hospital located in a middle-class urban community. The majority of participants were white middle-class women with careers. I attended that group for two months. The second group was held at a public county hospital located in a poor urban community. Almost all of the participants were low-income uninsured women and women with Medicaid, the federal- and state-financed health insurance program for poor and low-income women and children. The majority of women who attended the support group were African American, a significant minority were white women, and an equally significant number were immigrants from Asia and Eastern Europe. I attended that group for more than two years. The third group, which I attended for two and a half months, was organized by an independent suburban community cancer center that served both men and women. The support group I observed was attended primarily by white, college-educated, suburban, middle-class and upper-middle-class women. The fourth and final group, which I attended for more than two years, was organized by a feminist community cancer center. The vast majority of members of this support group, which had been meeting for several years, were white, highly educated, middle-class women with careers. I supplemented this observational research with approximately two dozen interviews and oral histories of support-group leaders and participants.

My research on support groups raised a number of questions about the clinical dimensions and public administration of breast cancer that required additional research. Thus, as my ethnographic research continued, I found myself spending more and more time investigating the history of breast cancer—or, more accurately, the history of the practices through which breast cancer had been medically managed in individual bodies (through screening, diagnosis, treatment, and rehabilitation) and publicly administered across populations (through cancer-education campaigns and the promotion of early detection). I read the work of sociologists, anthropologists, political scientists, and, especially, historians; articles in medical journals and journals of public health; congressional testimony; consensus statements and policy positions of the National Cancer Institute and the National Institutes of Health (NIH); and the illness narratives of breast cancer activists and patients.

Like others who studied the U.S. breast cancer movement, I discovered that a broad range of factors had shaped its development. These factors included the women's health movement, the AIDS movement, feminist and lesbian identities and communities, a network of support groups and patient advocacy organizations, good timing, savvy leaders, compelling claims, sympathetic victims, responsive politicians, the widespread awareness of rising cancer rates, the aging of second-wave feminists, the growing power and visibility of women's health advocates in medical and health-related institutions, the politically charged issue of gender equity in research funding, and the culturally charged meanings of women's breasts in U.S. society.[7]

At the same time, however, I discovered that when I examined the breast cancer movement through the lens of political process theory—which was then (and arguably still is) the dominant model of social movements in U.S. sociology—I inevitably experienced a deep sense of frustration and dissatisfaction. Yes, the "political opportunities," "framing processes," and "mobilizing structures" of political process theory were an important part of the story. These factors were real, they were important, and they justifiably drew the interest of scholars. But the longer I stayed in the field and the more research I conducted, the more I became convinced that the orientations and assumptions built into mainstream models were inordinately limiting because they inevitably led me to minimize, distort, and under-theorize some of the most powerful and compelling dimensions of the movement that I witnessed and experienced in my fieldwork.[8] Existing models, it turned out, were relatively useless when it came to mapping the dynamic relationship between the body politics of social movements and the biopractices of science, public health, and medicine—and it was this relationship, I came to believe, that held the key to a more satisfying, historically grounded understanding of the breast cancer movement.

I describe the weaknesses and limitations of mainstream models in greater detail in chapter 1, and I trace the path that led me to abandon them in a methodological appendix, so I will bracket that discussion for now. Instead, in the remaining section of this introduction, I briefly outline my perspective on the breast cancer movement and my approach to studying it.

## BODIES, DISEASE REGIMES, AND THE BIOPOLITICS OF SOCIAL MOVEMENTS

In the chapters that follow, I offer an alternative, poststructuralist approach to the study of health- and disease-based social movements, generally speaking, and a fresh perspective on the breast cancer movement in particular. Instead of focusing on the narrow arena of formal politics and policy making, this book heeds the call of feminist and poststructuralist critics to move "be-yond the state" in the study of social movements—that is, to move beyond a single-minded focus on the state, narrowly conceived.[9] It does so, first, by shifting attention to the regimes of practices—the *disease regimes*—through which breast cancer was medically managed in individual bodies and publicly administered in populations. It does so, second, by shifting attention to the San Francisco Bay Area *field of contention* and the three overlapping and interacting *cultures of action* that reshaped the local con-tours of breast cancer.

Part I of this book draws on secondary historical research, oral histories, and participant observation of cancer support groups to "renarrate" the story of breast cancer in the United States as a tale of two regimes. Although I am telling a story of historical change, I am not, by any means, writing a comprehensive history of breast cancer in the United States. I leave that daunting task to historians, several of whom have already produced richly detailed accounts of the social, cultural, political, scientific, and clinical histories of cancer and breast cancer in the United States.[10] What I *am* attempting to do in part I of this book, however, is to use the work of these historians, evidence from primary texts (articles in medical journals, gov-ernment reports, illness narratives, and so on), oral histories, and observa-tion of cancer support groups to tell a story about the development and transformation of the regime of breast cancer during the twentieth century and its implications for the emergence of new subjects, social groups, soli-darities, and social movements. In order to do this, I focus on those *tech-nologies of the body* that I believe were central to the social, spatial, temporal, visual, and emotional ordering of each regime. I focus, thus, on medical and public health practices, not medical professionals or research establishments.

In doing so, however, I necessarily ignore the complexity and diversity of women's experience of these regimes. If I did not do so, the first half of this book would become unmanageably large. To simplify, I compare the "ideal typical" trajectory of women with early-stage (locally confined) breast cancer and access to good health care in each regime. This is the group that experienced the greatest expansion in numbers during the twentieth century. It is also the group that experienced the most profound changes in clinical treatment. Finally, although women with advanced breast cancer have been leading organizers, activists, artists, and visionaries in the breast cancer movement—Breast Cancer Action, for example, was founded by women with metastatic breast cancer—the vast majority of women who are diagnosed with breast cancer in the United States these days are diagnosed with stage 0, stage 1, or stage 2 breast cancer, and the vast majority of patients who become activists do so before they experience metastatic (advanced) breast cancer.[11] Thus, because I could not portray the regime of breast cancer from the perspective of more than one group of patients, I chose the group that best illustrates the trends and transformations that were most consequential for the development of the breast cancer movement.

The first regime, which I conceptualize as the *regime of medicalization*, arose during the first few decades of the twentieth century and replaced an earlier era of therapeutic pluralism.[12] During the regime of medicalization, cancer treatment moved from the home to the hospital; surgeons were installed as the sovereign rulers of the kingdom; breast cancer was discursively constructed as a curable disease, and women exhibiting the "danger signals" of breast cancer were reconstituted as the new subjects of the regime; the Halsted radical mastectomy became the hegemonic treatment; and a new social script, dubbed the "sick role," was institutionalized. The sick role reinforced the paternalistic authority and knowledge monopoly of physicians, on the one hand, and the dutiful compliance and forced ignorance of patients, on the other. Finally, the sick role institutionalized a new architecture of the closet designed to ensure that "mastectomees" would be permanently invisible to each other and to the public.

During the 1970s and 1980s the first regime of practices gradually gave rise to a new configuration, which I conceptualize as the *regime of biomedicalization*.[13] The transition from the first to the second regime was marked by changes in the practices of cancer education, early detection, diagnosis, disclosure, treatment, and rehabilitation. Inside the walls of the cancer clinic, these changes in what Michel Foucault terms the "anatomo-politics of bodies" included the emergence of informed consent, the proliferation of surgical procedures, the growing use of adjuvant therapies, the rise of new discourses of risk, the redefinition of patient and physician roles and responsibilities, and the development of rehabilitation programs that diminished the isolation of breast cancer patients.[14] Moving beyond the walls of the cancer clinic, these changes in what Foucault terms the "biopolitics of populations" included the development of new screening practices, their expansion into asymptomatic populations, the reconstitution of normal, healthy women as asymptomatic, the virtually simultaneous reconstitution of asymptomatic women as risky subjects,[15] and finally, the gradual transformation of breast cancer from an either-or condition to an expansive *disease continuum* that included all adult women.

Although these changes did not improve breast cancer incidence or mortality rates during the 1970s or 1980s, they did transform the subjects and social relations of the disease regime, as well as its spatial and temporal dimensions. Importantly, the emergence of new subjects and social relations of disease facilitated the formation of new collective identities, social networks, solidarities, and sensibilities—new forms of what Paul Rabinow has termed "biosociality."[16] These new forms of biosociality, which revolved around shared experiences of risk, screening, diagnosis, treatment, and rehabilitation, were absolutely crucial to the development of the breast cancer movement.

Of course, changes in the regime of breast cancer did not magically "cause" the breast cancer movement to emerge, nor did they determine its content or character in different contexts and conditions. Thus, in part II, I trace the rise of the breast cancer movement and the configuration of movement boundaries, actors, and relationships that occurred in the San Francisco Bay Area. I do not, however, view the Bay Area breast cancer movement as a microcosm of the U.S. movement, nor do I view it as a minor tributary flowing toward Washington or the National Breast Cancer Coalition. Instead, I argue that we need to move away from images of social movements as pyramids with pinnacles or circles with centers. These images inevitably obscure the salience of place and the significance of different fields of contention that are key characteristics of institution-spanning, mass-mobilization social movements.

Rather than bracketing the significance of place by either ignoring it or controlling for it (which results in the same thing), I conceptualize the Bay Area as a distinct "field of contention" with its own history, culture, conflicts, players, and relationships.[17] Finally, I map the geography of this field by disaggregating the Bay Area movement into three overlapping and interacting *cultures of action* (COAs), showing how each COA embodied, enacted, emoted, and enunciated a different vision of what is and what ought to be, and how each COA influenced the others.[18]

Each COA, as I show in part II, privileged different discourses of disease, different body politics, different identities, different strategies, and different emotions. In addition, each COA constructed different relationships to heteronormative femininity, race and ethnicity, science and medicine, corporate capital, the state, and the pharmaceutical industry. The first COA, the *culture of early detection and screening activism,* focused its energies on the expansion of breast cancer screening into medically marginalized communities and on the diffusion of attractive, upbeat images of "breast cancer survivors," a new collective identity, in popular culture and the mass media. Hope, gratitude, the individual heroism of survival, and faith in the progress of science and medicine were foregrounded within this COA.

The second COA, the *culture of patient empowerment and feminist treatment activism,* focused its energies on providing direct services and resources to women with any kind of cancer (for example, medical information, social and emotional support, and practical assistance), amplifying the voices of women with cancer, changing the practices and priorities of the cancer research establishment, and building a vibrant subculture of "women living with cancer," a new collective identity. In this COA, anger was a common emotion—derived in part from a sense that women with cancer had been betrayed by the cancer establishment—but anger was complemented by expressions of compassion and support for women living with cancer.

The third COA, the *culture of cancer prevention and environmental activism,* focused its energies on reframing cancer in general, and breast cancer in particular, as an environmental disease; developing and promoting new policies to reduce exposures to carcinogenic processes and products; and advocating, designing, and participating in research exploring the links between cancer and the environment. This third COA shifted the emphasis from individual risk factors to toxic exposures, and from suffering patients to victimized communities. In this COA, anger was the dominant emotion. The diversity and interactions among these three overlapping cultures of action, as I show in part II, fed the dynamism and success of the Bay Area breast cancer movement.

The approach that I propose here, and elaborate in the chapters that follow, is heavily influenced by Foucault's genealogies of bodies and biopower and the "Foucauldian turn" in the study of science, public health, and medicine. I think of this approach, with a nod to Foucault, as *social movements without the sovereign.* The analysis of power is at the center of this approach, but it is nonetheless a poststructural analytics of *power without a center.* It is an approach that, as many feminists have long advocated,

XXX

INTRODUCTION

places the relationship between power and bodies at the center of the analysis. It does so in part by exploring the ways bodies figure not only as sites of organic suffering and targets for the inscription of power but also as sources of subjectivity, anchors of identity, and flexible, expressive symbols and signifiers of competing discourses and practices of health, normality, risk, deviance, disability, and disease. Above all, the social movements without the sovereign approach embraces the complexity of social movements, the diversity of the strategies they pursue, the myriad forms of participation they inspire, the multiple sites in which they act, the range of goals and successes they achieve, and the sometimes subtle and unexpected ways they shape our embodied experiences of health, illness, risk, disability, (ab)normality, beauty, death, and disease. As Donna Haraway reminds us: "The language of biomedicine is never alone in the field of empowering meanings, and its power does not flow from a consensus about symbols and actions in the face of suffering."[19]

This book thus offers an alternative account of the breast cancer movement, an account that is based, in part, on a different angle of viewing, a different object of analysis, a different set of experiences, and a desire to tell a different kind of story. I hope this book will contribute to ongoing efforts to understand the relationship between the management and marketing of health, risk, and disease and the ongoing transformations of our bodies, psyches, identities, relationships, practices, and beliefs.

## Organization of the Book

In chapter 1, I review the relevant scholarship on social movements, develop the core theoretical ideas that I've summarized above, and provide an overview—or preview—of how these ideas are further elaborated in parts I, II, and III. I encourage readers who are not interested in social theory or sociological debates about science, medicine, and social movements to skim or skip this chapter, as you please. The empirical meat of the book begins in part I (chapters 2, 3, and 4), where I trace the demise of the era of therapeutic pluralism, the rise of the regime of medicalization, and its transformation, during the 1970s and 1980s, into the regime of biomedicalization. In part II (chapters 5, 6, and 7), I examine the development and transformation of breast cancer activism in the San Francisco Bay Area, disaggregating the Bay Area field of contention into three overlapping COAs: screening activism, feminist treatment activism, and environmental activism.

In the final part of the book, part III, I move both inward and outward. First, in chapter 8, I adopt an individual, microlevel perspective by examining the illness narrative of one woman, whom I call Clara Larson, whose experiences within two different regimes of breast cancer help illustrate the impact of disease regimes and social movements on illness experience. Then, in chapter 9, I move outward and upward, highlighting recent developments in the regime of breast cancer and the COAs that continue to mediate, shape, and contest it during the twenty-first century. In the book's conclusion, I review key insights from parts I, II, and III and use these insights to theorize, more generally, about disease regimes and body politics of social movements.

# Social Movements
# without the Sovereign

In political thought and analysis, we still have not cut off the head of the king.

—MICHEL FOUCAULT, *History of Sexuality*

In the United States of a century ago, contagious diseases such as pneumonia, typhoid, and tuberculosis represented the greatest threat to human health and survival. Cancer was of only marginal importance, in both relative and absolute terms. By the 1930s, however, cancer and contagious diseases had switched places. Cancer had become the second-leading cause of death, and contagious diseases had moved several rungs down the ladder.[1] 3the second half of the twentieth century as age-adjusted cancer incidence and mortality rates continued creeping upward and the specter of life-threatening contagious diseases born by air, water, animals, and insects continued to recede. In 2005 cancer surpassed heart disease, becoming the number-one cause of death in the United States. Current estimates are that nearly half of the U.S. male population (46 percent) and more than one-third of the U.S. female population (38 percent) will be diagnosed with cancer before they die.[2]

Cancer, of course, is not one disease but many, and while the incidence and mortality rates of several types of cancer (for example, stomach, uterine, colon, and rectal cancers) actually decreased during the second half of the twentieth century, incidence and mortality rates for most types of cancer (including lung, breast, brain, prostate, and childhood cancers) continued to rise.[3] In the case of lung cancer, a consensus regarding the reasons for the dramatic increase emerged within a broad spectrum of "expert" communities.[4] In the case of most other forms of cancer, however, including cancer of the breast, no such consensus emerged. Between 1950 and 1990 the incidence of breast cancer increased by 53 percent.[5] During that same period, despite the development of new chemical therapies, refinements in radiation technologies, improvements in early detection, and the spread of population-based screening, breast cancer mortality rates increased by 4 percent.[6]

During the 1990s, breast cancer mortality rates finally began to decline. In 1990 the breast cancer mortality rate was 33.2 per 100,000. By the end of the decade the mortality rate had declined to 26.5 per 100,000.[7] The two factors most frequently credited with this improvement were the use of hormonal and cytotoxic chemotherapies and improvements in early detection. Despite these improvements, breast cancer remains the most common cancer diagnosed among U.S. women and the second-leading cause of cancer death (behind lung cancer). The United States continues to lead the world in breast cancer incidence and mortality.

Despite the preponderance of stories and images of young women with breast cancer that circulate in the media, the vast majority (approximately 77 percent) of women diagnosed with breast cancer are over the age of fifty. Age and sex are the two most important risk factors for the development of breast cancer (men constitute less than 1 percent of persons diagnosed with breast cancer). Despite popular perceptions, inherited genetic mutations in the BRCA1 and BRCA2 genes account for only a small proportion—between 5 and 10 percent—of women diagnosed with the disease.

Other known risk factors for invasive breast cancer—risk factors that are widely agreed upon and accepted among epidemiologists and biostatisticians—are low or late parity (childbearing), early onset of menstruation, use of hormone-replacement therapy, ductal carcinoma in situ, lobular carcinoma in situ, exposure to ionizing radiation (including medical radiation), intrauterine exposure to diethylstilbestrol (DES), consumption of alcohol, and postmenopausal obesity. Most of these risk factors, however, are quite weak, which means that they have a low predictive value and are commonly present, as well, in the population of women without breast cancer. The strongest risk factors (BRCA1 and BRCA2 mutations) are also the rarest. In the final analysis, however, all of these known risk factors added together can only account for somewhere between 50 and 70 percent f the incidence of breast cancer. Even the multiple-risk-factors model of breast cancer causality, in other words, has limited explanatory power.

Part of what makes breast cancer so threatening, although it shares this with many other forms of cancer, is the near absence of dependable strategies for avoiding it. Aside from having more babies at an earlier age and breast-feeding them for longer periods of time, there are very few things that women can do to significantly reduce their risk of breast cancer other than having their breasts removed prophylactically. The American Cancer Society (ACS) has identified several factors that appear to reduce the risk of developing breast cancer: maintaining a normal body weight, avoiding alcohol, exercising regularly, and avoiding hormone therapy. The bottom line, however, is that, with the exception of avoiding hormone therapy, the potential impact of these risk-reduction strategies is marginal at the level of populations and unknowable at the level of individual bodies. Thousands of women are diagnosed with breast cancer every year who have no known risk factors other than being a woman and growing older. On the flip side, millions of women are never diagnosed with breast cancer despite having a preponderance of risk factors. It is this stark fact, more than anything else, that underlies and animates the efforts of a growing number of groups to shift the focus of research scientists, medical clinicians, funding agencies, regulatory agencies, and health educators from a public health paradigm that privileges "lifestyle" risk factors to a paradigm that prioritizes the study and careful regulation of what are largely involuntary environmental exposures to toxic chemicals, processes, and products.

The position of African American women vis-à-vis breast cancer is particularly alarming. African American women suffer the second-highest incidence rates of breast cancer in the United States. They are more likely to be diagnosed at a later stage. They have shorter periods of disease-free survival. Finally, once diagnosed, they are more likely to die of this disease than Asian Americans, Native Americans, Latinas, or non-Hispanic white women. In other respects, however, the patterns of breast cancer incidence and mortality do not map straightforwardly onto social hierarchies. African Americans, Asian Americans, Latinas, and Native Americans, for example, have lower incidence rates than non-Hispanic white women. Asian Americans, Native Americans, and Latinas also have lower mortality rates than non-Hispanic white women.

Unlike most kinds of cancer and other life-threatening diseases, breast cancer is more common among white women than it is among any other group, and more common among well-educated, middle- and upper-class women than it is among poor or lower-income women with limited educations. White women are also, however, more likely to be diagnosed at an earlier stage; they are less likely to suffer metastases; and they experience longer periods of disease-free survival following their initial diagnosis. Finally, among all women diagnosed with breast cancer, white women are less likely than women from other racial or ethnic groups to die of the disease. In other words, white women on the whole receive better medical care and therefore benefit more from the medical care they receive than do women from nonwhite racial or ethnic groups.[8] Within *every* racial and ethnic group, however, poor women, women without insurance, and women with less education tend to be diagnosed later, suffer more metastases, and live for shorter periods of time following their initial diagnoses, and they are more likely to die from the disease.

The dramatic increase, beginning in the 1980s, in the diagnosis of preinvasive or noninvasive breast cancer adds a final twist to the story. Ductal carcinoma in situ (DCIS), a condition rarely diagnosed before the expansion of mammographic screening, has increased by more than 700 percent since 1980. Furthermore, lobular carcinoma in situ (LCIS), a condition that significantly increases the risk of developing invasive breast cancer in either breast, has increased by 400 percent during the same period of time.[9] A few decades ago, the standard treatment for LCIS was mastectomy.[10] Now, however, LCIS is typically treated by intensified surveillance: watch, wait, and see. The treatment for DCIS, on the other hand, mirrors the treatment of early-stage invasive breast cancer: surgery, often followed by radiation, and sometimes hormone therapy (usually tamoxifen) to reduce the risk of a recurrence of DCIS or the development of invasive breast cancer.[11] When the media and public agencies discuss breast cancer incidence rates, however, they are referring to the rates of invasive breast cancer. Women diagnosed with DCIS, LCIS, and other preinvasive conditions do not figure into these statistics. They are tracked by cancer epidemiologists, but they lead a shadowy existence in the public discussion—and the public's understanding—of breast cancer incidence. There are thus a significant number of women who have experienced the same medical treatments as women with invasive breast cancer but who are not counted as breast cancer patients. Women with noninvasive conditions, however, often see themselves, and in turn are often seen by other women, as part of the sisterhood of sur-vivors—a sisterhood that has grown to include well over two million women in the United States alone.[12] Women who have been diagnosed with "pre-cancers" of various types thus make up a crucial and rapidly expanding part of the breast cancer continuum.

This phenomenon is puzzling, if you stop to think about it. Mammo-graphic screening led to the creation of a new category of women at risk, or what I call "risky subjects," but this increasingly large category of "high-risk women"—women diagnosed with *noninvasive* breast cancer, or stage 0 breast cancer—did not thin the ranks of women with *invasive* breast can-cer. The diagnosis and treatment of thousands of women with "preinvasive" breast cancer is, in theory, supposed to diminish the number of women diagnosed with invasive breast cancer. In other words, if we were simply diagnosing women with breast cancer earlier, the number of women with invasive breast cancer would decline in direct proportion to the number of women diagnosed with preinvasive breast cancer. But this is not how it has worked. Instead, the number of women with DCIS has grown by leaps and bounds while the number of women with invasive breast cancer has barely declined.[13] It is as if mammographic screening simply created an entirely new category of patients. At the same time, it is worth remember-ing, as previously noted, that mortality rates have finally begun to decline, however modestly, even as more women are being fed into the treatment pipeline.

The improvement in mortality rates that began in the 1990s, however, had not yet been observed when the breast cancer movement emerged at the beginning of the decade. On the contrary, it was the *absence* of im-provement in mortality rates in the face of rising incidence rates that were being reported in the media. In turn, it was these media-publicized dis-courses of risk that breast cancer activists drew upon to frame their de-mands for an end to what the media had already labeled a "breast cancer epidemic."[14]

In fact, one of the main rallying cries of the breast cancer movement was the charge that breast cancer research had been neglected and medical progress had been stymied for decades because breast cancer is a women's disease. Surgery, activists pointed out, had been the first-line treatment for breast cancer since the invention of the Halsted radical mastectomy in the nineteenth century. Radiation, likewise, was nineteenth-century technology.

Cytotoxic chemotherapy, though of more recent vintage, had been used on women with breast cancer since at least the 1950s, which was the same decade that diagnostic mammography came on line. Granted, the use of mammography to *screen* for breast cancer was a more recent development, but even this much-ballyhooed technology, as activists accurately charged, failed to detect 10–20 percent of existing cancers and, even under optimal conditions, could not detect most breast cancers until they had been growing for six to eight years.

Activists directed their ire against what they saw as the male bias of elected politicians and the cancer establishment—the interlocking network of institutions, industries, public agencies, and private organizations that held complementary ideas about cancer policy and cancer research and whose staff, boards of directors, advisory committees, review panels, and financial investors rotated and overlapped.[15] Would men be satisfied with a technology that flattened their genitalia between vice-like plates and irradiated them? If breast cancer were a men's disease, would we still be stuck with such archaic and ineffective diagnostic technologies and treatments? Would we still be dying at such high rates if the burden of breast cancer was suffered in equal numbers by men? These were the sorts of largely rhetorical questions that breast cancer activists posed to politicians, the media, and the American public.[16]

Despite the intuitive plausibility of this argument and the popularity of this gender equity frame, the picture it painted was fundamentally misleading. The rising tide of women with breast cancer and the notable absence of progress in diagnosing and treating them were *not* the result of the cancer establishment's neglect of this disease compared to "men's cancers" or of the federal government's lack of investment in cancer research compared to its research investment in other kinds of life-threatening diseases. Part I of this book will develop this argument in much greater detail, but for now, a quick glance at the prioritization of breast cancer by key institutions will suffice.

Budgetary figures from the early 1980s, for example, reveal that a full decade before the National Breast Cancer Coalition achieved success in the lobbying arena, the federal government was funding breast cancer research at a higher rate than for other cancers of equal or greater significance (measured by rates of incidence and mortality).[17] In 1983, for example, breast cancer research received $47.7 million from the National Cancer Institute

(NCI). That may not seem like a lot of money by today's standards, but it was significantly more than the funding for any other type of cancer. For example, research on prostate cancer, which is obviously a men's disease, received just $10 million from the NCI despite the rough comparability of incidence and mortality rates for prostate and breast cancer. That same year, research on lung cancer—a disease that is diagnosed more frequently in men than women and that kills more people on an annual basis than breast cancer and prostate cancer combined—received just $35 million from the NCI.[18] By 1987 NCI funding for breast cancer research had grown to $70 million. Research funding for prostate cancer, on the other hand, had actually declined ever so slightly, to $9.9 million.

Budgetary figures, of course, are just one measure of a disease's importance, but a similar pattern can be found elsewhere. The number of consensus development conferences dedicated to a particular disease might plausibly serve as a rough measure of the importance of that disease in the eyes of the National Institutes of Health (NIH). Here again, however, breast cancer rises to the top of the list. Between 1977 and 1990 the NIH held more consensus development conferences to evaluate the diagnosis and treatment of breast cancer than it did for any other disease or medical condition.[19] In fact, the very first NIH consensus development conference, which was held in 1977, was designed to evaluate the safety and effectiveness of breast cancer screening by mammography.

Other measures of political salience and visibility lead to the same conclusion. The first major field campaign launched by the National Cancer Program (established by the National Cancer Act of 1971) was the Breast Cancer Detection Demonstration Project (1973–1978), which introduced millions of American women to mammographic screening. Finally, just to examine one more domain, between 1976 and 1985 three major congressional hearings were held on breast cancer. No other disease received this degree of congressional attention during that period of time—and this took place before the emergence of the breast cancer movement or the development of a breast cancer lobby in Washington, D.C.[20]

My point is a simple one: The scientific, medical, and political history of breast cancer prior to the 1990s was not a history of relative marginalization or neglect. As mobilizing frames and political claims, such characterizations are compelling. As historical insights, however, they are fundamentally misleading.

Let me pause for a moment to clarify what I am and am not arguing. First, I am not arguing that the institution of medicine has been particularly responsive to women and their health concerns. Not at all. The sexism, paternalism, and patriarchalism of the medical establishment—medical research and clinical medicine—during the twentieth century is a well-established fact.[21] Second, I am not arguing that the medical profession was particularly attentive to the needs of women with breast cancer. No indeed—as we shall later see. What was true of American medicine's treatment of women in general was also true of physicians' treatment of women with breast conditions. In other words, the medical profession's thorough investment in patriarchal forms of power, paternalistic practices, and sexist assumptions, which certainly carried over into physicians' treatment of breast cancer patients, is a well-established fact.[22]

This does not mean, however, that the disease of breast cancer or the women who were diagnosed with breast cancer were marginalized, overlooked, or neglected relative to other forms of cancer and other kinds of cancer patients, or that cancer and cancer patients were marginalized and overlooked by federal funding agencies relative to other life-threatening diseases. There is simply no convincing evidence of this. It is tempting to generalize from one set of experiences and conditions to another, but it is a mistake. Cancer, for example, was the first disease to inspire the establishment of a separate institute within the NIH (which occurred in 1937), and the NCI has always been the eight-hundred-pound gorilla of NIH agencies. More importantly, there is simply no evidence that women with breast cancer fared worse, were more neglected, or occupied a more structurally disadvantaged position in the medical or research establishments than other cancer patients.

If we were to focus on those groups that were systematically marginalized, neglected, or excluded from the concerns of cancer educators, researchers, and clinicians, women with breast cancer would not be at the top of list. This is even more true for women from the sociodemograhic group—white, middle-class, well-educated, and insured—that spearheaded the breast cancer movement. In fact, the list would be organized around a different set of categories altogether. People without insurance, low-income people, members of racial and ethnic minorities, immigrants, and the elderly would be at the top the list of groups that were systematically marginalized, neglected, and excluded from the concerns of cancer educators, researchers, and clinicians. The cancer movement that emerged during the 1990s, however, did not emerge from those groups. Like most of the health- and disease-based social movements and patient advocacy organizations that have emerged since the late 1960s, the breast cancer movement emerged from the white, urban, educated, insured, middle classes. This was not the most *marginalized* group of cancer patients but rather the most *medicalized*. Yet medicalization, according to the collective wisdom of medical sociologists and feminist critics, is a deeply depoliticizing and individualizing process. How can we make sense of this paradox? Hold that thought, and I will return to it in just a moment.

Whether or not breast cancer was neglected by the cancer establishment relative to other forms of cancer, and whether or not women diagnosed with breast cancer occupied a uniquely disadvantaged position in the pantheon of cancer victims, however, the fact remains that by the early 1990s the billions of dollars poured into cancer research by the federal government since World War II had yielded very little for most groups of cancer patients, including women with breast cancer.[23] My point, then, is not that women with breast cancer were sitting pretty, so to speak, but rather that no one was in particularly good shape. Why, then, after all this time, did women with breast cancer mobilize when other cancer patients remained socially isolated, silent, and invisible?

A satisfying answer to this question requires, first, that we abandon the popular origin myths of the breast cancer movement that frame this disease and its sufferers as particularly marginalized by and within the medical research and cancer establishments. It requires, second, that we rethink key assumptions in medical sociology and medicalization theory regarding the depoliticizing and individualizing effects of medicine. Finally, a satisfying explanation to this question requires that we move beyond the state-centered and economy-centered approaches that have guided the last few decades of research on social movements, but that we do so without abandoning an analysis of the influential practices of powerful institutions.

In the next section I provide a brief overview and critique of the state- and economy-centered models that have guided structurally oriented research on the development of social movements since the 1980s. Both models, I argue, are cracked at their foundation because neither offers an adequate conceptualization of power in its contemporary guises and manifestations. An alternative approach, which I outline in the subsequent sections, provides a more adequate theorization of power and its relationship to bodies, (bio)-medicalization, and social movements. I conceptualize this alternative approach as *social movements without the sovereign* and show, in the second half of this chapter, how it enables new angles of viewing and new insights into the development and diversity of the breast cancer movement.

## The Structural Origins and Development of Social Movements

During the last three decades, two main approaches have dominated scholarship on the structural influences and origins of social movements. The first, political process theory (PPT), grew out of a tradition in North American scholarship known as resource mobilization theory. Charles Tilly, Mayer Zald, Doug McAdam, John McCarthy, and Sydney Tarrow are key architects of this research program, which has dominated social movements scholarship for more than two decades. The second, new social movements theory (NSMT), grew out of a European tradition of Marxist analysis and critical theory. Alberto Melucci, Jürgen Habermas, Jean Cohen, Alain Touraine, and Claus Offe are key architects of NSMT. Although these research programs have yielded a number of important insights and a mountain of case studies, the empirical blind spots, intellectual aporias, and misguided assumptions (discussed below) of both paradigms have become increasingly problematic. PPT and NSMT continue to influence the work of many scholars, but there is a growing consensus that the foundations of these research programs are cracked and sinking.

Dissatisfied with these structural paradigms, scholars have increasingly abandoned them in favor of social constructionist approaches that emphasize the agentic dimensions of social movements. This was always an important research tradition, but it became stronger during the 1990s as researchers incorporated insights from the sociology of culture, gender, emotions, and identity.[24] As a result of this social constructionist turn, we now have a much stronger understanding of the expressive, emotive, discursive, interpretive, identity- and solidarity-building activities in which social movement actors engage.[25] Thus, the degeneration, in the Lakatosian sense, of the structuralist research program has in many respects provided impetus for innovation in social constructionist approaches to the study of social movements.[26] This is a wholly positive development, in my opinion, but I nonetheless believe that it would be a mistake to abandon the effort to think structurally about social movements, even as we embrace the social constructionist turn.

Social movements are prime examples of voluntary action and collective agency, of course, but they are also shaped by structural forces. Structural forces, to put it simply, are elements that cannot be wished away or avoided. Structural forces impose themselves on us whether we like it or not and whether we realize it or not. They shape the external world "outside," and they shape the internal world "inside"—the world, that is, that is *us* as *subjects*, as *selves*. These structural forces are not confined to the state, the economy, or any other institution, and they do not feed or facilitate the development of only one type of resistance or social movement.

Below, I provide a brief overview of PPT and NSMT. I paint these paradigms in broad strokes in order to highlight their major claims and weaknesses. Following my overview of these paradigms, I propose a new approach that I contend is better suited to studying the structural dimensions of social movements.

*Political Process Theory*

Political process theory, as previously noted, grew out of a tradition of scholarship known as resource mobilization theory (RMT), which focused on "the critical role of resources and formal organization in the rise of social movements."[27] The political process model added political opportunities to the list of necessary resources, "stress[ing] the crucial importance of expanding political opportunities as the ultimate spur to collective action."[28] There have been many versions of PPT over the years, but the one thing on which its main architects seemed to agree, at least until recently, was that the primary enabler, suppressor, and target of social movements was the nation-state, conventionally understood.

What I am calling the "strong program" of PPT posited that political opportunities were a necessary ingredient in the development and success of social movements. According to the logic of the strong program, political opportunities do not directly *cause* social movements, but social movements do develop in response to political openings and opportunities and do not succeed without them. Although the strong program was popular a decade or so ago, no one at this point, as Charles Kurzman has recently observed, seems willing to defend it.[29]

The "weak program" of PPT, where many of the architects of the strong program can now be found, is considerably less grandiose in its ambitions and considerably more restrained in its generalizations. The weak program extends the list of key resources by explicitly incorporating into its model of social movements David Snow's concept of "framing processes," which Doug McAdam, John McCarthy, and Mayer Zald define as "the conscious strategic efforts by groups of people to fashion shared understandings of the world and of themselves that legitimate and motivate collective action."[30] The inclusion of framing processes in the model was a response to widespread criticisms that resource mobilization and political process theorists had underestimated the causal importance of cultural factors such as ideas, perceptions, and sentiments in the development and success of social movements. Although framing processes, in the hands of McAdam, McCarthy, and Zald, constituted a rather minimalist and mentalistic interpretation of culture, theirs was a step in the right direction. Still, though, there was a reason that PPT did not change its name, and that reason is that the state remained the main actor and the punch line of the theory.

More recently, in response to a growing chorus of criticism that PPT grossly overestimated the primacy of the state as the *target* of social movements, leading figures in this research program have redefined their object of study and further restricted their claims to what they term "contentious politics."[31] PPT, they explain, was never intended to serve as a general model of *all* social movements, only of movements that engage in contentious politics. Contentious politics, they argued, have the state as their primary target. The study of other kinds of social movements, they conceded, would of course demand other kinds of theories. Political process theorists nonetheless suggested that it might be best if social movements scholars restricted their focus to the study of social movements that fit the PPT criterion. We can thus think of the theory of contentious politics as the weakest program—weakest in the sense that the claims of PPT have been further scaled back and reduced.

Recent work by Nella Van Dyke, Sarah Soule, and Verta Taylor, however, calls into question the empirical claims of even the weakest version of PPT.[32] Van Dyke, Soule, and Taylor point out that there is an abundance of scholarship (outside the citation networks of PPT) showing very clearly that social movements that engage in contentious politics target a wide variety of institutions—work, medicine, education, religion, the military, and the media. To make their point in the strongest possible terms, Van Dyke, Soule, and

Taylor undertook a quantitative analysis of the targets of contentious politics across social movements. Analyzing newspaper coverage of all "protest events" between 1968 and 1975, they demonstrated that protest events—which certainly qualify as contentious politics—were associated with a wide variety of social movements, including the civil rights, environmental, peace, international, human rights, women's, and gay and lesbian movements, among others. Their results clearly demonstrated that although public protests and other forms of contentious politics often targeted the state, they also often targeted other audiences and institutions. Furthermore, as they pointed out, although public protests and other forms of "contentious activism" constituted the most visible and easy-to-measure evidence of movement activity, protest events are just one small part of a much larger repertoire of political action engaged in by social movements.

In addition to the problem of PPT's unsupportable empirical claims, there is the larger issue of its blind spots and aporias. One of the most dissatisfying aspects of this research program, in my view, is that it ignores the causes and experiences of suffering and injustice that inspire and animate social movements. According to the logic of PPT (and RMT, for that matter), since injustice and suffering (experiences of pain, loss, domination, marginalization, inequality, exclusion, and the like) are omnipresent and endemic in modern societies, these experiences cannot provide explanatory purchase on the development of social movements. PPT thus brackets, at the level of theory, what social movements scholars antiseptically call "grievances" in order to focus its analytic lens on the mobilizing structures, framing processes, and political opportunities that are drawn upon and mobilized by social movements. One of the most unfortunate outcomes of this approach is that after thirty years of case studies, PPT has generated no theoretical insights into the relationship among suffering, subjectivity, and social movements. The deep structure of assumptions that undergirds PPT systematically erases the possibility of posing, much less pursuing, this line of questioning.

This does not mean that the study of political structures, processes, and opportunities is unproductive or that it is irrelevant to the development of the breast cancer movement. There are, in fact, a number of important studies of the breast cancer movement that grew out of the tradition represented by PPT. In "Breast Cancer Policymaking," for example, Carol Weisman convincingly argues that a combination of good timing and skill in strategically exploiting political openings and opportunities enabled the breast cancer movement to score significant policy achievements during the 1990s.[33] Unlike proponents of mainstream PPT, however, Weismann wisely does not generalize from federal policy making to the entire movement, nor does she mistake the one for the other. Instead, Weisman uses PPT to show how expanding political opportunities fed the success of breast cancer advocacy in the policy-making arena. This is what PPT does best. Nothing more. Nothing less.

Likewise, in *The Politics of Breast Cancer* Maureen Hogan Casamayou focuses on the lobbying successes of the NBCC in the federal arena of science policy making and research funding. Casamayou, a political scientist, explains the NBCC's success as the result of a "triple alliance," which she defines as a political structure "composed of protective congressional representatives with important committee posts, skillful executive agency personnel, and aggressive and resourceful interest group supporters."[34] Casamayou's "conventional political approach," however, as Ulrike Boehmer argues, has both advantages and disadvantages. It is an effective approach for understanding "traditional lobbying tactics," "power-broking in Washington," and the "multiple access points used by the NBCC to influence breast cancer policy."[35] It does so, however, as Boehmer argues, at the cost of ignoring important conflicts and differences within the breast cancer movement, including conflicts over the very definition of cancer activism, the importance of environmental research and alliances, relationships with corporate America and the pharmaceutical industry, and so on. Focusing on political insiders and lobbying tactics, Boehmer suggests, leads to a partial and distorted view of the larger movement. Boehmer's claims are consistent with a 1996 article by Verta Taylor and Marieke Van Willigan in which they argue that the breast cancer and postpartum movements challenge the gender order in ways that remained unrecognizable and incomprehensible from within the confines of conventional social movements theory.[36]

Finally, Jennifer Myhre's exemplary study of science activism, science policy, and the NBCC delivers the coup de grâce to PPT and its claims regarding contentious politics.[37] First, Myhre argues that although the breast cancer movement employed the conventional tactics associated with contentious politics (public rallies, protests, petitions, and so on), it was the *consensus-building* character of the NBCC's style of engagement that fed its success in the national policy-making arena. Myhre concludes that although contentiousness may attract the lion's share of attention in the media and the scholarship on social movements, we should pay more attention to the consensus character of social movement strategies and tactics. Second, and relatedly, Myhre argues that the emphasis on educating its constituents and providing advanced training in science literacy (through Project LEAD) was a key to the NBCC's success. Science education increased breast cancer activists' credibility among scientists and science-policy communities and ensured the reproduction of lay expertise. Third, Myhre argues that gender structured activists' encounters with the communities of policy makers, scientists, and physicians in ways that both helped and hindered.

Although Myhre's work suffers from the occupational hazard of generalizing from one organization to the movement as a whole—in this case, using the terms "the NBCC" and "the breast cancer movement" as if they were synonymous—her larger contribution to social movements theory is unassailable. In her words: "The scholarly emphasis on *contention*—protest and violence—and on *politics*—interactions with the state—fails to account for the nature and impact of breast cancer activism." Finally, Myhre argues that "gender not only shapes the arenas in which social movements act but also the very ways in which scholars conceptualize and theorize those arenas and actions."[38] Political process theory, as Myhre argues throughout her study, has been hampered by its androcentric bias—what Myhre terms its "masculinist" assumptions.

For these reasons and others there is a growing sense of dissatisfaction with PPT's limited vision, even among figures who were integral to its development. There is a growing consensus, in the words of Jeff Goodwin and James Jasper, that the main strands of PPT are, depending on how they are understood, "tautological, trivial, inadequate, or just plain wrong." In my view, the scholarship on women's movements clearly demonstrates that not a single core claim of PPT theory can hold up under scrutiny. At best, as Goodwin and Jasper argue, PPT "provides a helpful, albeit limited, set of 'sensitizing concepts' for social movements research."[39] These sensitizing concepts, however, have more than served their purpose. The state and the political environment are no longer terra incognita to social movements scholars. It is now time, in the words of Van Dyke, Soule, and Taylor, to "move beyond a focus on the state"—or rather, to move beyond a single-minded focus on a narrow band of activities that target the state, narrowly conceived.[40]

Again, to restate the point: I am not arguing that the state is unimportant or that scholars should ignore it. I am arguing that we need to move beyond the political process model of the relationship between states and social movements because (1) it brackets the question of suffering; (2) its androcentric bias marginalizes less-contentious forms of activism—including the construction of new forms of identity, cultural expression, and community, as well as the development of lay expertise, patient empowerment, social support, and practical services; (3) it lacks a (useful) theory of how power operates in wealthy Western democracies; (4) it relies upon a narrow, utterly simplistic conceptualization of the state; (5) it fails to take account of two of the most important developments of the last fifty years: the phenomenal growth in the power and scope of science and medicine and the ever-increasing "interpenetration," in the words of Steven Epstein, of the state, science, medicine, and social movements.[41]

*New Social Movements Theory*

New social movements theory, unlike political process theory, did not bracket the causes of conflict and suffering in its model of social movements. In fact, NSMT sought to explain the rise of what it called "new social movements" by analyzing the emergence of new sources of conflict and suffering in late capitalist or postindustrial societies. Why, new social movements theorists wondered, were Marxist expectations regarding the revolutionary role of the working class so, well, wrong? Why did so many new movements emerge instead from the middle classes? Why did they foreground issues of identity but not of class? Why, in the language of Nancy Fraser, did the "politics of recognition" overtake (or so NSMT maintained) the "politics of redistribution"?[42] Finally, NSMT strove, in its careful study of social movements, to uncover new insights about the forms of conflict and suffering produced by the macrostructural transformations that they observed in advanced capitalist societies.

Whereas PPT looked to the domain of formal politics for answers to its questions, NSMT argued that unlocking the mysteries of the new wave of postwar social movements required a better understanding of large-scale transformations in advanced, (post)industrial capitalism. NSMT argued that the new social movements of the 1960s and 1970s—the student movement, the environmental movement, the civil rights movement, the peace movement, the women's movement, the lesbian and gay movement, and so on—revealed that a shift had taken place in the "core" conflict of advanced capitalist societies. NSMT argued that the expansion of the state into the private sphere and the rationalization of life—the colonization of the "lifeworld," in Habermasian terms—had produced new sources of domination and hence new social movements.

NSMT did, in fact, put its finger on a number of important transformations in the functioning and forms of domination in late-capitalist societies. The problem with NSMT was that, like PPT, it tried to explain everything according to one logic, one teleology, one variable. Consistent with the long tradition of Marxist thinking, it sought to identify the one essential conflict at the core of transformations in late capitalism that could explain the logic of "new social movements."

Whereas PPT argued that social movements targeted the state and emphasized its policy-oriented goals and activities, NSMT made the opposite claim: Contemporary social movements, NSMT argued, were marked by a pronounced tendency to eschew the state and policy-oriented action in favor of lifestyle issues and the creation of space for the expansion and expression of new identities. NSMT's claims, however, were just as one-sided as PPT's characterizations. Most social movements of any size and longevity necessarily engage in both instrumental and expressive action, target the state and other institutions, and pursue a politics of recognition *and* redistribution.

A second problem with NSMT was that, unlike PPT, which was frustratingly ahistorical at the level of theory, NSMT made specific historical claims that upon closer examination (that is, upon consulting the work of historians) turned out to simply not be true. As historians of public health and medicine well know, for example, middle-class movements organized around health, disease, and the body were hardly an invention of the 1960s—or even, for that matter, of the twentieth century. The pre-1960s history of the United States is chock-full of health- and disease-related social movements of both minor and major significance, including the antituberculosis movement, the public hygiene movement, the temperance movement, the birth control movement, antivaccination and antifluoridation movements, and many others.[43] This does not mean that there were no significant differences in the movements that emerged before and after the 1960s, but these differences cannot be understood in terms of the rise of supposedly noneconomic issues such as health or in terms of the salience of identity. Thus, core empirical claims of NSMT, just like core empirical claims of PPT, were simply wrong.[44]

NSMT was not alone in exploring the relationship between collective identity and social movements.[45] What was original about NSMT's contribution, however, was that it strove to link the development of new collective identities to macrostructural changes in late capitalism. NSMT overestimated the necessity of a tight coupling between new identities and economic transformations, but it was right to draw attention to the relationship between historically shifting practices of power, the emergence of new identities, and the development of social movements. NSMT's efforts to theorize and map the relationship between historically shifting macrostructures and the development of new identities was nonetheless an important contribution to social movements theory, and it continues to generate innovative research.[46]

The Italian theorist Alberto Melucci, whose work exemplifies the best of this tradition, offered an elegant theory of the relationship between macrostructural changes in "post-industrial society" and the new collective identities constructed and mobilized by new social movements. Like many others, Melucci argued that macrolevel changes in advanced capitalism made certain sites of production, such as science, medicine, and other forms of expertise, and certain sites of appropriation and consumption, such as the body, health, and identity, key loci of domination, conflict, control, and resistance.[47] Melucci, for example, argued that "in comparison with the industrial phase of capitalism, the production characteristic of advanced [capitalist] societies require[d] that control reach beyond the productive structure into the areas of consumption, services, and social relations."[48] As a result, he theorized, these macrolevel changes created new sources of conflict and reorganized the social terrain on which they operated. According to Melucci, this reorganized terrain facilitated the development of new collective identities and identity-oriented social movements.

Melucci argued that collective identities are socially constructed, unfixed phenomena that emerge out of face-to-face negotiated interactions and the creation of new "cultural codes" and social practices. These processes transpire in what he called the "submerged networks" and "cultural laboratories" that constitute the "invisible pole" of contemporary social movements. Ultimately, then, Melucci believed that the link between macrostructures and movement identities was mediated by constellations of submerged networks that emerged in response to macrolevel changes in the structure and functioning of capitalism. The new collective identities and the social movements they fed were therefore both structurally produced and socially constructed.

But just how do macrostructural changes in capitalism congeal into the subterranean social networks that serve as the cultural laboratories of new collective identities and social movements? What are the actual practices and structural mechanisms that produce these effects? To these questions, neither Melucci nor other new social movements theorists provide an answer.

The breast cancer movement provides an excellent example of both the strengths and the weaknesses of Melucci's framework. The economy-centered approach of NSMT directs us to look at how macrolevel changes in capitalism facilitated the development of new collective identities. In the case of breast cancer, this proves to be a promising line of vision because the forty years preceding the rise of the breast cancer movement were years of tremendous growth and expansion in the medical-industrial complex, generally speaking, and the cancer establishment in particular.[49] Indeed, from this perspective, cancer would seem to be a key site around which, or from which, we would expect to witness the development of new social movements.

But if the expansion of the medical-industrial complex and the cancer establishment created the facilitating conditions for collective action, why were some diseases but not others politicized? Why did some diseases but not others generate social movements? Why, for example, did these macrolevel changes at the level of cancer science, cancer industries, and cancer medicine produce such inconsistent effects among people with cancer? Why was it breast cancer—instead of lung cancer or prostate cancer or children's cancers or women's cancers or, even more logically, cancer in general—that catalyzed a mass movement for change?[50] Why was it women with breast cancer who constructed new identities, new communities, and new discourses of disease? Why was it women with breast cancer who suddenly refused, in the words of Susan Sontag, to be "exiled" to this "kingdom of the ill"?[51] Equally important, why was this movement so readily embraced by healthy women and other strangers to this kingdom?

The weakness of this body of theory is that system-level changes—even when they are as clear-cut as the dramatic growth of the medical-industrial complex and the cancer establishment—are still so murky, so macro, and so general that they lack explanatory punch. There is no doubt that changes in advanced industrial capitalism fed and were fed by the growing power and scope of science, medicine, and the health care industry. There is also no doubt that the body became a key site of capitalist production, consumption, conflict, control, contestation, and challenge. But how do we get from the increasingly powerful and individualizing institutions of science and medicine to the emergence of new health- and disease-based social movements? The question still remains: How did a set of historical shifts that enhanced the power and scope of the medical-industrial complex lead to a mass-participation breast cancer movement that mobilized hundreds of thousands of women?

Melucci advances toward a poststructuralist understanding of culture, power, and bodies and dances with it provocatively before retreating to the more familiar terrain of Marxist-style Manichaean thinking. He argues, for example, that collective action "is shifting more and more from the 'political' form, which was common in Western societies, to a cultural ground."[52] He singles out the body as "an object upon which the concerted integrative and manipulative efforts of the system of domination are focused" and argues that the body is the "cultural locus of resistance and desire."[53] He identifies health, illness, death, and deviance as "critical points" for mobilizing collective action.[54] But after moving in this promising direction, Melucci backs away from these insights and returns to the conceptual terrain of economic structures and power-possessing classes. He ultimately argues, for example, that "the *dominant class* is attempting to 'psychologize' and 'medicalize' the social realm in order to drain all potential for conflict and collective action stemming from problems of identity."[55] It is therefore necessary, according to Melucci, "to show that these problems are what are really at the heart of *the new class conflicts*."[56]

Examining medicalization is a promising line of thinking. Examining the relationship between medicalization and social movements solely through the lens of class conflict, however, is not. The lesson we should take from the weaknesses and limitations of NSMT and PPT, however, is not that we should abandon the study of structures entirely, but that we should abandon the modernist, masculinist theories of power on which they were erected.

Instead of adopting an aerial view of macrolevel changes—focusing on the nation-state and advanced capitalism—we need to examine the *structuring practices* that shape social movements. What is called for is an approach that looks from the bottom up and laterally; an approach that examines multiple sites rather than privileging the center; an approach that pays attention to historically specific regimes of practices rather than fixating on political opportunities or controlling classes. Finally, we need an approach that puts the body at the center of the analysis. I outline this approach, which I conceptualize as "social movements without the sovereign," in the next three sections through the elaboration of three conceptual tools: disease regimes, fields of contention, and cultures of action.

## Social Movements without the Sovereign

More than thirty years ago the social theorist and historian Michel Foucault challenged the assumptions embedded in popular images and theories of power. We still picture power, Foucault argued, as if it were centralized in the state or the economy, possessed by particular groups or classes, and wielded like a club over others. Foucault used the metaphor of "sovereign power" to describe this centralized and repressive power that, he argued, originated in the rule of kings.[57] Although this form of power has not disappeared in modern societies, it no longer serves as their organizing principle.[58] The notion of sovereign power, Foucault argued, is increasingly incapable of decoding modern power and serving as its "system of representation."[59]

"Biopower" is the name Foucault gave to the new technologies of power that arose in the West at the end of the eighteenth century and fed the development, rationalization, and proliferation of modern institutions and populations, also known as "modern subjects." The "bio" part of this term indexes the growing involvement of modern institutions in managing the lives and even the biological processes of modern subjects. Biopower, in this sense, is "life power." Unlike the centralized sovereign power that it gradually colonized from below, biopower is exercised through dispersed, portable, flexible, and continuous technologies of the body that constitute and control modern subjects through the interlocking and overlapping practices of discipline, surveillance, and knowledge production. Unlike sovereign power, whose exercise is characterized by heavy-handed domination and repression, biopower is constructive, dynamic, optimizing, and enabling—albeit of social control and productivity, not of the liberation that humanists and theorists of modernity envisioned.

Importantly, Foucault argued that if we want to understand this new form of power "within the concrete and historical framework of its operation," we must first "break free" of the old-fashioned and anachronistic models that conceive of power as centralized, state-centered, and repressive.[60] These models are not only inadequate; they are red herrings that distract us from the real business at hand: mapping the exercise of biopower and its effects on modern subjects.

In a 1987 essay on methods, Foucault argued that the target of the researcher's analysis should not be institutions, theories, or ideology. The "target of analysis," Foucault argued, should be "regimes of practices" that "possess up to a point their own specific regularities, logic, strategy, self-evidence, and 'reason.'"[61] Foucault's focus on biopower and historically specific regimes of practices did not mean, as he insisted on dozens of occasions, that the state is unimportant. But "one of the first things that has to be understood," he argued, "is that power isn't localised in the State apparatus," and, further, that the "relations of power, and hence the analysis that must be made of them, necessarily extend beyond the limits of the State."[62] To the extent that we remain wedded to frameworks that rely upon state-centered theories of power, Foucault argued, we fail to recognize that technologies of power are employed "on all levels and in forms that [include but] go beyond the state and its apparatus." In political thought and analysis, Foucault argued, "we still have not cut off the head of the king."[63]

In mapping historically specific regimes of practices, Foucault insisted that the analysis of power should begin "with the question of the body and the effects of power on it."[64] The human body, as Foucault's genealogies of public health, medicine, madness, sexuality, deviance, and discipline so provocatively revealed, is not a transhistorical object but a culturally and politically invested product of specific regimes of practices.[65] The body is not solely the object and product of specific regimes of practices, however; it is also the material means by which human beings become historical subjects. "The individual," Foucault argued, "with his [or her] identity and characteristics, is the product of a relation of power exercised over bodies [and] multiplicities."[66]

Biopower circulates and operates via discourses and practices—biopractices—aimed at "the subjugation of bodies and the control of populations."[67] Analytically, Foucault mapped biopower and its regimes of practices along two axes. The first, what Foucault termed the "anatomo-politics of the human body," are exercised through biopractices that target individual bodies, optimize their capabilities, and enhance their functioning.[68] The second, what Foucault termed the "biopolitics of populations" consist of biopractices that operate at the level of populations, making possible their social control and regulation while enhancing their biological and social functioning and productivity.[69] The genealogy of anatomo-politics can be traced to the rise of scientific medicine, or what Foucault termed the "clinical" or "medical gaze" (both translations are common). The genealogy of biopolitics can be traced to the modern apparatus of public health, or what we might call the "epidemiological gaze." Thus health, for Foucault, is a particularly dense point of transfer within the modern circuitry of power.

Foucault's theorization of biopower and his genealogies of madness, sexuality, deviance, criminality, public health, and medicine have had a deep and lasting impact on many fields of inquiry. Among these, medical sociology and interdisciplinary studies of science, medicine, and technology have been particularly receptive to Foucault's contributions. The positive reception and integration of Foucault's work in these fields occurred in large part because Foucault's analyses of power and his focus on the body, science, public health, and medicine meshed both substantively and politically with core questions and research programs in these fields.[70] The focus on the body, for example, was clearly not a new idea to feminists. In many respects, second-wave feminism grew out of women's embodied experiences. The slogan "The personal is political" encapsulates this idea, as does the iconic image of feminist activists as "bra-burners." Likewise, as feminist scholars indicated, it was women's embodied experiences of medicine—medical knowledge, physicians, technologies, and practices—that launched the women's health movement.[71] In addition, not surprisingly, Foucault's insistence on moving beyond state-centered and economy-centered analyses and his insistence that science, public health, and medicine are core elements in the modern organization of power were readily embraced by feminists, medical sociologists, and interdisciplinary scholars of science, medicine, and technology, who had already reached the same conclusion.

What Foucault brought to the table, however, was a new theory of power that made visible the historically specific *construction* of bodies, identities, and subjectivities through the material and discursive practices of science, public health, and medicine. Foucault's focus on practices, his theorization of bodies, and his insights regarding the paradoxically productive and regulative character of modern power changed the way medicine, medical sciences, medical practices, medical power, medical technologies, medical patients, and processes of medicalization were conceptualized and studied by many feminists, historians, sociologists, and anthropologists. Thus, unlike macrostructural theorists of social movements, who held fast to their state-centered and economy-centered conceptualizations of power, a significant number of feminists and other scholars of medicine, science, and technology increasingly abandoned them and incorporated Foucauldian and poststructural understandings of power into their analyses. Below, I provide an overview of medicalization theory, its incorporation of Foucauldian and poststructural insights, and its relevance to my conceptualization of disease regimes.

## Theorizing (Bio)Medicalization

In an influential essay published in 1972, Irving Zola claimed that "medicine [was] becoming a major institution of social control." The "medicalizing of society," as Zola understood it, was "an insidious and often undramatic phenomenon accomplished by 'medicalizing' much of daily living, by making medicine and the labels 'healthy' and 'ill' relevant to an ever increasing part of human existence."[72] The extension of medical concepts, authority, jurisdiction, and practice, as Zola argued, had accelerated during the previous decades. Twenty years later Peter Conrad synthesized the copious literature on medicalization and clarified its core concept. Medicalization, he argued, "consists of defining a problem in medical terms, using medical language to describe a problem, adopting a medical framework to understand a problem, or using a medical intervention to 'treat it.'"[73] In other words, "medicalization" refers to the process through which diverse phenomena are "made medical."

Over the last few decades, countless case studies have illuminated the seemingly infinite ways in which vulnerable groups—children, women, and a wide variety of "social deviants"—were systematically dominated and controlled through the process of medicalization.[74] One group of scholars, versed in labeling theory and with strong ties to the sociology of deviance, trained their lens on the medicalization of socially problematic behavior, which they termed the "medicalization of deviance." Scholars working in this tradition examined the medicalization of a wide variety of nonnormative behaviors such as madness, drunkenness, same-sex desire, and the mistreatment of children.[75] Later studies examined the medicalization of children's learning difficulties, spousal abuse, eating too much or too little, gambling, shopping, promiscuity, and so on.

A second group of scholars, versed in feminist theory and with ties to the women's health movement, focused their attention on the medicalization of women's psyches and bodies, or what we might call the "medicalization of normality." Their studies, like the women's health movement in general, focused on the medical control of women's reproductive bodies by imperious physicians, misogynist technologies, the male-dominated institution of medicine, and the pharmaceutical industry. Over the last few decades feminists have examined the medicalization of childbirth, pregnancy, contraception, motherhood, menstruation, menopause, aging, sexuality, and unhappiness.[76] More recent work in this tradition has shifted toward an examination of the medicalization of men's bodies.[77]

During a second wave of medicalization studies, many researchers shifted their attention to the ways people actively negotiated the process of medicalization—at times resisting, at times willingly participating in the medicalization of their suffering.[78] The second wave of studies, then, emphasized that medicalization is rarely an issue of "medical imperialism" asserted over "feckless patients," nor is it a simple issue of "wannabe" patients strong-arming physicians.[79] Catherine Kohler Riessman's work was both pioneering and exemplary in this regard. In an essay on the medicalization of women's reproductive bodies, weight, and mental health, Riessman argued that "both physicians and women have contributed to the redefining of women's experience into medical categories." Whereas physicians seek to medicalize experience because of their beliefs and economic interests, middle- and upper-class women have collaborated in the medicalization process "because of their own needs and motives." It is a "tenuous and fraught" collaboration, Riessman argued, and women have "both gained and lost through the process of medicalization."[80]

Depending on their theoretical interests and empirical focus, scholars identified the main forces driving medicalization (the medicalization of life, the medicalization of deviance, and the medicalization of women's bodies) as medical imperialism, patriarchal domination, unrestrained capitalism, intraprofessional competition, economic entrepreneurialism, modern societies' growing reliance on scientific knowledge and expertise, and the efforts of suffering people to obtain medical recognition and relief. Despite the diversity of opinions on the question of causality, there was near-universal agreement regarding the consequences of medicalization: Medicalization privatized, individualized, and depoliticized suffering and social problems.

As Foucault's influence seeped in, medicalization scholars increasingly utilized a new vocabulary to describe the dynamics of medicalization: Discourse dislodged ideology, subjects supplanted patients, and medical practices stole the limelight from physicians.[81] As this occurred, critiques of medicalization as a form of professional, patriarchal, capitalist, or techno-rational domination—of women and a wide variety of social "deviants"—were increasingly joined by analyses of how medical categories, bodies, and subjects are actually constituted within the discursive and material practices of biomedicine and its allied sciences, industries, and professions.[82] "Medical work," as Monica Casper and Marc Berg argued, is simultaneously "a principal locus for the construction and reconstruction of (usually human) bodies" and "a crucial site of control over bodies and lives."[83]

Increasingly, as scholars such as David Armstrong, Robert Castel, Deborah Lupton, and Alan Petersen argued (drawing on Foucault), epidemiology and the practices of public health have exported the "medical gaze" to the private and public spaces that exist beyond the medical clinic. And increasingly, as many scholars have argued, it is through the discourses and practices of risk that modern bodies and subjects—embodied subjects—are being constituted.[84]

The work of these scholars is part of a larger shift in theorizing "risk society" that is commonly associated with the work of Anthony Giddens and Ulrich Beck.[85] In the conditions of late modernity, as Giddens, Beck, and many others have shown, the calculation of risks is linked to strategies for intervening in, capitalizing on, and controlling the various outcomes mapped by its algorithms—and developments in statistical techniques, information technologies, and computing over the course of the last several decades have accelerated what can be called the "riskification of society." Paradoxically, as Giddens and many others have argued, the colonization of chaos and the expansion of scientific knowledge—or what Ian Hacking refers to as the "taming of chance"—seems to have increased collective and individual experiences of risk-based anxiety. This sense of vulnerability feeds a growing distrust of scientific authority and expertise. Thus, as Beck has argued, the core conflicts of wealthy industrial societies are increasingly located in the definition and distribution of risks rather than in the production and distribution of wealth (although the generation of wealth is itself dependent on technologies of risk management and assessment). Accordingly, the evaluation, management, regulation, administration, and communication of risk—what we can call the "biopolitics of risk"—has become one of the most complicated, controversial, and consequential activities of modern institutions, including science, the state, public health, and biomedicine.

Whereas Giddens and Beck tied the emergence of risk society to grandiose structural transformations in late capitalism, however, poststructural theorists of science, medicine, and public health have tried to put flesh and blood on the bones of abstract theorizing.[86] David Armstrong, for example, showed how the discourses and practices of risk-based surveillance medicine dissolved the distinct clinical categories of healthy and ill as it attempted "to bring everyone within its network of visibility." In so doing, it fundamentally remapped the spaces of illness.[87] In another study, Armstrong traced the emergence of different regimes of public health and showed how they gave rise to different historical subjects. The "new public health" and its risk-factor epidemiology, Armstrong argued, has created neoliberal subjects charged with the responsibility of knowing the risk factors (for any given disease), avoiding risky behaviors, and continuously surveilling themselves and each other.[88]

In 1992 Paul Rabinow introduced the term "biosociality" to conceptualize the link between the emergence of new groups and identities, on the one hand, and new practices of science and medicine, on the other. Biosociality, Rabinow explained, referred to the formation of "new group and individual identities and practices arising out of [the] new truths" of genomics research—an arena of truth production in which the discourses and practices of risk are deeply implicated. Writing during the early years of the Human Genome Project, Rabinow argued that these new forms of biosociality were brought into existence in large part by the development and use of tests to screen for and identify carriers of genetic mutations. Rabinow predicted that these new groups "will meet to share their experiences, lobby for their disease, educate their children, redo their home environment, and so on."[89] Although Rabinow explicitly linked the concept of biosociality to genomics research and clinical consequences, the concept is used more loosely in the work of many other scholars to signify the ways in which the practices of science, public health, and medicine enable the formation of new subjects and social groups. It is this broader sense of biosociality that I draw upon in this book. Since the term was coined in 1992, the concept of biosociality has traveled far and wide. Although it is routinely invoked by scholars of science, public health, and medicine, however, the nature of the relationship between medicalization, biosociality, and social movements has received very little attention.

In 1996 Simon Williams and Michael Calnan argued that it was time to formally revisit and update medicalization theory to reflect key developments in social theory and key transformations in health and medicine such as the growing significance of risk in the management of health and disease, the growing involvement of the media in health affairs, and the "re-skilling of the lay populace" through the growth of self-help groups, access to information formerly monopolized by experts, and critiques of medical authority that had become part of mainstream culture.[90]

In 2003 Adele Clarke and her colleagues revisited and expanded the issues raised by Williams and Calnan in 1996. In an extraordinarily wide-ranging synthetic essay, Clarke and her colleagues proposed the term "biomedicalization" to signal what they called a "second transformation" of American medicine.[91] Biomedicalization, they argued, involved the "increasingly complex, multi-sited, multidirectional processes of medicalization, both extended and reconstituted through the new social forms of highly techno-scientific medicine." The theory of biomedicalization they put forward brought together key insights from the Foucauldian turn in studies of science, medicine, and technology described above (the medicalization of risk, new medical technologies, transformations in the production and distribution of biomedical knowledge and expertise) with empirically grounded work on the economic, institutional, and political reorganization of the U.S. medical-industrial complex.[92] In addition, they emphasized that biomedicalization reproduced the "dual tendencies" of medicalization. Building on the earlier work of Barbara and John Ehrenreich, they argued that biomedicalization was "a stratified process" that was simultaneously expansionist and exclusionary. The white middle and upper classes were primarily subject to expansionist and "co-optative" medicalization, whereas poor people, people without insurance, and people of color were systematically excluded from fully accessing the practical and symbolic resources of medicine.

Drawing on three decades of scholarship, then, this is what we now know about medicalization.[93] Medicalization can occur on at least four different levels.[94] (1) At the conceptual level, (bio)medicalization consists of the use of a medical model or vocabulary to identify or define a problem, even in the absence of the involvement or endorsement of medical professionals. (2) At the institutional level, medicalization consists of the involvement of a potentially wide range of organizations, industries, and institutions (including from science; medicine; public health; the state; the pharmaceutical industry; the health insurance industry; providers of health care services; the self-help and therapy industries; the body-enhancement, fitness, and weight-loss industries; private foundations; corporate philanthropies; health voluntaries; advocacy organizations; and patient groups) in the legitimation, definition, and treatment of phenomena *as* medical problems. (3) At the interactional level, medicalization consists of the social interactions and relationships through which phenomena are converted into medically meaningful conditions. The interactional level consists of patients' interactions with physicians, with other medical personnel, and with other patients. It also includes interactions with family, friends, coworkers, lovers, and even strangers—each of whom can reinforce or refuse to recognize the validity of a particular condition as a medical concern. Finally, it includes patients' relationships to and interactions with a wide assortment of medical technologies, including screening, diagnostic, treatment, and rehabilitative technologies. (4) At the individual level, medicalization consists of the subjective, lived experience of individuals vis-à-vis the medicalization of various desires, physical conditions, body parts, behaviors, and forms of suffering. The lived experience of these subjects, of course, is powerfully shaped by the conceptual, institutional, and interactional dynamics of medicalization.

In addition, we know that medicalization can occur on one or more levels, that its operation and effects are socially stratified, and that it is not an absolute or irreversible process. We also know that although the medical profession is usually involved in the process of applying and extending medical frames and definitions, in some cases the medical profession is only marginally involved in, or even resistant to, medicalization.[95] In fact, these days the impetus for medicalization often originates in the pharmaceutical industry or among self-constituted groups seeking recognition of and relief from their suffering. Regarding the latter, "Life's troubles," as Conrad points out, "are often confusing, distressing, debilitating, and difficult to understand," and medicine offers one way of making sense of human suffering.[96] It also, as many researchers have pointed out, serves as a gateway to both practical and symbolic resources—access to treatment, occupational therapy, disability benefits, Social Security benefits, legal redress, social legitimacy, sympathy, accommodation, and recognition.[97]

We know, further, that the process of medicalization involves collective organizing and strategic claims-making across multiple arenas and that it is a process engaged in and contested by a wide variety of social actors and their organizations, including patients, activists, advocacy organizations, researchers, physicians, universities, pharmaceutical companies, government agencies, employers, managed care organizations, corporations, health voluntaries, public health departments, and private foundations, just to name a few. We know that, increasingly, it is through the discourses and practices of risk and the promotion of health that (bio)medicalization is both expanding and intensifying. The discourses and practices of risk, however, are not limited to the asymptomatic, at-risk, prediagnosis populations but, rather, extend into the lives of postdiagnosis populations of people who are members of the remission society and people who are living with chronic disease.

Finally, although this has not been adequately emphasized or theorized in the literature, we know that medicalization is an ongoing process, not a one-time event. That means that medicalization, like other social processes, must be continuously reproduced. At the same time, because it is continuously reproduced, the practices involved in the medicalization of behaviors, processes, and conditions tend to disappear into the background once they have succeeded, becoming part of common sense and the ordinary, everyday world. Because medicalization is an ongoing process, however, it is also a process that changes over time. Thus, behaviors, processes, and conditions that are initially medicalized via one set of practices are always subject to being medicalized in a different way, at a later time, through a different set of practices. "The unique process of inscribing bodies as healthy or diseased," as Elizabeth Ettorre remarked, "is performed by authoritative discourses and scientific practices, including the pressing of technology into the service of medicine."[98] Thus, as technologies change, so do the inscribed bodies and subjectivities. This is an important point to remember, and I will return to it shortly, in my discussion of disease regimes.

It is also important to note that, while drawing on Foucault's essential insights, many scholars have criticized and moved beyond some of the limitations of Foucault's contributions. Foucault has been criticized, and rightly so, for occluding the deeply gendered exercise of power in biomedicine, for failing to account for the unevenness of power and its effects, for portraying the exercise of power in overly totalizing terms, for bracketing the lived experience of the subjugated, and for wholly dissolving the materiality of the body into the play of power.[99] Foucault has also been criticized, and rightly so, for his remarkably underdeveloped theory of resistance. Although Foucault repeatedly claimed that "where there is power there is resistance," there is little evidence of individual resistance in his writings and no theorization of collective action or social movements. The subjects who populate Foucault's genealogies of modern power are portrayed in unremittingly isolating, individualizing, and passive terms. Like Jeremy Bentham's Panopticon, which so captured Foucault's imagination, Foucault's image of modern society is one in which individuals are separated from one another by soundproof, windowless, impenetrable walls and condemned to isolation. Thus, although Foucault succeeded in "cutting off the head of the king" in political theory, he failed to take the next step. He failed, that is, to explore the terrain of social movements without the sovereign.

This terrain has grown increasingly crowded during the last few decades with the remarkable proliferation of patient organizations and health-, disability-, and disease-based activism.[100] The mother of contemporary health movements is without a doubt the U.S. women's health movement of second-wave feminism. A steady stream of cascading effects and "spillover" movements were fed by the women's health movement, with fast-churning pools forming around the reproductive rights movement in the 1970s and 1980s, AIDS in the 1980s and 1990s, and breast cancer activism during the 1990s and into the present, as well as around the environmental health and disability rights movements.[101] These mass mobilizations, however, are just the largest and most visible. Numerous smaller, less visible groups of patients have organized around a growing number of contested illnesses, including postpartum depression, chemical sensitivity disorder, chronic fatigue, fibromyalgia, Gulf War syndrome, and sick-building syndrome, just to name a few.[102] Others have organized to contest the ways well-established diseases and health conditions are scientifically investigated, medically managed, publicly administered, and culturally conceptualized. These organizations range across a vast territory, including everything from the Juvenile Diabetes Association to the National Association to Advance Fat Acceptance to the Genetic Alliance, an advocacy organization of people living with genetic conditions. It is no exaggeration to claim that the last few decades of the twentieth century witnessed the proliferation of patient groups for virtually every disability, disease, and health condition, old or new.

These health-, disability-, and disease-based social movements—what Phil Brown and Steve Zavestoski have conceptualized as "embodied health movements"—are challenging not only the programs and priorities of governments but the practices of scientific research, public health, and clinical medicine.[103] In addition, these social movements are both challenging and allying themselves with pharmaceutical companies and corporations engaged in cause-related marketing and other forms of corporate philanthropy. Among scholars of health, disability, and disease-based social movements there is thus a growing awareness of the increasingly hybridized and boundary-blurring relationships among the state, science, medicine, big pharma, corporate philanthropy, and social movements.[104] Clearly, the languages of science, public health, and medicine have become extremely powerful and popular media for the subjects of late modernity to communicate their suffering, distress, demands, and senses of injustice and entitlement.

But how do the new processes of biomedicalization enable new forms of embodied subjectivity? How are the embodied experiences of these subjects linked to new forms of identity and biosociality? How are these, in turn, linked to new forms of health-, risk-, and disease-based collective action?

In the next three sections I introduce the concepts of disease regimes, fields of contention, and cultures of action. My approach is heavily indebted to the work of Foucault and the scholarship on embodied health movements and (bio)medicalization referenced above. These concepts, I believe, help illuminate the complex relationships among processes of (bio)medicalization, historically distinct forms of embodied subjectivity, and the development of health-, risk-, and disease-based collective action.

## DISEASE REGIMES

Although diseases can and do have real effects on all of us, as embodied subjects, regardless of how we respond to them and what we think of them, it is equally true that diseases as social facts do not exist, as medical historian Charles Rosenberg has written, "until we have agreed that [they do], by perceiving, naming, and responding to [them]."[105] In my formulation, disease regimes consist of the institutionalized practices, authoritative discourses, emotional vocabularies, visual images, and social scripts through which diseases are socially constructed, medically managed, publicly administered, and subjectively experienced. The concept of disease regimes encompasses all four levels of medicalization but shifts the analytic focus from levels to practices.

The concept of disease regimes is designed to help illuminate the relationship between the practices through which breast cancer is (bio)medicalized, the forms of embodied subjectivity that these practices produce, and the emergence of new forms of biosociality. Here, in a nutshell, is the logic of that link. First, different regimes of practices produce different subjects and social relations of disease, as well as different spatial, temporal, and visual dimensions. Second, disease regimes can both enable and inhibit the formation of disease-based identities, social networks, and solidarities. Third, these forms of biosociality are crucial ingredients in the development of social movements.[106]

The underlying point here is that the practices of disease regimes are neither fixed nor automatic. Scientific discourses of disease can change over time; screening practices can rise and fall; diagnostic categories can expand and contract; new technologies can be invented; old technologies can be abandoned; the utilization of existing technologies can change; physician and patient scripts can be tightened, relaxed, and rewritten; and public health campaigns can target different groups, promote different ideas, and teach different practices. The important point is that changes in the practices of a disease regime can alter the spatial, temporal, and visual dimensions of disease and lead to the production of new subjects and social relations of disease.

In studying disease regimes, we can map them along the two axes of biopower that Foucault specified.[107] The first, the "biopolitics of populations," includes the discourses and practices of public health—public health education, screening campaigns, health promotion, health-behavior research, population surveillance, epidemiology, and environmental health sciences. I refer to the operation of these biopolitical technologies, in shorthand, as the *public administration of disease*. The second axis, the "anatomo-politics of individual bodies," includes the discourses and practices of clinical medicine—screening, diagnosis, treatment, rehabilitation, and clinical research, especially clinical trials. For shorthand, I refer to the operation of these practices as the *medical management of disease*. Some practices operate along both axes. Screening procedures, for example, are often part of the biopolitics of populations, but because screening practices are typically performed on individual bodies, they are also often part of the anatomo-politics of individual bodies. Likewise, biostatistics, clinical epidemiology, and preventive medicine straddle the two domains.

The voluntary subjects of disease regimes are the scientists, physicians, health care professionals, technicians, administrators, and others who have voluntarily chosen to involve themselves in the regime of practices. My analysis, however, focuses on the involuntary subjects—those who are involuntarily recruited and incorporated into the regime through its discourses and practices. "Involuntary," however, does not necessarily mean unwilling. On the contrary, disease regimes are most effective when their involuntary subjects are willing and able to participate in their own subjectification. All of us are subjects of, and subject to, disease regimes (and health regimes) of various compositions and degrees of intensity. As subjects of disease regimes we have agency, but it is an agency that is shaped and bounded by the regime's discourses and practices.

Disease regimes do not, of course, wholly determine the experiences of their subjects—and this is where my conceptualization is informed by the critiques of Foucault's work previously mentioned. First, disease regimes are not totalizing because they do not saturate social space. All of us, all of the time, are subjects of and subject to multiple regimes of practices—gender regimes, race regimes, sexuality regimes, political regimes, health regimes, and disease regimes, just to name a few. In fact, it is this radical multiplicity, as numerous theorists of modernity and postmodernity have argued, that most distinguishes modern industrial and postindustrial societies from earlier social formations.

These regimes of practices do not simply reinforce one another. They change in different ways and at different rates—often in response to the new groups and social movements that arise within them. Thus, as people live within and move between different regimes of practices—occupying different subject positions, embodying different forms of subjectivity, enacting different social scripts—we are shaped by different technologies of power. As this occurs, we develop different cultural, emotional, practical, and intellectual capacities and limitations. The capacities and limitations that we acquire in one domain are not abandoned at the door of another. Rather, we bring them with us as we move between and live our lives in multiple regimes.

Second, disease regimes do not penetrate equally into all parts of society. Breast cancer screening, for example, penetrated the bodies and psyches of middle-class white women in their forties, fifties, and sixties more thoroughly than it did any other group of women. Likewise, access to medical treatment for any given disease or health condition in the United States has always been a question of privilege rather than entitlement. The concept of "stratified biomedicalization" put forth by Adele Clarke and her former students encapsulates the persistent reality of unequal access to culturally appropriate health care, preventive care, and health education in the United States.[108]

Third, even similarly positioned people do not necessarily respond in the same way to the practices of disease regimes. Why? Because people are different and our differences matter. It makes no sense to claim otherwise. Disease regimes are not totalitarian forms of governance. Individual differences will out. Admittedly, the concept of disease regimes is not designed to highlight individual differences. It is nonetheless important to recognize that individual differences exist and that they affect the ways people who occupy similar or identical subject positions in a given regime respond to its practices.

Fourth, although Foucault tends to portray the exercise of power in gender-, class-, and race-neutral terms—as if the social identities and group memberships of the subjects of a regime were irrelevant—the evidence clearly points in the opposite direction. In my conceptualization of disease regimes, the social identities of the people exercising power are often quite relevant to the actual exercise of power. The class, gender, and racial identities of surgeons during the first regime of breast cancer, for example, reinforced their power in the medical setting. It is no coincidence that the rapid entry of women into the medical profession during the 1970s coincided with the growing power of patients, the reconceptualization of patient–physician relationships, and the articulation of new social scripts for both patients and physicians.

Fifth, diseases themselves, like people, often resist efforts to shape, manage, and control them. The biology and physiology of disease and the materiality of the body cannot simply be dissolved into the play of power. Many diseases do respond to humanly created technologies and interventions, but they also act within the bodies of their subjects according to a logic that often exceeds our understanding and our best efforts to manage the disease. This means that the capacity of disease regimes to shape disease is, almost inevitably, partial and incomplete. Although it is impossible to gain access to the disease itself—the disease unaltered by human ways of seeing—it is nonetheless important to remember that the disease itself, whatever that may be, is also an actor on the stage of human history.

We turn now, to a brief overview of the application of the concept of disease regimes to the case of breast cancer.

## BREAST CANCER IN TWO REGIMES

I characterize the first regime of breast cancer, which took shape during the first few decades of the twentieth century, as the *regime of medicalization* because it was during this period that scientific medicine consolidated its jurisdiction over breast cancer and supplanted the *era of therapeutic pluralism* that preceded it. The medicalization of breast cancer was neither easy nor automatic. It took several decades to complete, and it was initially resisted by ordinary women and physicians. The medicalization of breast cancer, which I explore in chapter 2, can be mapped along both axes of biopower: the biopolitics of populations and the anatomo-politics of bodies.

The biopolitics of populations (the public administration of disease) proceeded via cancer education campaigns that recruited new subjects to the regime by encouraging ordinary women who exhibited the "danger signals" of breast cancer to consult physicians. The anatomo-politics of breast cancer (the medical management of disease) took place inside physicians' offices and hospital operating rooms, where dangerous and endangered women were reconstituted as symptomatic subjects, a subgroup of whom were then surgically reconstituted as "mastectomees"—a medical category, not a social identity. Medical norms of nondisclosure and the absence of informed consent ensured that women diagnosed and treated for breast cancer were rarely told the whole truth about their diagnoses.

Accompanying the rise of the regime of medicalization, a new social script, dubbed the "sick role" by Talcott Parsons, was institutionalized. The sick role was a set of institutionalized mechanisms that, in the words of Talcott Parsons, "channels deviance [that is, sickness] so that the two most dangerous potentialities, namely, group formation and successful estalishment of the claim to legitimacy, are avoided."[109] The sick role by definition entailed the segregation of "the sick" from the "nonsick" and required the isolation of patients from each other. With the advent of the sick role, Parsons wrote, "The sick are tied up, not with other deviants to form a 'subculture' of the sick, but each with a group of non-sick . . . above all, physicians." Thus, as Parsons makes clear, one of the most important functions of the sick role was that it "deprived" patients "of the possibility of forming a solidary collectivity."[110] The sick role was a temporary role that, in the case of breast cancer, required new mastectomees—women who had undergone a radical mastectomy—to exit the sick role via the architecture of the closet (death was the only other option) and return to their normal lives and duties.

The anatomo-politics of individual bodies thus proceeded via the technologies of diagnosis and treatment, new social scripts for patients and physicians, and the architecture of the closet, which ensured the invisibility of former patients and mastectomees. Although the subjects of the disease regime were enclaved behind the walls of the medical clinic, the social relations of disease—via the architecture of the closet—extended beyond the confines of the clinic: isolating mastectomees from one another, segregating mastectomees from the "normal" (nonsymptomatic) population, and ensuring their silence and invisibility throughout the body politic. The formation of disease-related identities, solidarities, social networks, and other forms of biosociality was thus heavily constrained by and within the regime of medicalization.

During the 1970s and 1980s new practices arose within the regime of medicalization, practices that, taken together, led to the emergence of a new regime with its own "specific regularities, logic, strategy, self-evidence, and 'reason.'"[111] I characterize the second regime of breast cancer as the *regime of biomedicalization* to signal the emergence of new forms of medicalization connected, in large part, to new investments and developments in biomedical research and cancer epidemiology. Within the regime of biomedicalization, the discourses and practices of risk moved to the fore. Like the regime of medicalization, the regime of biomedicalization can be mapped along both axes of biopower. Chapter 3 examines the public administration of breast cancer, focusing on the biopolitics of screening. Chapter 4 examines the medical management of disease, focusing on the anatomo-politics of diagnosis, treatment, and rehabilitation.

Through the biopolitics of screening, breast cancer was reinvented as an invisible risk and symptomless disease that required continuous bodily vigilance and surveillance. Breast self-exam, clinical exam, and mammo-graphic screening were heavily promoted and discursively constructed as the moral duty of every woman. As this occurred, the temporary sick role for symptomatic women was replaced by a permanent "risk role" for all women. The regime of biomedicalization thus reconstituted healthy, asymp-tomatic women as risky subjects and transformed the disease from an either-or condition to a breast cancer continuum.

Inside the medical clinic, as I show in chapter 4, diagnostic and treat-ment options multiplied, norms of nondisclosure were replaced by legal standards of informed consent, and the space of patient decision making expanded. The Halsted radical mastectomy was eliminated, adjuvant ther-apies proliferated, treatment expanded into new parts of patients' bodies, the complexity and longevity of treatments dramatically increased, and the sovereign authority of surgeons was replaced by the more diffuse and less absolute authority of health care teams. Finally, new forms of patient support and rehabilitation were institutionalized, further undermining physicians' monopoly on information and reducing the social isolation and (imposed) ignorance of breast cancer patients. Upon finishing their treat-ment, breast cancer patients were channeled by the risk role into what Arthur Frank has termed the "remission society," the members of which, in Frank's words, are "effectively well but could never be considered cured."[112]

The growth of new practices within the regime of biomedicalization did not immediately eliminate the practices of the earlier regime, but it fore-grounded a new logic and constructed new subjects, social relations, tem-poralizations, spacializations, and visual experiences of disease. In doing so, it gave rise to new forms of biosociality—new social networks, solidarities, and shared sensibilities. Within this new regime of practices there was greater transparency and communication among the involuntary inhabitants, yet at the same time there was a heightened sense of uncertainty and risk and a greater awareness of the limitations of medicine. Taken together, changes in the diagnosis, treatment, and rehabilitation of women with breast can-cer made possible the development of cancer-related identities, solidarities, and sensibilities. These new forms of biosociality, in turn, constituted the preformations and facilitating conditions of the breast cancer movement.[113] Table 1 provides a brief overview of salient differences between the regimes of medicalization and biomedicalization.

These are ideal types, of course, and this typology cannot begin to capture the experiences of different groups of patients. It does, however, capture important changes over time in the regimes of practices through which breast cancer was constituted and experienced by a significant portion of white middle-class women—the group that spearheaded the breast cancer movement. Table 1 portrays the typical treatment regime faced by women diagnosed with stage 1 or stage 2 breast cancer.

The regime of biomedicalization, of course, neither caused the development of the breast cancer movement at the beginning of the 1990s nor determined the precise content or character of activism. It did, however, create fertile conditions for the development of new forms of biosociality

TABLE I    Breast Cancer in Two Regimes

|  | *Regime of medicalization* | *Regime of biomedicalization* |
|---|---|---|
| Subjects | women exhibiting "danger signals" | all symptomatic and asymptomatic women |
| Script | sick role | risk role |
| Biopolitics of populations | "Do not delay" (medicalization of danger signals) | "Go in search" (continuous screening of asymptomatic women) |
| Anatomo-politics of bodies | surgical hegemony | therapeutic choice and complexity |
| Temporal dimension | short-term treatment; temporary sick role | prolonged treatment; permanent risk role |
| Spatialization | rigid, dense, and narrowly circumscribed boundaries of the regime; isolation and segregation of mastectomees | increasingly soft, blurry, transparent, and expansive boundaries of the regime; new forms of biosociality in and outside the medical setting |
| Visual dimension | silence and invisibility of mastectomees | proliferation of discourses of disease; growing visibility of images and voices of women with breast cancer |
| Social relations of disease | architecture of the closet | breast cancer continuum |

and collective action among the "risky subjects" of the new regime—asymptomatic women, women with liminal diagnoses and ambiguous symptoms, women in treatment, women at risk of recurrence, and permanent members of the remission society.[114] These fertile conditions, as the next two sections explain, fed the development of three cultures of action in the Bay Area field of contention.

## Cultures of Action and Fields of Contention

When I began my research on breast cancer activism in 1994, I expected to find feminist cancer groups in the San Francisco Bay Area mobilizing behind the NBCC and, for example, gathering signatures for its well-publicized petitions. Much to my surprise, however, I discovered that the NBCC— the group repeatedly identified by itself and by the mass media as the voice of the breast cancer movement—was nearly invisible, organizationally speaking, and discursively marginal. Even more surprisingly, instead of developing a stronger presence over time, the NBCC seemed to fade further into the distance. During the second half of the 1990s, while the NBCC consolidated and extended its hegemony within the national arena of breast cancer policy making, the San Francisco Bay Area crystallized into a separate field of contention.

My conceptualization of the Bay Area as a "field of contention" draws explicitly on the work of sociologists Raka Ray and Nick Crossley. The work of both Ray and Crossley, in turn, is deeply indebted to Pierre Bourdieu's conceptualization of fields as dynamically structured environments in which individuals, groups, and organizations interact both cooperatively and competitively in ways that shape their strategies, identities, and orientations. Drawing on Bourdieu's understanding of fields, Crossley introduced the term "field of contention" to help map and explain important changes over time in the mental health movement in the United Kingdom.[115] Ray extended Bourdieu's understanding of fields into the terrain of the women's movement in India, showing how regional variations in the political fields of Bombay and Calcutta shaped the strategies, identities, and orientations of social movement organizations in each field.[116]

In *Fields of Protest* Ray developed a typology of political fields—fragmented, segmented, hegemonic, and pluralist—and showed how the type of field, as well as an organization's position within it, affects its goals, strategies, and mobilization of identities. Although Ray's definition of political fields is too narrow for my purposes (the players are limited to the state, political parties, and social movement organizations), my analysis of the Bay Area field of contention is heavily indebted to Ray's work on political fields and her insights regarding and the significance of regional variation. Crossley's term "field of contention," however, is more inclusive and is thus more suited to analyzing the wider array of actors involved in the breast/cancer movement in the San Francisco Bay Area.[117]

The geographic specificity of some fields does not mean that the activities and alliances of the field's actors are geographically circumscribed. A wide variety of programs, campaigns, and coalitions that percolated within the Bay Area field of contention, for example, adopted a local or regional focus, but an equally large number of projects extended beyond these geographic limits to include the state of California, the United States, the international community, or the planet. Furthermore, many organizations active in the women's breast/cancer movement in the Bay Area participated in more than one field of contention. The Women's Cancer Resource Center, for example, was involved at one point in a network of feminist and lesbian cancer resource centers scattered across the country, and Breast Cancer Action routinely collaborated with the National Women's Health Network and other extralocal and national organizations. So too did many of the environmental health organizations that participated in the Bay Area breast/cancer movement.

The point is that there are fields within fields, and fields within fields within fields. It is fields all the way down, so to speak. My argument is not that local or regional fields are necessarily the most important organizational dimension in any given social movement. I suspect that subnational, geographically based fields are not always the most relevant unit of analysis and that the most important relationships between social movement organizations in many areas of the country are those linking local chapters to national headquarters. It is impossible to know for certain, however, when and where this is and is not true, because research on social movements typically brackets the question of subnational, geographically based dynamics and differences.

In the case of the U.S. breast cancer movement, there are at least three major hubs of women's breast/cancer activism that in no way mirror the actors or agenda of the breast cancer movement in Washington, D.C. The first field of contention is the Long Island area. The second is the

Cambridge/Boston area. The third, the focus of my research, is the San Francisco Bay Area. The Bay Area field of contention, to use Ray's typology, was a "fragmented" field when I began my research—a field in which power was relatively widely dispersed, political culture was heterogeneous, and there was no consensus about the boundaries of the field or the rules of the game. In a fragmented field, as Ray explains, domination of the field is always "partial and tenuous" and "a multiplicity of organizations and ideologies can co-exist."[118] In contrast, the Washington, D.C.–centered political field in which the NBCC dominated could more accurately be characterized as a "hegemonic" political field in which power was concentrated among a relatively small number of established players who shared a common understanding of the field and its rules of engagement. In hegemonic fields, as Ray explains, the dominant groups are more dominant and less tolerant of diversity.

Although I have insisted throughout this chapter—and I will continue to insist throughout the book—that the state is not the be-all and end-all of social movements, I nonetheless want to emphasize the important role that state actors and agencies did indeed play in the development of the breast/cancer movement. One of the most significant events in the development of the movement in California, for example, occurred when the Breast Cancer Act of 1993 was signed into law by the governor of California. The California Breast Cancer Act levied an additional two-cent tax on the sale of cigarettes and designated that the tax revenue be used to establish breast cancer research and screening programs. The first, the California Breast Cancer Research Program (BCRP), provided funding for California scientists and (later) community-based organizations to conduct research on breast cancer. At the time of its creation, the BCRP was the largest state-funded cancer research program in the country and one of the largest publicly funded breast cancer research programs in the world. The second, the California Breast Cancer Early Detection Program (BCEDP), provided funding for free clinical breast exams and screening mammograms to poor and low-income women who were uninsured or underinsured. The BCEDP, like the BCRP, was the largest breast cancer program of its kind in the country.[119]

The Breast Cancer Act of 1993 was a truly pioneering piece of legislation. It originated in 1991 in the office of Congresswoman Barbara Friedman, who invited San Francisco activists Susan Claymon (cofounder of Breast Cancer Action) and Andrea Martin (founder of the Breast Cancer Fund) to cowrite the legislation. The involvement of Claymon and Martin helped ensure that a permanent role for breast cancer activists was written into the final language of the legislation, and the involvement of a wide assortment of groups across the state contributed essential political leverage to the legislation's eventual success (which was an uphill battle).[120]

The Breast Cancer Act of 1993 occurred in the early days of the California breast cancer movement. Not only did it precede the rapid growth of the movement during the second half of the 1990s, but it fed that growth in a number of interesting ways. The implementation of the Breast Cancer Act, for example, created a slew of new committees, organizations, roles, and positions, many of which were filled by breast cancer educators and activists. These women volunteered on program advisory committees and scientific review panels. They worked as paid staff and consultants. They joined BCEDP regional partnerships and served as liaisons to various communities. In addition, beginning in 1997, the BCRP began funding community-based research projects that provided opportunities for established (often university-based) scientists to collaborate with community-based organizations. Many of these projects were initiated by local breast/cancer advocacy organizations.

The BCEDP and the BCRP thus illustrate the usefulness of Mark Wolfson's notion of the "interpenetration" of states and social movements. In order to understand the significance of the Breast Cancer Act of 1993, however, we need to pay attention to the various ways in which the programs it established were implemented in particular fields of contention. The Breast Cancer Act of 1993 contributed to the development of the Bay Area field of contention, for example, but not in a simple or straightforward manner. Furthermore, the implementations of the BCEDP and the BCRP were deeply shaped—at the state, regional, and local levels—by the actions of breast/cancer educators and activists.

The regional identity of breast/cancer activists and organizations in the San Francisco Bay Area was also fed by the Bay Area's growing reputation, during the second half of the 1990s, as the "breast cancer capital of the world."[121] This reputation was in large part the result of the rapid growth of cancer epidemiology and tumor registries during the previous two decades and the Bay Area's inclusion in the Surveillance, Epidemiology, and End Results (SEER) Program of the NCI. That breast cancer incidence rates were measurably higher in the Bay Area than elsewhere made it the "breast cancer capital of the world," but if the area had not been designated as a SEER site, it would never have been labeled or identified in this manner. Once the label was assigned, however, Bay Area activists strategically mobilized it to help generate a sense of urgency among Bay Area dwellers. Living in the Bay Area, activists argued, was an environmental risk factor that demanded urgent attention. The Bay Area's identity as the breast cancer capital of the world was thus, at one and the same time, externally imposed and strategically mobilized.

The Bay Area field of contention was also shaped by preexisting social movements, preexisting cancer organizations, and new trends in corporate philanthropy. These, however, are better addressed through an examination of their influence on specific cultures of action. As part II of this book shows, and as I briefly outline below, the Bay Area field of contention was shaped, above all, by the development of three intersecting cultures of action.

## THREE CULTURES OF ACTION IN THE BAY AREA FIELD OF CONTENTION

The term "culture of action" is a heuristic device for conceptualizing and mapping patterns of similarity and difference within social movements. COAs are collectively produced by the individuals, groups, agencies, organizations, councils, corporations, and coalitions that participate in them. They are held together—sometimes tightly, sometimes loosely—by a density of shared goals, assumptions, discourses, interactions, allies, opponents, sources of support, constituencies, and collaborations. The boundaries of COAs are sometimes fuzzy and permeable, sometimes clear and rigid. Furthermore, individuals and organizations can, and often do, participate in more than one COA—wearing different hats, playing different roles, and foregrounding different identities in each.

Cultures of action, as the name implies, are dynamic. They change over time in response to multiple influences: the actions of their members, the impact of their activities, their relationships to other organizations, their interactions with other COAs, the shifting structure and dynamics of the fields in which they are embedded, and the discourses and practices of the regimes they seek to change. COAs are not simple constellations of ideas, frames, cognitions, or identities. Rather, they enact, embody, emote, and articulate (visually and verbally) particular visions of what is and what ought to be.

During the 1990s three COAs took shape within the Bay Area field of contention. Each COA, as I show in part II of this book, foregrounded a different experience and understanding of breast/cancer. As such, each COA privileged different discourses of disease, different alliances, different identities, different body politics, different emotions, different priorities, and different agendas. Each COA drew upon and deployed different discourses of gender, race, class, and sexuality. Each COA developed different relationships to these same social groups and communities (women, men, racial and ethnic groups, class sectors, sexual minorities, and the heterosexual mainstream). Each COA developed different relationships to, and understandings of, science and medicine, capitalism, corporate philanthropy, the state, and the pharmaceutical industry.

The first COA, the culture of early detection and screening activism, complicated widespread assumptions about clear boundaries between the state, the private sector, and social movements. The culture of early detection and screening activism included public health agencies, private corporations, corporate foundations, cancer charities, health voluntaries, professional associations, and conventional social movement organizations. The culture of screening activism drew primarily upon the mainstream discourse of early detection but extended and refashioned it to foreground issues of access for medically marginalized women.

This COA constructed "breast cancer survivors" as the privileged identity, emphasized individual agency and responsibility, connected breast cancer survival to heteronormative femininities, created an emotion culture of caring gestures and uplifting feelings, and mobilized hope and faith in mainstream science, medicine, and the cancer establishment. Pink ribbons were the most easily identifiable and omnipresent symbol of this COA. Consensus politics were its strength. Corporate-sponsored, mass participation fund-raising events were its signature. Lack of breast cancer awareness and barriers to screening were its enemies. The public faces of this COA are explored in chapter 5 and crystallized in Table 2 by the annual Race for the Cure, sponsored by the San Francisco chapter of the Susan G. Komen Breast Cancer Foundation.

The second COA, the culture of patient empowerment and feminist treatment activism, drew upon the organizational and discursive resources of feminism, the women's health movement, the lesbian community, and AIDS activism. It constructed a feminist discourse that emphasized patient empowerment and treatment activism. Feminist breast/cancer organizations in the Bay Area criticized and attempted to reform the breast cancer research establishment, but Bay Area organizations also emphasized the needs of women living with breast/cancer—access to mainstream, alternative, and complementary therapies, clinical trials, scientific research, medical information, practical services, social support, community spaces, political activism, and cultural expression.

This COA linked breast cancer to other women's cancers and constructed a new collective identity: "women living with cancer." The culture of patient empowerment challenged the mainstream discourse of early detection and its normalizing practices, created an emotion culture that legitimized the expression of emotions, such as sorrow and anger, that were banished by the culture of early detection and aggressively challenged the practices and priorities of the cancer establishment and associated industries. One-breasted women, bald women, and buttons proclaiming "Cancer Sucks" symbolized the spirit of this COA. Coalition politics were its strength. Challenging established authority was its signature. The cancer establishment and the "pinkwashing" of breast cancer were its enemies. The public faces of this COA are explored in chapter 6 and are represented in Table 2 by the Women and Cancer Walk in San Francisco.

The third COA, the culture of cancer prevention and environmental activism, drew upon the organizational and discursive resources of feminist cancer organizations and the environmental health and justice movements. This COA broadened the focus of feminist cancer activism to include people—both men and women—with cancer, people suffering from environmental illnesses, and people living or working in toxic communities. The Toxic Links Coalition, for example, discursively represented breast cancer as both a product and a source of profits for a global cancer industry, mobilized outrage against corporate malfeasance and environmental racism, and replaced the emphasis on biomedical research and early detection with demands for corporate regulation and cancer prevention. Industrial chemicals, smokestacks, garish images of death and deformity, and contentious politics characterized the most visible face of this COA.

Not all environmental breast/cancer activists, however, were comfortable with the contentious style of the Toxic Links Coalition, and as a result the culture of environmental activism was more internally fractured than the other two COAs, though it was fractured in a way that seemed to expand its scope rather than diminish it. Different (sub)cultures of action appealed to different audiences, recruited participants from different places, and made inroads in different kinds of terrain. Some organizations, for example, pursued a more cooperative strategy, working with rather than against local politicians, corporations, and mainstream cancer organizations. Others, like the Toxic Links Coalition, maintained a rigid separation between itself and its opponents. The public faces of this COA are explored in chapter 7. Table 2 summarizes the more contentious face of this COA, as represented by the Toxic Tour of the Cancer Industry.

TABLE 2    Culture of Action in the Bay Area Field of Contention

|  | Early detection | Patient empowerment | Cancer prevention |
|---|---|---|---|
| Public culture | Race for the Cure | Women and Cancer Walk | Toxic Tour |
| Privileged identity | breast cancer survivors | women living with cancer | victimized communities |
| Representative symbol |  |  |  |
| Definition of the problem | lack of awareness of and access to screening | entrenched, male-dominated cancer establishment committed to "business as usual" | profit-driven global cancer industry |
| Attitude toward science | trusting, respectful, committed | critical, unintimidated, participatory | critical; strategic use of science |
| Emotion culture | hopeful, grateful, upbeat, positive, celebratory | public anger but private compassion and support for women with cancer | unmitigated anger targeted at the cancer industry |
| Body politics | "normal" bodies: fit and feminine; prostheses and reconstruction | "deviant" bodies: bald, bold, one-breasted, and unashamed | "macabre" bodies: gruesome images, deformities, skeletons |
| Public political culture | consensus politics | coalition politics and contentious politics | contentious politics |

Table 2 provides a snapshot of some of the salient differences among these three cultures of action, emphasizing the dominant trend within each. The table could be expanded to twice its length, but the axes of comparison that it includes depict essential differences that can be captured by a word or phrase. Chapters 5, 6, and 7 develop a more in-depth look at these three COAs, as well as their interactions, relationships, history, and development. Emphasizing their differences necessarily minimizes and occludes their overlaps and similarities, but I do so in order to highlight important differences within the movement that has been de-emphasized in the published literature and popular media. In arguing that we need to pay greater attention to the role of difference in the breast/cancer movement, I am not making a normative argument about the importance of appreciating diversity. Rather, I am arguing that if we fail to pay attention to the role of difference, we are fundamentally misunderstanding the dynamics, ambitions, and achievements of this movement. We turn now to an examination of the prehistory of the breast/cancer movement: breast cancer in two regimes.

PART I

# BREAST CANCER IN TWO REGIMES

# chapter 2

# The Regime of Medicalization

> Silence itself—the things one declines to say, or is forbidden to name, the discretion that is required between different speakers—is less the absolute limit of discourse, the other side from which it is separated by a strict boundary, than an element that functions alongside the things said, with them and in relation to them within over-all strategies.
>
> —MICHEL FOUCAULT, *History of Sexuality*

Egyptian papyri from the eighteenth dynasty (1587–1328 BC) describe the medical treatment of breast diseases by surgery and other medical techniques, including the application of plasters, incantations to the gods, and the use of magical formulas.[1] Curiously enough, women living in the United States during the nineteenth century, the era of therapeutic pluralism, encountered a similar repertoire of treatments: surgery, the application of plasters, incantations to the gods, and the use of magical formulas sold as patent medicines. During this period, women with painful or troubling breast conditions could consult with orthodox, "regular" physicians. They could also seek relief from homeopaths, phrenologists, mesmerists, hydrotherapists, botanists, Eclectics, folk practitioners, and religious healers, among others. In addition, they could purchase secret potions by mail order or buy them from traveling saleswomen and men.

It was not until the first few decades of the twentieth century, however, that orthodox physicians achieved a virtual monopoly over the medical management of women with breast cancer in the United States. As this occurred, the vast array of medical sects, healers, and sellers of cancer cures were marginalized and pushed underground. The sectarians, or "irregulars," were demonized as quacks, denied medical licenses, excluded from medical societies, and denied hospital privileges. Simultaneously, new laws prohibiting foreign commerce and the interstate transport of improperly labeled foods and drugs cut into the brisk trade in secret nostrums and patent medicines sold as cancer cures.[2]

Although cancer of the breast had been medicalized in the past, in the sense that women with painful or distressing breast conditions often consulted a variety of medical doctors, it was not until the twentieth century that breast cancer came to reside exclusively within the domain of scientific medicine. Among the new breed of scientifically trained physicians, it was surgeons—formerly a relatively low-status group within medicine—who claimed the authority not only to treat but to cure cancer of the breast and other "female cancers." Thus, in the new regime, the regime of medicalization, it was surgeons who ascended the throne and crowned themselves the sovereign rulers of the kingdom. With new rulers came new subjects. The new subjects of the disease regime were women who exhibited what the American Society for the Control of Cancer (ASCC) termed the "danger signals" of cancer. Within the anticancer campaigns of the ASCC, these marked, or "signifying" women were, first and foremost, endangered by what these physical signs portended. On another level, however, they were discursively positioned as dangerous—to themselves, their spouses, and their children—if they did not behave responsibly and heed the early warning of these danger signals.

The repositioning of these dangerous and endangered women—or symptomatic subjects—within the jurisdictional domain of surgeons, however, did not happen overnight or automatically. It was the outcome, first, of a series of struggles between scientific medicine and its main competitors, the "irregulars." It was the outcome, second, of a series of campaigns designed to convince ordinary physicians to refer their symptomatic patients to surgeons. It was the outcome, third, of a series of campaigns designed to teach ordinary women to identify the "danger signals" of cancer and seek prompt medical attention from a regular, licensed physician.

This chapter examines the rise of the first regime of breast cancer. It focuses on the creation and diffusion of new discourses of disease, the institutionalization of new treatment technologies, the articulation of new physician and patient roles and relationships, the construction of new disease subjects and social relations, and the reorganization of the temporal and spatial dimensions of disease. The involuntary subjects of the regime of medicalization were the relatively small number of women who exhibited the "danger signals" of breast cancer and responded by consulting a physician. A subgroup of these endangered women became, at the hands of surgeons, mastectomees.

In the context of breast cancer, the temporary sick role identified by Talcott Parsons coconstituted the imperial authority of surgeons and the isolation and obedience of breast cancer patients. The architecture of the closet that greeted mastectomees when they exited the hospital thus complemented and reinforced the practices of normalization and isolation mobilized by the sick role script.

In order to illuminate the scale and scope of the changes wrought by the regime of medicalization, this chapter begins with a brief overview of key characteristics of the era of therapeutic pluralism that preceded it.

## THE ERA OF THERAPEUTIC PLURALISM

American medicine traces its lineage, through European lines of descent, to Hippocratic medicine. Within Hippocratic medicine, illness was conceptualized as a systemic disturbance, the result of an imbalance among the four humors—blood, phlegm, yellow bile, and black bile—which were linked to the four elements of the universe—earth, air, water, fire.[3] In medical treatises attributed to the Greek physician Hippocrates (born 460 BC), cancer appears as *karkinos* and as *karkinoma* in Latin, the language of modern medicine.[4] In this medical system, no matter where in the body cancer appeared, it was the result of an excess or congestion of black bile.[5] Cancer in the breast was different in location but not in kind from cancer in other parts of the body.

In Hippocratic medicine the treatment of people with cancer was designed to rebalance the four humors within the bodily system. Surgery was sometimes used, but only as one part of an ensemble of techniques designed to work at the systemic level by unblocking the flow of black bile and purifying the body of its excess. One text, for example, specified that surgery be preceded by a "general detoxification of the body . . . by purging and by administering theriac . . . and other draughts, or warm blood of a goose or duck." This "general detoxification" was followed by the administration of poultices and dietary restrictions.[6] Thus, even when surgery was used, it was part of a systemic, not a localized, approach to treatment that was designed to detoxify and rebalance the system.

Until the eighteenth century, the humoral tradition served as the foundation of European medicine. As in ancient times, treatment aimed at "dilution of the stagnating, inspissated or coagulated juices, whatever their nature or provenance, and at restoration of their normal flow within the affected breast."[7] A lively debate over how to categorize, identify, and treat various types of cancer in the breast extends from the time of Hippocrates through the late nineteenth century. Throughout these more than two thousand years, however, the dominant tone was one of caution with regard to the treatment of breast cancer and skepticism with regard to the use of surgery.

A major shift in medical conceptualizations of the human body, health, and disease occurred during the eighteenth and nineteenth centuries as humoral medicine gradually gave way to "scientific medicine," which was founded upon new technologies of seeing—the microscope, anatomical dissection, and, most importantly, what Foucault termed "the clinical gaze." Scientific medicine also gave rise to new conceptualizations of cancer. In this new paradigm, cancer of the breast gradually became a distinct disease, different from the cancers that appeared in other parts of the body. No longer the result of a systemic imbalance, breast cancer came to be seen as a disease of distinctly local origins and a disease that could potentially be vanquished with a local solution. Surgery—a local treatment—thus came to be seen in a more favorable light.

Since breast cancer is generally painless in its early stages, however, patients could rarely be convinced to undergo surgery. Operations during the latter stages of breast cancer, on the other hand, were viewed as unwise and ineffective since the cancer, having spread to distant organs, was no longer considered a local disease amenable to surgical extraction.[8] Writing in the late eighteenth century, for example, the influential physician Alexander Monro argued that surgical treatment for breast cancer should only be attempted on young and healthy women with "occult" cancers that had been caused by bruising or some other external cause. Even then, according to Monro, "an operation should only be proceeded to at the earnest request of the patient who had had the danger of relapse clearly explained to her."[9] There are no reliable postoperative statistics prior to the twentieth century, but a report written by Monro and published in 1781 suggests that conservatism with regard to surgery was more than warranted. Out of sixty cases of cancer that Monro treated by surgery, only four patients appeared to be alive without signs of disease after two years.

The absence of an effective anesthesia not only discouraged patients from enduring the procedure, it also inhibited the development of surgical methods. In the absence of anesthesia, only those breast surgeries that were deemed absolutely necessary were performed, and they were performed as quickly as possible, in the form of "a few short razor strokes."[10] A letter written in 1751, for example, recounts the story of a famous surgeon who assured his patient that he would not need more than one minute to amputate the patient's breast. The patient's directive to him, as recounted in the letter, was to "take four [minutes] and make a good job of it."[11]

One of the only accounts of surgical treatment written by a breast cancer patient during the nineteenth century was that of the English writer Fanny Burney. In letters to her kin, she described in vivid detail the breast amputation that she endured in her home in 1811. Burney was fully conscious during the operation, having had nothing but a glass of wine beforehand to prepare her for the twenty minutes of "utterly speechless torture" that ensued. In a famous passage, Burney wrote, "When the dreadful steel was plunged into the breast—cutting through veins—arteries—flesh—nerves— I needed no injunctions not to restrain my cries. I began a scream that lasted unintermittingly during the whole time of the incision—& I almost marvel that it rings not in my Ears still! so excruciating was the agony."[12]

American medicine, at least the sect that achieved a legal monopoly and cultural hegemony during the twentieth century, traces its lineage through this European line of descent. A famous painting by the artist Thomas Eakins offers a glimpse of the growing acceptance of surgical approaches to the treatment of breast cancer in the United States. In *The Agnew Clinic* (1889), Eakins painted a breast amputation in progress. Three surgeons and a nurse are shown in the foreground of the amphitheater, bent over the prone body of a woman on an operating table. All three doctors and the nurse are wearing clean, white surgical attire and the patient's body is draped, except for her torso, which remains uncovered. Two male surgeons brace the patient, who we can assume has been anesthetized, while the third surgeon puts a knife to her breast. At a slight distance, Dr. Hayes Agnew, the chair of surgery at the University of Pennsylvania, observes the progress of the three surgeons. Surrounding the surgical scene, male medical students pack the amphitheater, their attention riveted by the performance taking place front and center. The surgical field is brightly lit and seems to positively glow with the light of science. Unlike an earlier Eakins painting, *The Gross*

*Clinic* (1873), which is somewhat dark and foreboding, *The Agnew Clinic* clearly shows that by 1889 the antiseptic principles of Joseph Lister had been incorporated into the practice of surgery.[13]

A straightforward reading of *The Agnew Clinic* would suggest that by the late nineteenth century breast cancer had been successfully claimed by surgeons and incorporated into the domain of scientific medicine. If we were to move outside the medical amphitheater, however, we would see that surgeons' jurisdictional claims over breast cancer were not widely recognized either by the lay public or by ordinary physicians. This is hardly surprising, given that even a famous surgeon like Dr. Agnew expressed serious reservations about the benefits of surgery: "Indeed, I should hesitate," he acknowledged, "with my present experience, to claim a single case of absolute cure where the diagnosis of carcinoma had been verified by microscopic examination."[14]

Outside the operating amphitheater, surgeons competed with regular physicians and the so-called irregulars—homeopaths, hydropaths, Eclectics, Thomsonians, and many others. They also competed with religious healers, folk practitioners, domestic guides to medicine, and patent medicines sold by mail and by traveling salesmen and women. If any sector dominated the treatment of cancer, it was probably the brisk trade in mail-order cures and patent medicines.

From the colonial period until the end of the nineteenth century, the practice of medicine in America was notable for its stunning variety. Whereas in England medical guilds enforced categorical distinctions between the higher-status physicians and the lower-order surgeons, no such structure of medical estates existed in the colonies.[15] Instead, because orthodox physicians lacked the ability to enforce categorical distinctions and jurisdictional domains, not only were the boundaries between general physicians and surgeons blurred indiscriminately, but medicine itself, as Paul Starr has pointed out, was taken up "by all manner of people."[16]

The regular physicians of the nineteenth century were a diverse lot. Some regular physicians, especially in the urban centers of the Northeast, were trained at the best medical schools in Europe. The practice of medicine in the eastern cities of the United States was dominated by regular physicians, typically middle- and upper-class white men. Others were barely literate, with degrees from makeshift medical schools. The majority were somewhere in between.

The number of regular physicians who were women increased steadily after 1850.[17] By 1900 women made up at least 10 percent of the enrollment in eighteen regular medical schools across the country, reaching a high of 18 percent in Boston and other select East Coast cities, and made up nearly 6 percent of the total enrollment in medical schools, 75 percent of which were "regulars."[18] But these women, according to Carol Weisman, "met with hostility from many of their male colleagues, and they were excluded from membership in the AMA (American Medical Association) and from many local medical societies, hospital positions, and hospital-based training programs."[19]

Sectarian medicine offered a more hospitable environment for women to practice, especially middle-class white women, and the second half of the nineteenth century was the heyday of sectarian medicine. There were numerous medical sects during this period of time, each with its own training programs and medical schools—some with their own hospitals and institutions. Because of their minimal cost, prerequisites, and training requirements, proprietary medical schools were accessible to a much broader range of students. Also unlike many of the regular medical schools, they welcomed women.[20] Thomsonian medicine, for example, which was characterized by a botanical approach to treatment, developed a particularly wide following among women. Perhaps, in part, this was because Thomsonian medicine promoted a democratic and commonsense medicine for the people and a political philosophy based on a critique of the elitism of regular medicine. Irregular schools of medicine also included homeopathy, hydropathy, and Eclecticism, to name just a few. The nineteenth-century medical marketplace was one in which, according to Naomi Rogers, "regulars and sectarians competed, practiced, and worked with each other—therapy and principle at times rigid and defining, at times flexible."[21]

In addition to regular and irregular physicians, people in the nineteenth century turned to domestic guides, patent medicines, and folk traditions. These options were particularly popular among groups outside the upper and middle classes of the eastern cities. Guides to domestic medicine written by physicians began circulating widely in the eighteenth and nineteenth centuries. These guides strengthened the self-help approach to medicine that was practiced by necessity, narrowed the distance between domestic and professional medicine, and contributed to the democratization of medical

knowledge and practice.[22] The popularity of these guides testifies to the
strength of domestic medicine, which was the province of women.

According to Paul Starr, until the late nineteenth century "lay practitioners and folk healers flourished in the countryside and towns, scorning
the therapies and arcane learning of regular physicians and claiming the
right to practice medicine as an inalienable liberty comparable to religious
freedom."[23] The work of Susan Cayleff suggests that there were probably
as many kinds of folk medicine as there were regional, racial, and ethnic
cultures.[24] According to Cayleff, these diverse folk traditions had at least
three things in common: a component of self-help, oral transmission, and
a worldview congruent with the patient's. Both women and men were folk
practitioners, but women supplied the medical therapies within their homes
through remedies, food preparation, and prayer.[25]

The popularity of folk medicine, like that of domestic medicine, contributed to an "ecology of medical practice" that tended to diminish the
social boundaries between practitioners and patients.[26] Even within regular medicine, where the most elite stratum of practitioners was found, the
distribution of power between patients and physicians was practically the
reverse of what it later became. Physicians usually visited patients in their
homes, for example, and listened while they gave voice to their symptoms.
This orientation toward symptoms, according to Nicholas Jewson, "reflected
a consultative relationship in which the patient was the more powerful
figure."[27] During the nineteenth century the doctor in America, in the
words of Paul Starr, "was more of a courtier than an autocrat."[28]

Given this "ecology of medical practice," an interesting picture emerges
with regard to the management of breast cancer during the second half of
the nineteenth century. According to James Patterson:

> Unorthodox cancer cures flourished because many Americans were afraid to
> confront the reality of the disease. To consult a [regular] doctor about a lump
> or discharge was to risk an unpleasant diagnosis—and possibly surgery. The
> promise of relief from pain was then and always one of the strongest draw-
> ing cards of unorthodox practitioners. Some people shrank from consulting
> physicians because they did not want anyone to know they had the disease.
> They were sure that cancer was unmentionable—perhaps contagious, per-
> haps hereditary, surely insidious and fatal. Better to face one's fate in private,
> or to treat the illness oneself with potions available by mail or vendor.[29]

There are no definitive data on the help-seeking practices of women with breast cancer during the era of therapeutic pluralism, but Patterson notes that physicians who practiced "heroic" medicine were avoided by a significant portion of the population. This made a world of sense given that regular practitioners "asserted the virtues of surgery," whereas "quacks promised to help people escape pain."[30]

In short, women who sought treatment for painful breast conditions during the era of therapeutic pluralism could, depending on their means and geographic location, consult physicians from a variety of medical traditions, as well as faith healers, folk healers, domestic guides to medicine, and patent medicines advertised as cures. The tremendous commercial success of these medicinal "cancer cures" provides additional evidence of the popular distrust of, and distaste for, regular physicians.[31] Therapeutic choices were no doubt shaped by class and cultural factors and constrained by the distribution of practitioners, but the treatment of cancer in the nineteenth century was not monopolized by any one tradition, and it was not dominated by surgery.[32]

## THE REGIME OF MEDICALIZATION

The shift from the era of therapeutic pluralism to the regime of medicalization was made possible by a revolution in medicine that developed first in France, at the end of the eighteenth century, and then spread through Europe and the United States during the nineteenth and early twentieth centuries. Underlying the rise of scientific medicine was the emergence of a new form of medical perception, or what Michel Foucault, in *The Birth of the Clinic,* termed "the clinical gaze."

The clinical gaze was not simply a form of perception but rather was a mode of objectification that involved specific practices of seeing, speaking, touching, listening, and representing. It was this insistent, revolutionary gaze that opened up living bodies and human corpses to new kinds of investigation and new modes of objectification. "The clinician's gaze," as Foucault described it, became "the functional equivalent of fire in chemical combustion."[33]

It was the clinical gaze, according to Foucault, that led to the transformation of medicine, patients, and physicians. The details of this transition need not concern us here. What it is important to know, for our purposes, is that the rise of scientific medicine in the United States coincided with three interrelated developments: the consolidation of power by regular physicians and the rising status of surgeons, the reform of medical education, and the building of a vast network of hospitals.

Prior to this transformation, hospitals functioned as warehouses for the poor, as places of death and contagion, and as destinations of last resort for people with no other options. Through what Foucault termed "the sovereign power of the empirical gaze," however, both hospitals and patients were transformed.[34] Hospitals became factories of knowledge production and cure-oriented medical treatment rather than warehouses for the sick and dying, and patients became the key resource, or raw material, for the production of medical knowledge. Hospitals made possible the multiplication of observations, the recording of these observations in the form of "cases," the accumulation of vast amounts of data for comparison and evaluation, and the development of new forms of treatment. As the work of Charles Rosenberg, Rosemary Stevens, Paul Starr, and many others makes clear, "the rise of hospitals was a precondition for the formation of a sovereign profession."[35]

The clinical examination changed the relationship between practitioners and patients. The consultative relationship between patients who narrated their own stories and physicians who listened was transformed into a relationship in which the power of interpretation shifted to the physician and the patient's narrative was narrowed and muted.[36] Previously, patients had remained clothed during medical consultations. Now their bodies were exposed, touched, and examined by physicians, who adopted a stance of scientific detachment.[37] Only by abstracting the disease from the patient could the physician render a diagnosis. Thus, according to Jens Lachmund, the introduction of diagnosis by physicians "was a cultural project which involved the creation of new meanings of illness, a reorganization of treatment schemes and changing modes of social interaction."[38] All of this was premised upon "the shift from the patient's narrative to the body's interior."[39]

In revolutionary France the clinical gaze emerged at the end of the eighteenth century and was quickly institutionalized. Across the ocean, however, the context and conditions of medical practice were quite different. In the United States the rise of the new clinical gaze and the transformation of hospitals, physicians, and patients occurred later and more gradually. Between 1870 and 1910, however, according to Starr, "hospitals moved from the periphery to the center of medical education and medical practice."[40]

Johns Hopkins Medical School was the leader in the transformation of American medicine. According to Paul Starr, the significance of Johns Hopkins Medical School lay in the new relationships it established: "It joined science and research ever more firmly to clinical hospital practice. While apprentices had learned the craft of medicine in their preceptor's office and the patient's home, now doctors in training would see medical practice almost entirely on the wards of teaching hospitals."[41]

Before the twentieth century, the occupation of physician did not, according to Starr, "confer a clear and unequivocal class position in American society" because "the inequalities among physicians paralleled the class structure." The social position of physicians was not low, but it was "insecure and ambiguous" and depended "as much on his family background and the status of his patients as on the nature of his occupation." Between the 1870s and the early 1900s "the social distance between doctor and patient increased, while the distance among colleagues diminished as the profession became more cohesive and uniform." This occurred through licensure laws, the restructuring of the profession, the consolidation of power through the vehicle of the AMA, and the reform of medical education.[42]

As part of the modernization of medicine and the professional dominance of physicians, the AMA made a concerted effort to tighten medical-school licensing laws, eliminate the "less respectable" schools, and duplicate the system of medical education pioneered by Johns Hopkins Medical School, which brought together science education, medical research, and hospital medicine—all within one institution.[43] The stringent requirements and high costs of the remaining medical schools limited the access to medical education for students from the lower and working classes, and most of the schools that accepted women, Jews, blacks, and students of limited means were closed. Fourteen of the seventeen medical schools for women closed their doors, for example, and the coeducational medical schools that remained limited the enrollment of women to a quota of about 5 percent. Out of seven medical schools for blacks, only two survived.[44]

The reform of medical education enhanced the professional authority, political strength, social status, and market position of orthodox physicians while the exclusion of women, blacks, immigrants, and students of modest means strengthened the social cohesiveness of the medical profession. The growing homogeneity and elitism of the medical profession widened the social distance between physicians and their patients, exaggerating the

disparity in power introduced by the modern clinical method.[45] Homeopathic and Eclectic physicians—the two largest sects—were gradually
absorbed into the institutional structure of orthodox medicine; the other
sects were denied entry, and over time, many of them disappeared. Some
sects, for example osteopaths, Christian Scientists, and chiropractors, maintained a parallel, but marginal, presence outside organized medicine.

A book by Annie Riley Hale, one of the many irregulars, or "cultists"
(her term), who were pushed to the margins of the medical marketplace and
labeled "quacks," provides a fascinating glimpse of the rise of scientific
medicine and the marginalization of the irregulars from the perspective of
one of the many practitioners who lost their livelihood in the process. In
*These Cults,* which was originally published in 1926, Hale used the term
"physician politicians" to describe the AMA, a reference to the social, cultural, and political power of this organization of orthodox physicians.
According to Hale, the AMA's "physician politicians . . . manned [literally]
all the health-boards, dictated all the health legislation, and framed all the
medical practice acts," which "determine[d] who shall and who shall not
minister to the sick."[46] Key to the AMA's success, as Hale noted, was its
"publicity machine."

The AMA, according to Hale, "fostered in the laity a blind trust in its
teachings, and consistently fought and hounded every other school of healing." In the United States this "monopolistic control," in Hale's words,
was accomplished "by the development and perfection of the most colossal,
the most all-inclusive publicity machine ever known, never surpassed—if
equaled—by any political party in the world."[47] Finally, drawing a picture
of "misery and ill-health" among the masses, Hale argued that "the most
dreaded and devastating diseases" had grown more fatal while orthodox
medicine exerted its "monopolistic control of the therapeutic situation."
Among the "most dreaded and devastating" diseases that had "grown more
fatal" during orthodox medicine's watch, cancer was at the top of her list.

Thus, as scientific medicine was institutionalized within the United
States, orthodox physicians gained a monopoly over the right to treat cancer patients, and medicine became an elite profession whose practitioners
were almost exclusively white, Christian, upper-class men. The rise of scientific medicine and the medicalization of breast cancer, as the next few
sections make clear, thus reorganized the social relations of the disease.
Within this new regime of practices, a new social script for patients was

institutionalized that simultaneously coconstructed the power and authority of male physicians and the compliance and isolation of female patients.

This new social script, the sick role, entailed the patient's transfer of
authority over her body to the physician, the obligation to "comply" with
the doctor's orders, and the obligation to make every effort to "get better"
and return to normal.[48] In exchange, the patient was entitled to receive the
temporary benefits of the sick role—compassionate treatment within a safe
and segregated enclave, sympathy from friends and family, and the sus-
pension of regular responsibilities until she recuperated from surgery. Because physicians—especially surgeons—were almost always men, and breast
cancer patients, with only rare exceptions, were women, the new regime of
breast cancer reinforced and reproduced the dominant gender order. We
turn now to an examination of the sick role in the context of breast cancer
patients and their surgeons. We begin with a discussion of the "invention"
of breast cancer as a curable disease.

## Inventing a Curable Disease

By the end of the nineteenth century, according to historian David Cantor, much of the framework of twentieth-century oncology had been laid:
"'True' neoplasms were distinguished from inflammatory lesions, cysts,
tubercles, and the many other swellings with which they had been grouped
for over two thousand years. Pathologists treated tumours as having a cel-
lular nature: they originated in normal cells and tissues of corresponding
types . . . [and they] could either be 'malignant' or 'benign.'"[49] Most importantly, instead of being viewed as a systemic disease, cancer was reconceptualized as "a localized disease that spread centrifugally in a slow, ordered
manner."[50] If local diseases could be removed through local procedures,
breast cancer could, in theory, be excised from the body. Breast cancer was
reconceptualized within medical journals and textbooks as a disease for
which radical surgery, if performed early enough, could be curative.[51] Breast
cancer, in the provocative words of Barron H. Lerner, was "invented" as a
curable disease.[52]

It was primarily surgeons who invented this new disease, and foremost
among them was William Stewart Halsted, the high priest of breast cancer surgery.[53] During the 1880s Halsted synthesized the work of European
surgeons into a coherent theory of breast cancer and helped refine a surgical procedure that became known as the Halsted radical mastectomy.[54]

However, Halsted was not only the head of surgery at Johns Hopkins, the premier medical school in the country; he was also a tireless and charismatic crusader on behalf of this surgical innovation. By the time of his death in 1922, former students of Halsted were spread throughout the country, many of them heading their own departments of surgery.[55] By the early years of the twentieth century, the Halsted radical mastectomy had become "the treatment of choice" among surgeons.[56] "All this," according to historian Joan Austoker, "was in the absence of any historical evidence that the introduction of the radical technique significantly improved on the survival rates achieved by more conservative measures in the pre-Halstedian era."[57]

The growth of hospitals and medical training programs in the early twentieth century—and the key role played by Johns Hopkins in the reform and standardization of medical education—made the Halsted radical mastectomy hegemonic among American surgeons. It remained so until well into the 1970s, and old-school surgeons continued performing the operation well into the 1980s.[58] Despite the hegemony of the Halsted radical mastectomy, it remained a relatively rare procedure in individual hospitals until well into the twentieth century.[59]

The Halsted is a radical procedure that involves the removal of all of the breast tissue (in the affected breast), as well as the chest muscles and lymph nodes in the region. Its consequences were quite serious. Women who underwent this procedure were typically left with a deformed, concave chest. In addition to the loss of strength that resulted from the removal of the pectoral muscles, women who underwent this procedure were prone to the development of lymphedema, a chronic and sometimes severe and painful swelling of the arm that further inhibited physical strength and mobility.

Although the technical components of the new regime of breast cancer (hospitals, surgical technique, trained surgeons, anesthesia, sterile operating environments) were in place for the urban, white, upper and middle classes by the early part of the twentieth century, the existence of a relatively select group of well-trained surgeons making claims about the curative value of the Halsted radical mastectomy, as noted earlier, did not mean that other physicians were immediately convinced of the merits of radical surgery and were willing to refer their patients for surgery, or that women diagnosed with breast cancer were willing to undergo this procedure.

The growing use of anesthesia and antiseptic procedures made patients more willing to undergo surgical procedures and surgeons more willing to perform them, but this did not translate easily or automatically into a belief in the surgical cure for breast cancer (and justifiably so).[60] The diffusion of the Halsted radical mastectomy was dependent upon the willingness of women to undergo the procedure and the willingness of physicians who were not trained in this procedure to refer their patients to surgeons who were. The institutionalization of the procedure within American medicine was, in large part, the result of the creation of a new health voluntary, the American Society for the Control of Cancer, and the campaign it conducted during the first half of the twentieth century—a campaign designed to convince potential patients and physicians that cancer of the breast, if diagnosed early, could be cured by surgery.

## DANGER SIGNALS AND DANGEROUS/ENDANGERED WOMEN

In 1905 the AMA appointed a committee to prepare a report on cancer mortality. The committee made two recommendations. First, it recommended that physicians be educated about cancer. Second, it recommended that the public, especially women, be educated as well. In 1912, at a meeting of the American Gynecological Society in Baltimore, Maryland, a series of papers was presented on cancer of the cervix, which posed a much greater threat to women in the early twentieth century than cancer of the breast. In response to these papers, a committee on cervical cancer was formed. The committee, in turn, resolved to form an organization "for the purpose of putting before the public the necessity of taking steps to reduce the number of deaths from cancer."[61]

In 1913, the Thirty-eighth Annual Convention of the American Gynecological Society was held in Washington, D.C., along with the Congress of American Physicians and Surgeons. The entire second day of the convention was devoted to the subject of cancer control. Frederick Hoffman, an actuary with the Metropolitan Life Insurance Company, gave a talk in which he argued that cancer mortality rates were increasing and that the increase was "not primarily due to improved medical diagnosis and more accurate methods of death certification." He concluded his speech with ten recommendations.

The number one priority on his list was to organize "an American Society for the study and prevention of cancer, primarily for the purpose of educating the public at large in the absolute necessity of operative treatment at the earliest indication of cancerous growths." He also recommended "the

immediate preparation and widest distribution of a concise outline of accepted cancer facts, showing the disease in all cases to be of local origin, that
the chief danger to the patient lies in the tendency toward a rapid extension of cancerous growths, that the only certain remedy known to science
is the complete surgical removal of the affected parts at the earliest possible indication of the disease, and that when this is done the outlook for a
cure in the accepted meaning of the term is decidedly hopeful, but that to
the contrary delay and neglect or refusal to submit to operative treatment
are practically certain to result fatally within a comparatively short period
of time." Shortly thereafter, another meeting was held at the Harvard Club.
At this meeting the ASCC was formed.

In 1913, in the same month the ASCC was founded, the *Ladies Home
Journal* published an article titled "What Can We Do about Cancer?" that
was inspired by the committee of the American College of Surgeons that
founded the ASCC. This article caused a stir, according to Walter Ross,
"because it discussed a taboo subject in lay language for a mass audience."
The author concluded with several "truths," including the statement, "If the
development of cancer be determined in the early stages, the patient can
probably be cured by operation, but not by any other method."[62]

The importance of the ASCC to the institutional history of cancer in
the United States cannot be overestimated. More than any other private
organization or public agency, the ASCC shaped public and professional
practices and perceptions of cancer in general and of breast cancer in particular. The ASCC was, in large part, responsible for moving women with
breast cancer into the jurisdiction of surgeons. During the regime of medicalization the ASCC launched a wide array of cancer-education campaigns
that targeted both physicians and the lay public, especially women. Cancer
education, not cancer research, remained the ASCC's sole purpose until
the post–World War II era.

During the early years of the twentieth century, according to numerous
sources, the medical profession as a whole did not accept the idea of cancer control and was extremely reticent about referring their patients to surgeons.[63] In the words of Lester Breslow and Danile Wilner, "Each physician
would see ordinarily only an occasional case of cancer and a high proportion of such patients would die. The outlook was dismal, both in the eyes
of most medical practitioners and in the view of the general public, which
tended to look upon cancer as a loathsome and hopeless disease."[64] Many

doctors "remained more frightened and pessimistic about the disease," according to historian Walter Ross, "than their patients."[65] In order to move breast cancer into the jurisdictional domain of surgeons, ordinary women and their physicians had to be convinced that cancer could be successfully treated by surgery.

The first major campaign launched by the ASCC carried the following message: "Do Not Delay" if you discover one of the "Danger Signals of Cancer." The number and definition of these danger signals have varied over time, as has the wording of the message, but the cancer campaigns of the ASCC (later the American Cancer Society) have been organized around a discourse of early detection throughout the century. As historian Robert Aronowitz has argued, the apparent wisdom of this message has become so ingrained in contemporary culture that we mistakenly assume that the "Do Not Delay" injunction was based upon epidemiological or clinical studies demonstrating a relationship between a woman's delay in seeking medical attention and the outcome of her treatment. It was not. Only in recent decades, as Aronowitz has noted, has medical evidence in the form of observational studies and clinical trials "served as the rationale for specific clinical and public health practices and ideas."[66]

Nevertheless, in 1920 the ASCC produced its first motion picture, *The Reward of Courage,* and in 1921 the ASCC began organizing an annual National Cancer Week during which it stepped up its cancer education campaigning and media outreach.[67] In 1929 a booklet entitled *What Every Woman Should Know about Cancer* was prepared in English and translated into Yiddish, Italian, Spanish, Polish, French, and Russian. Over 650,000 copies of the booklet were distributed through a network of women's clubs and women's groups and by the Metropolitan Life Insurance Company. A second pamphlet, *The Danger Signals of Cancer,* was published in twenty-two languages.[68] The danger signs included "any lump, especially in the breast."[69] These pamphlets, like the smaller-scale efforts that came before them, adopted a twofold strategy. First, the pamphlets reconstituted specific bodily signs as signifiers, or symptoms, of cancer. Second, the pamphlets provided instructions regarding the appropriate action to be taken upon discovery of "danger signals." The instructions were clear: Consult a physician immediately.

Results from two surveys conducted by the Pennsylvania Medical Society thirteen years apart, in 1910 and 1923, indicate that by 1923, at least in that part of the country, the ASCC's double-pronged "Do Not Delay" campaign had already achieved an impact. According to these surveys, between 1910 and 1923 the delay between a patient's "discovery of the first symptoms . . . and the first call on the physician" decreased from 18 months to 14.6 months. Over that same period, physicians "learned the importance of prompt action" and reduced the "interval" between the patient's first appearance and the "institution of treatment" from 13 months to 4.5 months for "superficial cancer" and from 12 months to 3.9 months in "deep seated cancers."[70]

In an article from 1926, published in the lay-oriented medical journal *Hygeia,* which was launched by the AMA in 1923 to disseminate its views to the public (and did so through an impressive distribution network that included doctors' offices, public schools, newspapers, private homes, and state legislatures), the author endeavors to instruct the reader on the appropriate action to take if she discovers a lump in her breast. The article, which I quote at length below, communicates the position of the ASCC, which the AMA fully supported. The author first explains that "tumors are at first a local growth, limited to the spot at which they make their appearance" and that only after time and prodding do they spread to "distant parts of the body":

> As regards cancer of the breast, the question arises as to why the transfer of the disease from one organ to another should be so extensive, and it has been concluded that when a woman discovers a lump in her breast she feels it perhaps a half dozen times and then asks the opinion of her mother, who likewise feels it two or three times to be certain it is a lump; then she consults neighbors and friends, who, after considerable manipulation, tell her what she already knew in the first place, that it is a lump.
>
> It must be realized that cancer is exclusively a medical problem and that the neighbors and friends, the parents and relatives, who have no medical training, are in no position to make a differential diagnosis . . . but beyond this must be taken into consideration the fact that with laboratory animals, when it is desired to spread tumors rapidly and to see how extensively it can be done, the tumors are massaged.
>
> If a woman has a lump in her breast she should understand that to feel it once is all-sufficient. Her next step should be to go to the best possible physician, one in whom she has implicit confidence, and to abide by his decision. She should not shop around from doctor to doctor, because each in turn

must make an examination, and no matter how gently an examination is made there must be some manipulation, and the less of this the better for the patient, so far as preventing the spread of cancer is concerned.[71]

As this passage makes clear, women who discovered the danger signals but did not follow the sick role script precisely as it was written by the ASCC and endorsed by the AMA could be held responsible for the deadly spread of their cancer—not just indirectly, through delay, but also directly, through repeated touching and massaging of the "lump."

In "Cancer of the Breast," a 1930 article published in *Hygeia,* the author goes one step further, counseling women to "beware of the physician who is not able to make a diagnosis and requests the patient to return week after week . . . which means a lost opportunity for possible cure by early treatment." Such doctors, the author insists, should be viewed as "dangerous advisors" and dealt with by seeking a consultation with "a specialist in breast diagnosis"—that is, a surgeon.[72] Consistent with the discourse of the ASCC, the articles in *Hygeia* are directed at women who discover a lump in their breast—one of the "danger signals" of cancer—and it scripts a clear line of action and attitude for these newly constituted subjects of the regime, these dangerous and endangered women. "By 1930," according to historian Kirsten Gardner, "the ASCC had published thousands of copies of pamphlets on cancer, distributed *The Great Peril,* and encouraged dozens of magazines, newspapers, and radios to teach the public about cancer. Moreover, it had worked to inform women that lumps in the breast . . . might indicate cancer." Furthermore, among cancers specific to women, "breast cancer received the most attention."[73]

In the late 1930s the Federal Art Project, which was the visual arm of the Works Progress Administration (President Roosevelt's New Deal antipoverty program of public works), created a series of cancer posters in conjunction with the ASCC and the U.S. Public Health Service. "More Women Die of CANCER Than Do Men," one poster began, followed by the hopeful message that "70 percent of the 35,000 women who die annually of cancer of the breast and uterus could be saved if treated in time." A second poster stated, "STOP CANCER NOW. Delay Reduces the Chance for Recovery." In this poster, a figure of a woman is posed next to a chart that juxtaposes "Percent Cured When Treated Early" with "Percent Cured When Treated Late" for cancer of the uterus, breast, mouth and lip, skin, rectum,

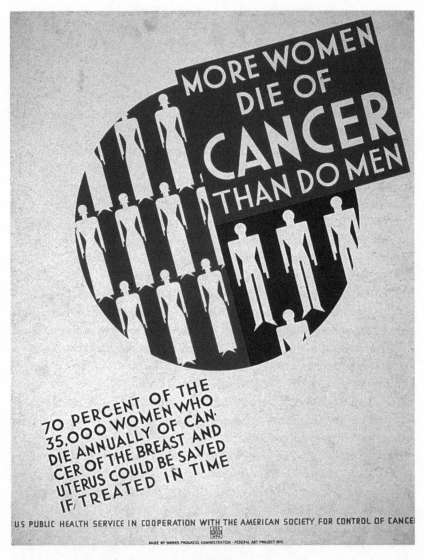

More women die of cancer than do men. Library of Congress, Prints and Photographs Division, WPA Poster Collection, reproduction number LC-USZC2-1009.

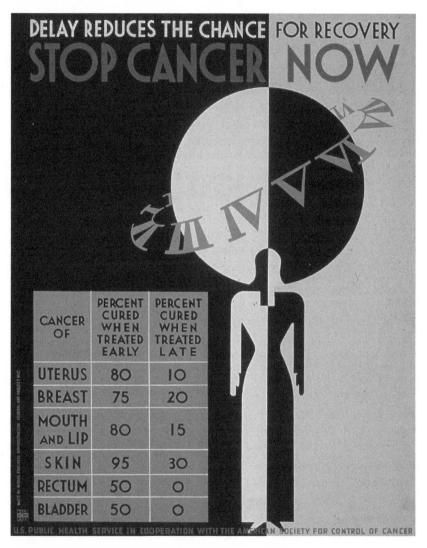

Delay reduces the chance for recovery. Library of Congress, Prints and Photographs Division, WPA Poster Collection, reproduction number LC-USZC2-1120.

and bladder. Breast cancer treated early, according to this poster, led to a 70 percent cure rate, whereas breast cancer treated late resulted in a cure rate of only 10 percent. Other posters proclaimed "DON'T FEAR CANCER—FIGHT IT!" and "Don't Fight Cancer Alone." Another series of posters promoted "surgery, radium, and x-rays" as the treatments offered "by reputable physicians" and cautioned that "other methods of treatment are experimental or quackery."

In the early 1930s the ASCC expanded its campaign of public and professional outreach and education. Clarence Cook Little, the new managing director of the ASCC (appointed by the board of directors) divided the United States into four regions and hired one physician to communicate the ASCC's cancer control message to physicians in each region. These ASCC-affiliated physicians organized exhibits, spoke at medical meetings, distributed literature written by the ASCC for physicians, and gave lectures at medical schools.[74]

Little also approached the General Federation of Women's Clubs to "enlist their members in a public-education campaign."[75] In his earlier travels to Europe, Little had come away with the impression that European physicians were strongly opposed to cancer-education campaigns directed at the lay public. They, and subsequently Little and the ASCC, were concerned "that a superficial program of lay publicity would only lead more patients to cancer phobia, quacks, and disillusionment." After working with volunteers from the General Federation of Women's Clubs for several years, Little "completely reversed his position" and came to the conclusion that the time was right for a "widespread and intensive campaign" to inform the public about "the prevention of cancer."[76] According to Walter Ross, "The Society's need for more volunteers to carry out public education, and for new sources of money, forced it to broaden its volunteer base. The ASCC Executive Committee decided that women would make the best public-education volunteers for a number of reasons: The campaign would go into people's homes, where tact and patience would be essential; it would require a good deal of time, which many women could more easily spare in the mid-1930s than could their husbands; and the emphasis would be on cancers that affected women."[77] Thus, in 1936, the Women's Field Army (WFA) was born.

The Women's Field Army, in the words of Ross, "was a quantum leap forward in volunteer power."[78] According to Little, "In 1935 there were fifteen thousand people active in cancer control throughout the United States. . . . At the close of 1938, there were ten times that number. This growth [was] due to the Women's Field Army."[79] The tremendous success of the WFA enabled the ASCC, for the first time, to reach substantial numbers of women outside the white middle and upper classes of the Northeast.[80] Posters and handbills recruiting volunteers for the WFA featured a flaming sword and the proclamation "There shall be light! Enlist in the Women's Field Army!" During its first year of existence, women's field armies were established in twenty-five states.[81] The organization of the WFA was loosely modeled after that of the army. At the top of the command structure was the national commander, who issued orders to state commanders and captains. Members of the army—volunteers dressed in brown WFA uniforms—conducted door-to-door campaigns designed to "carry the message of early detection and medical intervention into every home in the land."[82]

Articles about the WFA appeared in such mass-circulation magazines as *Elks Magazine, Women's Home Companion, Good Housekeeping,* and *American Legion Monthly.* In addition, the ASCC enlisted the support of the major news outlets—*Time, Life,* and *Fortune*—which showed stories on cancer as part of their newsreel series.[83] The WFA successfully recruited the Association of American University Women to its cause and worked extensively with the General Federation of Women's Clubs, which mobilized its membership in support of cancer education. In fact, the commander of the WFA, Marjorie B. Illig, was recruited from the General Federation of Women's Clubs, where she served as the chair of the Public Health Division. The WFA raised money from public donations to subsidize its educational and outreach activities and to subsidize "needy" cancer patients' travel to diagnostic and treatment centers. The WFA also encouraged the public to donate money to hospitals, clinics, and laboratories.[84] The WFA eventually grew to approximately 700,000 officers and troops—by far the largest division of the ASCC.[85] The WFA, in the words of Kirsten Gardner, "epitomized women's involvement in the ASCC, devotion to cancer awareness, and particular concern for women and cancer." However, as Gardner emphasized, "the limits of the female cancer awareness campaign were ignored . . . cultivating a sense of false optimism that assured women that early detection would lead to a cure."[86]

In 1946 a palace coup restructured the ASCC, which was renamed the American Cancer Society (ACS). Led by Mary Lasker and her husband

Albert, an advertising tycoon who made his fortune working for the tobacco industry, this "beneficent takeover" transformed the ASCC from a small-scale, weakly organized, fiscally conservative, physician-dominated organization into a high-powered, hierarchically structured, bureaucratic philanthropy organized around the principles of modern management, salesmanship, and advertising. From that point on, the ACS leadership included business and advertising professionals with a knack for marketing and fund-raising. The "modernization" of the health voluntary included a new focus on medical research. The ACS also became "a potent lobby" for cancer research within the federal government.[87]

The WFA was first scaled back by the new leadership of the restructured ACS and then eliminated altogether in 1951. Over the years, according to Breslow and Wilner, the WFA had come to be regarded as "too independent and frequently unmanageable."[88] Furthermore, their support of cancer patients of limited means threatened the ASCC's hands-off approach to cancer patients. In several states the WFA provided assistance to destitute cancer patients. These services were independent of the national structure of the ACS, however, and these were exactly the kinds of activities that made the medical profession, and hence the ACS leadership, uneasy about the WFA.[89]

The reorganized ACS continued its campaign of medicalization through the development of early detection campaigns that supported the interests of private physicians by channeling more women into the diagnostic and treatment pipeline. A new campaign was launched in the 1950s called "Every Doctor's Office a Cancer Detection Center." This slogan perfectly captures the ACS's dual focus on transforming symptomatic women into cancer patients and integrating ordinary doctors into the larger regime of practices. This campaign was designed with detection technologies for cervical cancer more than for breast cancer in mind. Unlike for breast cancer, which required a surgical biopsy to confirm a diagnosis, the diagnostic test for cervical cancer—a Pap smear—could actually be performed in the doctor's office, although the "smear" had to be analyzed in a pathology laboratory.[90]

At the same time, the ACS launched a new campaign that extended early detection further into the domestic sphere. In 1949 the ACS created an instructional video that taught women how to systematically examine their breasts on a regular basis in the privacy of their homes. Between 1949 and 1953, over six hundred copies of this film were distributed, and more than three million women attended screenings sponsored by local ACS chapters.[91] A newspaper photograph taken in South Bend, Indiana, showed a remarkable scene unfolding. A throng of women gathered outside a movie theater beneath a banner that read "Cancer Program 10 AM Today for Women Only!" The caption beneath the photograph indicates that four hundred women were turned away because the 2,500-seat theater was already filled to capacity.[92] Building on this momentum, articles encouraging women to examine their breasts began appearing during the 1950s in mainstream women's magazines such as *Ladies Home Journal, Good Housekeeping,* and *Women's Home Companion.*

## THE TEMPORARY SICK ROLE AND THE ARCHITECTURE OF THE CLOSET

Outside the doctor's office, discourses of early detection circulated in women's magazines, in the pamphlets distributed by women's clubs and ACS volunteers, in the media campaign known as National Cancer Week, in newsreels and news magazines, and in the breast self-examination (BSE) film screenings that were held during the 1950s. Through these discourses of early detection healthy women exhibiting danger signals were reconstituted as responsible, well-informed subjects actively pursuing the medicalization of their condition. Once they entered the doctor's office, women exhibiting danger signals were reconstituted as symptomatic women. From there, if the consulting physician deemed it necessary, symptomatic women became subjects of, and subject to, the sovereign gaze of the surgeon.

Just as the regime of medicalization invented breast cancer as a curable disease, it invented breast cancer patients as potentially curable patients. As subjects of the regime of medicalization, women diagnosed with breast cancer were shaped, first and foremost, by their experiences of diagnosis and treatment; second, by the norms of nondisclosure that governed physicians' interactions with cancer patients; and third, by the normalizing practices through which "cured" women—the temporary subjects of this regime— were taught to return to their normal lives and pass as "normal" women. This was a deeply gendered and patriarchal regime of practices in which the sovereign rulers were male surgeons who wielded absolute power in the medical setting over breast cancer patients and demanded total obedience from their subjects.

During the regime of medicalization, breast cancer was diagnosed by means of a surgical biopsy and treated by means of the Halsted radical mastectomy. The Halsted, as mentioned earlier, was a deforming, often debilitating procedure that involved the removal of the chest muscles and surrounding lymph nodes as well as the breast tissue. Instead of separating the surgical biopsy from the surgical treatment, however, surgeons combined the two procedures into one operation. First, a surgical biopsy was performed by the surgeon and analyzed by a pathologist present for the procedure. If the pathologist diagnosed cancer and the surgeon agreed, an immediate radical mastectomy was performed while the patient remained unconscious.

From the surgeon's perspective, the one-step procedure made perfect sense. It was safer for the patient because it avoided the risk of a second general anesthesia, and it was more efficient for both patient and physician because it avoided the added time and trouble of scheduling a second operation. The one-step procedure required that a patient sign in advance a consent form authorizing her surgeon to perform an immediate mastectomy if he determined that the tumor was malignant. Practically speaking, this meant that a certain percentage of patients who entered the hospital expecting nothing more than a surgical biopsy awoke to discover that they had been treated for breast cancer by radical mastectomy before learning of their condition.

Although the one-step procedure was the preference of surgeons, in practice many women underwent surgical biopsies in medical facilities without a pathologist on site. In this case the biopsy and surgery were separated while the specimen was sent to the nearest pathology lab and the surgeon waited to hear from the pathologist. In *Nothing's Changed: Diary of a Mastectomy*, Dorothy Abbott described the two-step procedure that she received in a small, southwestern town in 1978 and summarized the experiences of fourteen other women she interviewed in her town who were treated for breast cancer during the 1940s, '50s, '60s, and '70s. According to Abbot, one woman, who was diagnosed in 1945, was told by her physician, "Go to the Mayo Clinic in Rochester, Minnesota. As far as I know, that is the only place where there are facilities to test for cancer while the patient remains under sedation. The biopsy and the mastectomy, if necessary, can be accomplished in a single trip to the operating room." In the text, Abbott commented approvingly that "this would save Vera the dangers of a second anesthetic and the trauma of waiting for mastectomy."[93] The passage quoted thus suggests that the one-step procedure was viewed, at least by some women, as a desirable state-of-the-art treatment available only at top-notch medical facilities. In this instance, the two-step procedure was positioned as the lower-tech, small-town alternative to the high-tech, big-city procedure. During the late 1970s, however, feminist health activists across the country reframed the one-step procedure as a paternalistic, patriarchal procedure that deprived breast cancer patients of their right to be informed of their diagnoses and to participate in medical decision making regarding their treatment. Ironically, these activists demanded access to the old-fashioned, lower-tech, two-step procedure, which became a symbol of breast cancer patients' rights and, within relatively short order, the new standard of breast cancer care in high-tech, leading-edge medical centers.

In theory the two-step procedure, which was performed in towns without pathology facilities, could have opened up additional space for a dialogue between patient and physician and created the opportunity for greater patient participation in decision making. There were additional factors, however, that constrained the opening-up of this space during the regime of medicalization. The most important of these was the absence of treatment alternatives. During the regime of medicalization, it was the Halsted radical mastectomy or nothing. Although European studies suggested that less radical procedures were equally effective, these studies were soundly rejected by surgeons in the United States.[94] If surgeons informed anyone of a patient's diagnosis between the performance of the biopsy and the surgical "cure," it was typically the patient's husband, who inevitably authorized the surgeon to proceed.

Diagnosis thus occurred in tandem with treatment—and both typically occurred while the patient was under general anesthesia. When the patient awoke from the one-step procedure, she typically awoke not as a cancer patient but as a mastectomee who had been successfully treated for a condition that was not called by name, at least not in front of the patient. Women with early-stage breast cancer typically recuperated in the hospital for one or two weeks before returning home. Women with more advanced cancer—for example, cancer that had invaded their lymph nodes—were often treated with some form of radiation therapy, depending on the historical period in which they were diagnosed.[95] In order to sketch a general picture of treatment during the regime of medicalization, however, I will continue to focus on women with early-stage disease.

For most patients, the only source of information regarding their post-operative prognoses came from their surgeon or their family physician, after he (or she) consulted with the surgeon. It was up to the surgeon to show new mastectomees how to perform therapeutic exercises to regain physical strength and mobility or to arrange for a nurse to teach the patient. It was up to the surgeon to be responsive to the emotional needs of patients who had just suffered the trauma of an unexpected breast amputation. It was up to the surgeon to instruct family members, especially husbands, about the physical, sexual, emotional, and psychological impact of surgery. It was also up to the surgeon, who sometimes delegated this task to a nurse, to inform the new mastectomee where to find a corsetiere who could fit her with a "breast form" to help hide the evidence of her surgery. Surgeons were not trained in these matters, however; nor were they known for their bedside manner. Nurses could assist, but only at the discretion of the surgeon.

"Hiding the awful truth," to quote the words of James Patterson, meant teaching women who underwent "the operation" how to avoid crashing headlong into the public stigma and shame of breast cancer. It meant teaching them how to pass as "normal" women. As a general rule, it was the discourse of early detection that dominated the coverage of breast cancer in women's magazines, including instructions and drawings on how to perform breast self-examinations. The actual treatment for breast cancer, however, was rarely discussed or depicted in detail. During the 1950s, however, a small trickle of articles discussing the experience of breast loss and explaining the availability and importance of breast prostheses began to appear in women's magazines.[96]

A 1954 article published in *Good Housekeeping*, for example, was called "After Breast Surgery." This article raised the curtain on breast cancer surgery, however, only long enough to explain the importance of keeping it lowered. Most doctors, according to the author, would explain to their patients before "the operation" that "she will emerge from the operating room the same woman she was when she went in" and that "her life will be the same as it always was." The author emphasized that "no one outside the immediate family need know she has had the operation—just as she does not know that many women whose names are household words have undergone the experience."[97]

This article paints a vivid portrait of the normalizing practices to which women with breast cancer were subject: "No woman," the author wrote, "need look different after breast surgery than she did before." There are many kinds of devices "that will prevent any suggestion of malformation," the author reassured readers, and "doctors and nurses realize that restoring normal appearance is extremely important to health and recovery as well as to vanity and morale." As soon as possible after the operation, the author explained, "the doctor will suggest that the patient wear a brassiere." Thus, while still recuperating in the hospital, the postoperative patient acquires— although just how this acquisition occurs remains a bit of a mystery—a "special garment" with an opening that can be filled by the patient or nurse with cotton batting or lamb's wool. "When the patient gets out of bed, this makeshift bra helps her keep her balance. . . . But most important of all, the bra reassures the patient—when her husband or family come to visit her—that there is no noticeable, lumpy dressing or sagging negligée to re-mind anyone of the operation. The patient looks the same as she ever did. When she walks down the hospital corridor, no one can guess what has happened." Advocating the extension of this normalizing process into the everyday world outside the hospital, the author explained that "as soon as the doctor gives his permission, the patient should be fitted with a pros-thetic device" that should be worn to maintain the appearance of normal-ity every day.[98]

In providing advice and information about buying and wearing breast prostheses, women's magazines made the issue of mastectomy visible be-tween the covers of magazines while encouraging the erasure of flesh-and-blood mastectomees from the public sphere. These popular magazines taught women with mastectomies how to successfully "pass" as "normal" women and contributed to a public culture in which passing was expected. Thus, even as they contributed to the production and circulation of new discourses of breast cancer and helped build awareness of the material cul-ture (breast prostheses) of this disease, women's magazines helped design and maintain the architecture of the closet.

Consistent with this, the regime of medicalization positioned breast can-cer patients in one of two temporal positions. Either the diagnosis came too late and they were positioned as "hopeless cases," or the operation was a success and they were "cured" and sent on their way after surgery (and, in certain cases, radiation therapy). In either event, the subject position of "cancer patient" was a temporary one that rapidly dissolved upon the patient's brief foray into the world of medical treatment. As temporary subjects, women were enclaved behind the walls of the hospital. Within that enclosure, they were isolated from each other, constituted as individual patient-subjects, and visible *as cancer patients* only within the confines of the hospital. The regime of medicalization thus shaped breast cancer's social, spatial, and visual dimensions.

## NORMS OF NONDISCLOSURE

A second factor that limited women's ability to participate as agentic subjects in medical decision making regarding their treatment was the norms of nondisclosure that governed physicians' interactions with cancer patients. Despite the proliferation of discourses of early detection in public arenas, explicit discussions of cancer were avoided within the medical setting. Physicians, in the words of James Patterson, "conspired with frightened relatives to hide the 'awful truth' of cancer."[99] Hiding the "awful truth" involved everything from maintaining a studied silence on the subject, to using euphemistic language, to dexterously dissembling, to, if those all failed, bald-faced lying.

From a contemporary vantage point, the literature on physicians' practices of nondisclosure during the regime of medicalization is a bit shocking. Diagnostic dissembling was clearly the rule rather than the exception in the physician–patient relationship until well into the 1960s. In a 1946 article entitled "The Doctor, the Patient, and the Truth," for example, which was published in *Annals of Internal Medicine*, the author offers this advice to physicians when discussing their diagnoses with cancer patients: "Certainly, at the start of the interview," the author suggests, the physician "should avoid the words carcinoma or cancer. He should use cyst, nodule, tumor, lesion, or some other loosely descriptive word that has not so many frightening connections." The physician should divulge as little information as possible—just enough, the author indicates, to obtain the patient's consent for an operation. If, however, for some reason the patient shows signs of hesitation and the physician is unable to solicit "the husband's cooperation" in persuading his wife to consent, the physician should explain to the patient "that the lesion is in imminent danger of becoming a cancer and that a good chance of cure still remains if action is immediate."[100] As the scenario winds down, the patient, now fearing that any hesitation on her part will lead to cancer (not knowing that she is already, in fact, a cancer patient), agrees to what she believes is an operation to prevent the development of cancer.

Fifteen years later a survey of physicians' "truth-telling" practices showed that norms of nondisclosure still prevailed. According to the results of a survey of 217 physicians at Michael Reese Hospital in Chicago, 90 percent practiced some level of diagnostic dissembling.[101] A clear majority told their patients the truth "rarely, if ever," and *not one* of the physicians reported a policy of truthfully informing every patient of his or her cancer diagnosis.

Follow-up interviews conducted with the survey's respondents provided additional insight into the mind-set of the physicians surveyed and, more importantly, the meaning of their responses. When, for example, the small number of physicians who reported that they "often" told their patients the truth were asked to expound on what they meant by "telling the truth," they revealed that, to them, "telling the truth" meant that while they might use the word "tumor," they strictly avoided using terms like "cancer" and "malignancy." "These words were almost never used," according to the study's author, Donald Oken, "unless the patient's explicit and insistent questioning pushed the doctor's back to the wall."[102] Even in such situations, however, euphemistic speech was the accepted practice. These euphemisms ranged from "the vaguest of words ('lesion,' 'mass'), to terms giving a general indication that the process [was] neoplastic ('growth,' 'tumor,' 'hyperplastic tissue')." The euphemisms also included terms like "suspicious" or "degenerated" tumor. Oken explained, however, that the use of terms suggesting that the process was neoplastic were "often tempered by a false explicit statement that the process [was] benign."[103] In other words, truth telling—even among the small handful of physicians who reported telling cancer patients "the truth"—ranged from using euphemistic language to making deliberately false statements designed to give the patient the impression that the malignant tumor was benign.

In cases where major surgery or radiation therapy were required, Oken reported, especially if the patient was hesitant about proceeding, "recourse may be had to such terms as 'pre-cancerous,' or a tumor 'in the early curable stage.'" As Oken explained, "The modal policy" was "to tell as little as possible in the most general terms consistent with maintaining cooperation in treatment," but some physicians "avoid even the slightest suggestion of neoplasia and quite specifically substitute another diagnosis."[104] A cyst? A nodule? Heart trouble? The possibilities for misdirection were seemingly endless.

Finally, sealing any possible exit from this house of mirrors, Oken reported that "questioning by the patient almost invariably was disregarded and considered a plea for reassurance unless [it was] persistent and intuitively perceived [by the physician] as 'a real wish to know.'" But even then, Oken indicated, "it may be ignored." In sum, the vast majority of doctors simply "feel that almost all patients really do not want to know regardless of what people say."[105] Furthermore, regardless of what patients might have believed they wanted to know, and what patients might have believed was best for them, physicians were utterly convinced that the best thing they could do for their patients was to "sustain and bolster" their hope and "communicate the possibility, even the likelihood, of recovery."

It is difficult to know what, from the patient's point of view, was actually being communicated in these conversations. Is it possible that a woman who had just received a radical mastectomy actually believed her surgeon or family physician when they insisted that the tumor was benign? Yes. Is it possible that she suspected she was being lied to? Yes. Is it possible that patients understood what was going on when they heard the euphemisms tripping off the tongues of their physicians? Yes. But surely they also knew that the role scripted for them demanded their full participation in the performance.

## Conclusion

During the era of therapeutic pluralism cancer was conceptualized as a systemic disease whose symptoms might be alleviated but whose progression could rarely be arrested. Within the regime of medicalization breast cancer was reconceptualized in theory and reconstituted in practice as a disease of local origins that could be cured if detected early and treated by radical mastectomy. This "invention of a curable disease," in the words of Barron H. Lerner, had important consequences for the newly constituted subjects of this regime.

Through its "Do Not Delay" and "Every Doctor's Office a Cancer Detection Center" campaigns, the ASCC and, later, the ACS promoted public awareness of the danger signals of cancer and directed women to seek immediate medical attention if these signals were discovered. Women exhibiting danger signals were thus constituted as symptomatic subjects of the regime, as patients.

The one-step procedure collapsed the diagnosis and treatment of women with breast cancer into one operation. In practice, this often meant that patients were "cured" before they learned that they had been diagnosed with breast cancer, if indeed they ever did. The conventions of nondisclosure that organized relationships between physicians and cancer patients mitigated against the development of a "breast cancer patient" identity. Women treated for breast cancer became mastectomees—a secret subject position derived from a surgical procedure rather than a disease-based identity. Furthermore, the sick role required mastectomees, like other patients, to return to their normal lives, take up their normal duties, and pass as normal women. Discretion and breast prostheses were viewed as key elements in a patient's successful return to normality.

Women's magazines cooperated in promoting the private management of public appearance, the return to normality, and the invisibility of flesh-and-blood mastectomees. In this way they served as one of the key architects of the closet. Concerns about breast loss and blending in were certainly not invented by women's magazines or the regime of medicalization; nonetheless, this regime of practices did more than simply reflect or reproduce what already existed. It organized a new set of practices to shape, support, and sustain the isolation of breast cancer patients and the invisibility of mastectomees.

Even more important than the constitution of breast cancer patients as silent, obedient subjects was the construction and transformation of dangerous, or endangered, women into patients. The "Do Not Delay" discourse of early detection reconstituted ordinary women as conscientious interpreters of bodily signs, as women who responded proactively by seeking immediate medical attention, and as women who refused to have their concerns dismissed by physicians. These women were encouraged to demand that their doctors seriously investigate any suspicious signs of disease. At the same time, as Leslie Reagan observed, "their energies were contained within a medical model that granted authority to physicians and expected patients to be compliant."[106] Thus, in essence, this regime of practices sent a mixed message. On the one hand, women were encouraged to be proactive, independent, mature, and resourceful in reading the danger signals, seeking medical care, and finding a responsive physician. At the same time, they were channeled into a sick role that demanded their unquestioning obedience to the authority of surgeons, as well as their silence and invisibility.

Compared to the proliferation of discourses about breast cancer outside the clinic, the discourse of breast cancer inside the clinic was muzzled and muted. Physicians spoke to each other about their patients but did not speak straightforwardly to their patients about their diagnoses. It would not be entirely accurate, however, to characterize the discourse of breast cancer during the first seventy years of the twentieth century, as many do, as a "conspiracy of silence." It was through a *proliferation* of public and private discourses and practices, not a deficit, that breast cancer was constituted as a "hidden" disease and women with breast cancer were constituted as its invisible victims.

Inside the surgeon's office, the operating room, and the hospital setting, breast cancer patients were indeed surrounded by silence, lies, and dissembling. It is also true that the role scripted for mastectomees required that, upon leaving the hospital, they return to their normal lives and hide the evidence of their surgery. At the same time, however, discourses of breast cancer proliferated outside the medical setting through high-visibility cancer-control campaigns. Despite their abundance, however, these biopolitical campaigns reinforced the sovereignty of surgeons and the silence and invisibility of mastectomees. Thus, the regime of medicalization and its architecture of the closet protected mastectomees from the stigmatizing gaze of the public and simultaneously protected the public from witnessing the thousands of women with breast cancer living in their midst as neighbors, coworkers, family members, and friends.

# Biomedicalization and the Biopolitics of Screening

Without question, knowledge and authority are exerted through the surveillant techniques of disease management; however, certain bodies are systematically excluded from this gaze. One's identity is defined, in part, in terms of one's position within or on the margins of a social body composed through a visual apparatus. . . . Though medicine may control bodies and communities it images, it also offers imaging as a class and cultural privilege.

—LISA CARTWRIGHT, *Screening the Body*

During the 1970s and 1980s, new practices arose that gradually transformed the regime of sovereign surgeons and temporarily sick and symptomatic subjects. In this new regime of practices, the regime of biomedicalization, surgeons were dethroned, dangerous women were replaced by permanently "risky subjects," and women diagnosed with breast cancer played an increasingly active role in their increasingly complicated and prolonged regimens of treatment.[1] Changes in the regime of medicalization occurred simultaneously along both of its axes: the biopolitics of populations and the anatomo-politics of individual bodies. This chapter examines the first of these—the public health discourses and practices that expanded the regime of breast cancer into the healthy, asymptomatic populations and reconstituted adult women as risky subjects. More specifically, this chapter explores the biopolitics of breast cancer screening during the 1970s and 1980s, focusing on the development of new subject populations and the reorganization of the temporal, spatial, visual, and institutional dimensions of this disease.

During the 1970s and 1980s healthy, asymptomatic, presumably cancer-free women were incorporated en masse into the medical machinery of breast cancer. This mass incorporation of cancer-free women was achieved through the development and diffusion of screening discourses and practices. The expansion of breast cancer screening into the asymptomatic populations reconstituted healthy women as risky subjects saddled with the duty and responsibility to routinely and proactively search for hidden signs of disease. Healthy, asymptomatic women were incorporated into the regime of breast cancer as both subjects and objects of screening.[2]

The transformation of healthy women into risky subjects, however, like the earlier transformation of "dangerous women" into compliant patients and mastectomees, did not happen overnight or automatically.[3] The momentum behind this transformation, which was spearheaded by the American Cancer Society, was generated by the movement of the mammographic gaze into asymptomatic populations. The movement of the mammographic gaze into asymptomatic populations transformed a relatively clear either-or distinction into a more fluid, fuzzily bounded, and ambiguous *breast cancer continuum*. Instead of the temporary, either-or sick role of the earlier regime, the regime of biomedicalization created the "risk role" for its new subjects—a role that required that the regime's risky subjects take up permanent residence along the breast cancer continuum.[4] Breast cancer screening and surveillance technologies transformed the subjects and social relations of disease. It constituted—and simultaneously extended medical authority over—new domains of experience. The biopolitics of screening thus created new relationships to, and embodied experiences of, breast cancer as a regime of practices. In doing so, it created new subjectivities, sensibilities, and solidarities that fed the breast cancer movement of the 1990s.

This transformation did not, however, occur evenhandedly. As Lisa Cartwright points out, although medical screening and surveillance technologies function in part as technologies of social control, they also function, at least in the United States, as a form of "class and cultural privilege."[5] Whereas white middle-class women were successfully interpolated into the new disease regime, less privileged women were marginalized by the discourses and practices of breast cancer screening.[6] Thus, as the discourses and practices of breast cancer screening increasingly penetrated the social spaces, bodies, and subjectivities of the white middle classes, they skirted the edges of communities of color and took a wide detour around poor women and women without health insurance.

## THE RISE OF MASS SCREENING: RECONFIGURING ASYMPTOMATIC WOMEN AS *Risky Subjects*

In the regime of medicalization, "early detection" meant the absence of delay in consulting a physician if "danger signals" were observed by a symptomatic woman. It also meant the absence of delay by the physicians consulted in referring symptomatic women to qualified surgeons for diagnosis and treatment.[7] The campaign slogan "Every Doctor's Office a Cancer Detection Center" encapsulated this dual objective. During the 1970s, however, the discourse and practices of early detection underwent an important shift, transporting the medical gaze into asymptomatic populations and reconstituting asymptomatic women as permanent subjects of the disease regime. In this new regime, invisible, unpalpable risk replaced visible, palpable danger as the focus of attention. Mammographic screening was the means through which this occurred. Although the content of early detection campaigns changed over time, as Leslie Reagan has shown, the use of "gender conventions" to "get the message across" did not.[8]

Screening, which means examining asymptomatic people for signs of disease, was first used as a public health technology at the turn of the century to examine schoolchildren for signs of contagious disease.[9] By the 1930s screening had been used by antituberculosis societies to control the spread of disease, by private industry to identify and eliminate unhealthy workers, by the military to identify and eliminate unfit draftees, and by insurance companies to minimize their risks and maximize their gains.[10] In the domain of breast cancer, screening was introduced on a mass basis in the 1950s, when the ACS began encouraging women to examine their breasts for palpable abnormalities. During the 1970s, however, the ACS shifted gears and made breast cancer screening a top priority. This occurred, in large part, through their promotion of mammography as a new screening technology.

Mammography is an X-ray technology that uses ionizing radiation to create images of the breast's interior. It can be used both as a diagnostic tool, to examine suspicious lesions, and as a screening technology, to examine asymptomatic women. As a diagnostic tool, the use of radiation to image the breast dates back to 1913. It was not until the 1930s and 1940s, however, that surgeons in different parts of the world succeeded in improving the technology of breast imaging enough to make it a viable diagnostic tool.[11] The first radiological unit explicitly designed to image breasts was developed in 1951. "Dedicated" mammography machines—machines used only for imaging breasts—did not enter the market until 1967.[12] American surgeons were unenthusiastic about the technology, however, because they preferred to surgically biopsy suspicious masses and submit the specimens to pathologists, with whom they were accustomed to working in close collaboration. Surgeons viewed diagnostic mammography, a technology under the jurisdiction of radiologists, as a redundant measure.[13] In fact, even well into the 1970s, the majority of breast masses were not X-rayed prior to biopsy.[14]

Diagnostic mammography was still a rare procedure in 1960 when Robert Egan "revolutionized the diagnosis of breast cancer by adapting high-resolution industrial film to a mammographic technique."[15] Egan screened two thousand patients and reported in 1962 that, using this new technology, he had discovered fifty-three cases of "occult carcinoma" in women with no visible signs of disease.[16] Egan's technique proved reproducible and accurate and made it possible, at least in theory, to screen large numbers of women with relative ease. Shortly thereafter, the Health Insurance Plan of Greater New York (HIP) launched the first study to assess mammography as a screening technology.

The HIP study, which was funded by the National Cancer Institute, investigated the cost-effectiveness of screening large numbers of middle- and working-class women for breast cancer.[17] Between 1963 and 1966, the HIP conducted a randomized, controlled trial involving 62,000 women between the ages of forty and sixty-four. Half the subjects received mammographic screening and physical breast examinations, and the other half did not. After an interval of five years, women aged fifty to fifty-nine in the study group had suffered one-third fewer breast cancer deaths than those in the control group. In the HIP trial, women over the age of fifty-nine also benefited from screening, but the sample size was too small to reach statistical significance. Women under the age of fifty did not benefit from screening.[18] The HIP study was a major turning point in the use of X-ray mammography as a screening technology. The HIP study, in the words of Lisa Cartwright, "began to move mammography from private, experimental, almost random use into the public sphere."[19]

It was the Breast Cancer Detection Demonstration Project (BCDDP), however, which was inspired by the HIP study, that introduced the concept and practice of breast cancer screening to a national audience. It was the BCDDP that transformed mammographic screening into a mainstream, widely accepted, and heavily promoted public health technology. The BCDDP was a joint project of the American Cancer Society and the National Cancer Institute. It was also the first major field campaign of President Nixon's "war on cancer," which was launched by the National Cancer Act of 1971. The idea for the BCDDP, however, originated with the ACS, not the NCI, and developed out of discussions between Philip Strax, the lead investigator for the HIP study, and Arthur Holleb, the senior vice president of medical affairs at the ACS. As Holleb later wrote:

> The demonstration project was designed to find out if modern screening, including the teaching of breast self-examination, a clinical breast examination, a mammogram and a thermogram, in a variety of community institutions— such as university centers, major hospitals, smaller community facilities, specialized institutions—could discover unsuspected early and readily curable breast cancer. Ancillary questions were whether qualified institutions, and highly specialized radiologists, would participate; and whether enough [asymptomatic] women would volunteer and faithfully return for annual follow-up examinations.[20]

The original ACS plan called for twelve two-year clinics, at an estimated cost of $1 million per year, and was approved by the ACS board of directors in 1972. When Congress passed the 1971 National Cancer Act, which greatly expanded the NCI's budget, the ACS approached the NCI about joining the project. According to Holleb, John C. Bailar III, the NCI's deputy associate director of cancer control, was "totally disinterested [sic] and wanted no part of it." However, Frank Rauscher, the director of the NCI, agreed to put up 75–80 percent of the cost if the ACS would agree to supply volunteer recruiters, secretaries, and other personnel, as well as "expertise," to the cancer centers. With the NCI's funding, the length of the study and the number of sites more than doubled, and the number of subjects in the project's design quadrupled.[21]

The BCDDP was not, however, designed as a scientific study. For example, the study design did not include a control group. Instead, it was designed to assess whether hospitals and health care facilities could effectively conduct mass screenings and whether American women could be convinced to undergo breast cancer screening—and return for rescreenings on an annual basis—in the absence of "danger signs" or symptoms. The BCDDP was not simply designed to measure the existing level of women's willingness to voluntarily undergo screening, however; it was also designed as a public health intervention to promote breast cancer screening in asymptomatic women. Although most screening centers accepted any adult woman who wanted to enroll in the project, 99 percent of the participants were between the ages of thirty-five and seventy-four when they entered the program. The decision to enroll women under the age of fifty was problematic from the get-go, since the results of the HIP trial indicated that there was no mortality benefit to screening women under the age of fifty. Because the demonstration project was not designed as a study, there was no way of measuring the effectiveness of screening for women under the age of fifty or any other group of women, even if they had wanted to. As a member of the BCDDP Data Management Advisory Group wrote: "The Breast Cancer Detection Demonstration Project (BCDDP) was implemented to disseminate the techniques of early detection of breast cancer to both the public and the medical profession."[22]

The BCDDP began recruiting women in 1973, and by 1975 more than 280,000 women had enrolled in the program at twenty-seven locations throughout the United States. Most centers recruited approximately 10,000 women over a two-year period and had a mandate to screen each woman for five years and to follow her for an additional five-year period. The project was designed to screen the enrolled subjects on an annual basis using a combination of medical history, physical examination, mammography, and thermography. In addition to these four screening modalities, the clinical subjects were also taught BSE and were encouraged to practice BSE on a monthly basis. Screening was completed in early 1981, and a Data Management Advisory Group (DMAG) was appointed by the NCI to begin a descriptive analysis of the data base.[23]

There was some concern at the beginning of the program about the feasibility of recruiting 280,000 women with no symptoms of breast cancer to participate in a study that required them to return for five annual multimodality screenings and, at least ideally, perform BSE on a monthly basis. To that end, the ACS went all out to publicize the screening project. ACS volunteers "compiled lists of women to be contacted, spoke on radio and television, made presentations at meetings, and carried out a variety of other activities aimed at informing the public about the BCDDP and encouraging women to participate."[24] According to data collected in conjunction with the demonstration, by far the most important source of information about the project, and the most effective form of recruitment, was information gained from friends (44 percent)—word of mouth, in other words. Newspapers (29 percent), television (12 percent), and to a slightly lesser extent physicians (9 percent) were also important sources of information.[25] The BCDDP was, in many respects, one of the earliest and most significant instances of what is now termed "lay participation in science." In other respects, the reliance of the ACS on an army of female volunteers was simply the 1970s version of the Women's Field Army.

The demographic distribution of BCDDP subjects is unsurprising, but it is useful for illustrating the diffusion of screening technologies within the emergent regime of practices. As with other public health campaigns aimed at the "general public," the subjects recruited by the BCDDP's promotional activities were primarily white, non-Hispanic women (86 percent). Black women constituted only a small percentage of participating subjects (5 percent). Asian American and Native American women constituted an even smaller percentage. In addition, a higher percentage of black women dropped out of the program after one or two screenings than white, Hispanic, or Asian American ("Oriental") women. Exhibiting a pattern that continues to this day, women under the age of fifty responded in numbers far exceeding the proportion of breast cancer incidence accounted for by this age group. Half of the participants were under the age of fifty when they enrolled in the project, for example, even though that group accounted for only 32 percent of the cases of breast cancer diagnosed.[26] The household income of 76 percent of the participants was at or above the national median ($11,000). More than 40 percent of the subjects had attended some college (and half of those had attended college for four years or more).[27] The BCDDP subjects, in other words, tended to be white, well-educated, and middle-class.

The medical history of the BCDDP subjects was equally revealing. Only 3.2 percent of the participants reported that they had never received a breast examination by a physician, and 85.8 percent reported having received three or more clinical exams. On the other hand, 80.5 percent reported that they had never received a mammogram, and only 3.5 percent had received three or more mammograms. Breast self-examination was midway between these two extremes, with 35.9 percent reporting that they regularly examined their breasts for signs of cancer, another 44.6 percent reporting that they had done so a few times, and 18.3 percent reporting that they had never examined their breasts.[28] These descriptive statistics indicate (1) that women who enrolled in the BCDDP showed a greater-than-average familiarity with breast cancer screening, and (2) that a large number of educated, white, middle-class women and primary care physicians had already been converted to the logic of searching for nonobvious signs of disease in healthy, asymptomatic breasts.

In 1974 Betty Ford, the wife of then president Gerald Ford, was diagnosed with breast cancer. Forthright and public about her breast cancer diagnosis and mastectomy, the First Lady, who credited breast cancer screening with the early detection and successful treatment of her cancer, publicly promoted mammographic screening and encouraged American women to practice "constant vigilance." Maintaining a stiff upper lip, she also advised, "Once it's done, put it behind you and go on with your life."[29] Betty Ford's public disclosure was followed within a month by Happy Rockefeller's.[30] Both disclosures received extensive coverage by television and print media and generated a great deal of positive publicity for mammographic screening and early detection.

The impact of these disclosures was dramatic. Practically overnight the demand for mammograms skyrocketed, and recruitment for the BCDDP accelerated. Some mammography screening centers reported that their waiting lists were two months long.[31] The response was so strong that breast cancer incidence rates for 1974–1975 spiked upward before settling back down to a slower climb. The spectacular response to the disclosures would not have occurred if breast cancer had not been so heavily stigmatized and if women with breast cancer had not been so silent and invisible. It was the architecture of the closet, in large part, that generated such a dramatic response. Decades of early detection campaigns and stories in women's magazines had not changed the fact that flesh-and-blood mastectomees were completely absent from public life and everyday interactions.

It is often claimed that the disclosures by Betty Ford and Happy Rockefeller heralded the public "coming out" of women with breast cancer and the dismantling of the closet. This is misleading. The disclosures of Ford and Rockefeller were shocking but not contagious. The symbolic power of these public disclosures was significant, but they by no means launched a new trend. Ordinary women diagnosed with breast cancer continued to hide their disease diagnoses and treatment histories. The media buzz that followed the disclosures, however, provided a platform for a series of public debates about breast cancer screening, diagnosis, and treatment.

The first controversy erupted in the fall of 1975 when John C. Bailar III, a biostatistician and the deputy associate director of NCI's cancer control program, went public with his criticisms of the BCDDP after, according to Bailar, his criticisms were dismissed by authorities in the NCI.[32] On the basis of a recently completed study, Bailar claimed that for women under the age of fifty the risk of developing breast cancer as a result of repeated exposures to mammographic radiation might exceed the chance of finding an early cancer that could be successfully treated and would not otherwise have been found by physical examination alone. In his analysis of the radiation risks associated with screening mammography for younger women, which was published in *Annals of Internal Medicine,* Bailar wrote: "I regretfully conclude that there seems to be a possibility that the routine use of mammography in screening asymptomatic women may eventually take as many lives as it saves. . . . Screening by medical history and physical examination alone will probably provide much or more of the same benefit without risk from irradiation, at least in women under some fairly high age limit."[33]

Bailar's "ominous warnings" became national TV and radio news, generating front-page stories and editorials.[34] The impact of Bailar's bomb, like that of the disclosures of Ford and Rockefeller, was dramatic. The number of women examined each month dropped from 24,000 to 17,000.[35] Ironically, because the BCDDP was a demonstration project rather than a scientific study, the demonstration sites were not required to distribute consent forms to participants warning them of risks of radiation from mammograms.[36] In fact, not until after the Bailar controversy did the NCI draft a consent form to be signed by subjects participating in the demonstration project.[37] Controversy over the BCDDP did not begin or end with Bailar's bomb. Additional controversies erupted over the appropriate age to begin screening, the overtreatment of noninvasive, "precancerous" conditions, and "false positives" and the subsequent performance of unnecessary mastectomies.[38] According to historian Walter Ross: "Mammography became transformed almost overnight in the public's mind from a desirable examination into an unacceptable menace."[39]

These controversies pushed the NIH into the business of technology assessment in 1977, when it organized its first ever consensus development conference.[40] The NIH/NCI Consensus Development Meeting on Breast Cancer Screening was organized primarily in response to questions that had been raised in the BCDDP regarding the relative value of mammographic screening compared to the risks involved from exposure to ionizing radiation from mammography. The meeting focused on three topics: a review of the HIP study; reports of three working groups on the pathology, risks, and epidemiology of breast cancer screening; and a review of data from the BCDDP.

Among other things, the consensus conference concluded that the evidence did not support the use of thermography for any group of women or mammographic screening in women under the age of fifty. The panel recommended that the BCDDP continue screening women age fifty and older with a combination of mammography and physical examination but that routine mammographic screening of women between the ages of forty and forty-nine be restricted to women with a personal history of cancer and women whose mother or sister(s) had been diagnosed with the disease.[41] The panel also concluded that the amount of radiation to which participants in the demonstration project were exposed was not high enough to raise their risk of breast cancer to any significant degree. Finally, the panel examined the "practical and ethical considerations" of the BCDDP. Demonstration programs "by definition," according to the panel, "utilize proven and practical methods to project new information to the medical community." The BCDDP, on the other hand, "from [its] inception" had "incorporated certain practices of assumed but unconfirmed value."

The NIH/NCI panel asserted that, as a demonstration project with "investigational components," the BCDDP needed to "come to grips with several important ethical concerns" and recommended that informed consent forms include information on the radiation dosage and assurances that "all information gained through the program . . . [would] be disclosed to the screenee as well as to her physician." Finally, the panel recommended that two pathologists confirm every diagnosis of breast cancer and that "women who have been screened already and who have had a diagnosis of cancer . . . be notified promptly if the diagnosis has been changed." In other words, the panel recommended that women who had been mistakenly diagnosed and treated by mastectomy for breast cancer should be informed of their misdiagnosis.[42] Instead of notifying these women directly, however, the BCDDP left it up to the judgment of their physicians, many of whom did not inform their patients.

The BCDDP ignited a series of public controversies and debates, many of which are still with us. The NIH and the NCI, for their part, continued to revisit and revise their breast cancer screening guidelines during the 1980s and 1990s.[43] But by the time the BCDDP concluded in 1978, the idea that perfectly healthy women exhibiting no signs of disease should be regularly screened by mammography for breast cancer was a widely accepted approach to the public management of this disease. The BCDDP received both positive and negative publicity, but it also, and more importantly— probably in large part *because* of the volatile debates it engendered—introduced growing segments of the female population to the concept, and increasingly the practice, of screening for breast cancer. The BCDDP launched a new era in the discourse and practice of breast cancer early detection. This was its most powerful and enduring legacy.

By 1979, according to Christina Marino and Karen Gerlach, women's magazines were giving a great deal of coverage to breast cancer, and "breast cancer . . . had become one of the most frequently reported cancers in the media."[44] By 1980, according to the NCI's Office of Cancer Communications, 76 percent of the 1,580 women that were surveyed believed that cancer was their most serious health problem, and 58 percent "specifically mentioned breast cancer as the type of cancer most serious."[45] Prior to the BCDDP the principles and practices of early detection were embodied in the "Do Not Delay" discourse of public health campaigns. After the BCDDP the regime of practices was reorganized around the principles and practices of screening. A "Go in Search" orientation to early detection replaced the "Do Not Delay" message of the first three-quarters of the twentieth century. The new trilogy of technologies consisted of breast self-examinations, clinical breast exams, and screening mammograms.

In the late 1970s the ACS decided to reevaluate its physician recommendations for "cancer-related checkups."[46] The resulting guidelines—to which an entire issue of the ACS's journal, *CA: A Cancer Journal for Clinicians,* was devoted in 1980—received widespread distribution and discussion.[47] In its guidelines, the ACS recommended that women begin monthly breast self-examination at the age of twenty, that a clinical breast examination be performed every three years beginning at age twenty and every year beginning at the age of forty, that women receive a baseline mammogram between the ages of thirty-five and forty, that women under the age of fifty follow the advice of their personal physician with regard to mammographic screening, and that annual mammograms begin at age fifty.[48]

In issuing these guidelines, the ACS went to great pains to reassure private physicians that they were not suggesting that the government should get into the business of cancer screening. For example, in its introductory remarks the ACS defined early detection as "the use of tests in asymptomatic people on an individual basis," whereas it defined screening as "the search for cancer in a large population (not all of whom will necessarily be asymptomatic) through a centrally coordinated mass program." According to the ACS's verbal gymnastics, the guidelines—and the larger report in which they were embedded—described "the use of various tests and procedures for [the] early detection of cancer," not population-based screening, which would have raised the specter of government interference and infringement on their market.

In case any further clarification was needed, the ACS concluded with the following statement: "*These recommendations pertain to the early detection of cancer—the search for early cancer in asymptomatic people on an individual basis.* They are not recommendations for mass screening programs at public expense."[49] The title of the report, "Guidelines for the Cancer-Related Checkup," emphasized the individual physician–patient relationship and the private setting of the doctor's office, avoiding any hint of publicly financed screening clinics or government interference. In 1983 the ACS issued a new set of guidelines. This time the ACS recommended that all women between the ages of forty and forty-nine receive a mammogram every one to two years—no longer dependent on the judgment of individual physicians—and that they begin receiving an annual mammogram at age fifty.[50]

During the 1980s the screening of healthy populations accelerated. In the mid-1980s the ACS launched the Breast Cancer Detection Awareness (BCDA) project, a two-pronged campaign aimed at healthy women and primary care physicians. Both prongs emphasized what was increasingly viewed as the "holy trinity" of early detection—breast self-exam, clinical breast exams, and mammographic screening. The BCDA was developed in response to a 1984 survey of physicians in family practice, internal medicine, and obstetrics and gynecology that was commissioned by the Ohio

Division of the ACS. Unlike the BCDDP study published in 1982, which gathered information about the screening practices of women enrolled in the BCDDP, the BCDA study, conducted in 1984 and published in 1985, sampled the attitudes and practices of physicians.[51]

Nearly seven in ten physicians reported that they were "now doing more screening of asymptomatic patients for early detection of cancer" than they had been five years earlier. In terms of breast cancer, 97 percent of physicians (99 percent of obstetrician/gynecologists) reported that they conducted breast examinations on asymptomatic patients with no history of cancer, and 80 percent of the physicians reported exceeding or following the ACS guidelines. Ninety-two percent reported that they advised all of their adult female patients to do breast self-exams, 6 percent advised only their high-risk patients to do breast self-exams, and only 2 percent did not advise women to examine their breasts. Unlike mammographic screening, the promotion of BSE had been widely adopted by primary care physicians.

With regard to mammographic screening, however, the response was more mixed. Although nearly seven out of ten (68 percent) physicians ordered mammograms for asymptomatic patients, only 11 percent followed ACS guidelines for mammographic screening.[52] Only 41 percent of the physicians surveyed "agreed completely" with the ACS guidelines; an additional 27 percent "agreed partially," but a rather significant 32 percent simply "did not agree." Among physicians who did not agree completely with the guidelines for mammographic screening, expense was the most frequently cited reason for disagreement (39 percent cited the expense of the procedure). Other common reasons for disagreement were the belief that mammograms were not necessary for asymptomatic women, the belief that mammograms were not necessary every year, and concerns about radiation.

The BCDA program, which was conducted between 1986 and 1989, was the largest program for promoting awareness of breast cancer detection that the ACS had ever mounted.[53] Although it promoted all three screening technologies, mammographic screening received special emphasis. Since 40 percent of the breast cancers diagnosed through the BCDDP had been discovered by mammography alone, whereas only 10 percent had been found by clinical exam alone, the ACS was committed to the promotion of mammographic screening of asymptomatic women.[54] Furthermore, the ACS believed that follow-up studies conducted on the BCDDP outcome data, compared to the NCI's SEER (Surveillance, Epidemiology, and End Results) Program data, demonstrated a clear benefit of mammography screening for women age forty to forty-nine.[55] According to the BCDA program manual, the goal of the program was "to increase by 100 percent primary care physicians' use of high quality, low dose screening mammography for asymptomatic women age 35 years and older."[56] In addition, however, it was in conjunction with the BCDA program that the ACS launched its Special Touch program. Special Touch was a community-based program through which women were taught, in small group settings, to perform BSE and to teach other women how to examine their breasts.

BCDA projects were community organized and implemented, but they involved the resources, planning, publications, and financial support of the national ACS as well. At the community level, according to Diane Fink, the ACS's vice president for professional education, "important groups were recruited into the planning process, includ[ing] state radiologic groups, local and state health departments and medical societies, community organizations representing primary care physicians, provider organizations, and local experts to advise on program implementation."[57] In addition, working with local units of the ACS, state health departments *also* initiated community screening projects. According to medical anthropologist Patricia Kaufert, the format of these programs "was based on principles of community mobilization from the 1960s, shrewd marketing strategies, and elements of evangelical revivalism."[58] A survey of obstetrician/gynecologists conducted in 1989 showed that 37 percent of these physicians were now following ACS guidelines regarding mammographic screening—the doubling goal had been surpassed. In addition, a significantly higher percentage were recommending mammograms to asymptomatic patients, even if they did not precisely follow ACS guidelines.[59]

Another important development in the history of breast cancer screening occurred in 1985 with the founding of National Breast Cancer Awareness Month (NBCAM). NBCAM was created to "promote the importance of the three-step approach to early detection: mammography, clinical breast examination and breast self-examination."[60] Interestingly, NBCAM was not the brainchild of the American Cancer Society, the National Cancer Institute, the Centers for Disease Control and Prevention, or any other public health agency, medical society, or health organization. NBCAM was the brainchild of Imperial Chemical Industries (ICI), a British manufacturer of plastics, paints, pesticides, and pharmaceutical therapies, among other things. ICI's interest in breast cancer stemmed from its ownership of the drug tamoxifen (under the brand name Nolvadex), the best-selling breast cancer treatment drug in the world. ICI—later Zeneca Pharmaceuticals, now AstraZeneca—held the patent on tamoxifen, and the United States was their biggest market.[61]

The history of NBCAM can be traced to 1985, although in 1985 it consisted of a week, not a month, of activities designed "to fill the information void in public communication about breast cancer."[62] As part of this effort, NBCAM created a public service message featuring Susan Ford Bales and her mother, Betty Ford. The American Academy of Family Physicians and Cancer Care, Inc.—both sponsors of NBCAM—distributed brochures, spoke to news reporters, and testified before a U.S. congressional committee about the crucial need for widespread access to mammography.[63] The success of this series of activities led to the creation of NBCAM, which has taken place, with growing fanfare and sponsors, every October since. In a brochure distributed as part of its "consumer education" program on breast cancer, Zeneca Pharmaceuticals referred to NBCAM, not inaccurately, as "the nation's most widely acclaimed breast cancer education program."[64]

In addition, companies selling or manufacturing mammography equipment—such as General Electric, DuPont, and Eastman Kodak (manufacturers of mammography machines and the film they use)—initiated their own series of advertising campaigns during the 1980s. Full-page advertisements were placed in news weeklies and women's magazines, and commercials were broadcast during prime-time television.[65] One commercial that began running on network TV in 1989 showed a young woman examining her breasts in front of a mirror as a voice-over explained, "Mary Brodie won't feel the tiny lump in her breast for two years. But she'll discover it tomorrow after her first mammogram." The commercial, which was paid for by DuPont, a manufacturer of film for mammography machines, explained that the new X-ray film made it "safer to start early."[66]

One group of researchers who surveyed the industry argued that the marketing of mammography to younger women was driven by the oversupply and underutilization of dedicated mammography machines.[67] In 1981, for example, 134 mammography machines were installed across the country. Between 1981 and 1990, however, nearly 10,000 mammography machines were installed—concentrated on the coasts and in major metropolitan areas.

According to the analysis of this survey, 7,892 machines running at full capacity could screen the entire population of eligible women (based on NCI guidelines for eligibility), and 1,675 machines could handle the lowest estimate of actual demand.[68]

In addition to the mammography screening campaigns initiated by private companies and nonprofit organizations, dozens of bills expanding access to mammographic screening were proposed in state legislatures, and many of these bills were signed into law. In 1988 and 1989 mammography topped the list of new state mandates for health insurance benefits.[69] The push for state legislation mandating mammography coverage—and the lobbying effort that secured its passage in state after state—was spearheaded by the ACS, the American College of Radiology, and women lawmakers "operating under the banner" of the Women's Network of the National Conference of State Legislatures. By the end of the 1980s nineteen states had adopted legislation requiring private health insurance companies and managed care organizations to cover (or offer coverage) for routine mammographic screening, and by the end of 1991 that number had doubled again.[70] In 1990 Medicare, the federal health insurance program for the elderly and disabled, began covering mammographic screening for its beneficiaries—one every two years for women over sixty-five.[71] Embedding mammographic screening in state legislation was an important step toward institutionalizing and routinizing mammographic screening within the U.S. health care system.

Mammography extended the "early" part of early detection by allowing many breast cancers to be visualized long before they became palpable. But mammography, as Barron Lerner has argued, did not "reveal" breast cancer in a simple or straightforward manner. Rather, the ability to interpret mammograms required skill, practice, and extensive training during which radiologists "learned to identify mammographic findings" and assign them appropriate "names and meanings."[72] Radiologists, according to Lerner, "viewed mammography as a way to both help individual patients and solidify their professional role as breast cancer diagnosticians," and they helped turn mammography into an "obligatory passage point in the diagnosis of breast cancer."[73] Radiologists also, although this was not their intention, contributed to the reconfiguration of breast cancer from an either-or diagnosis to a breast cancer continuum.

As the imaging technology of mammography improved and as radiologists grew more adept at reading mammograms, they were able to identify—

and identify more frequently—a broader array of ambiguous breast conditions. On follow-up, the vast majority of these turned out to be benign conditions, but each abnormality required additional evaluation procedures. Thus, a growing number of perfectly healthy and asymptomatic women who walked through the door of a medical imaging facility or radiology clinic left with puzzling diagnoses of uncertain and ambiguous conditions that required further testing and evaluation.

Most women, if they received annual screenings, were eventually—and in many cases repeatedly—recalled for additional mammographic images, ultrasound procedures, and even biopsies. For every woman recalled for additional testing who received a positive breast cancer diagnosis, nine or more women were recalled for follow-up diagnostic procedures that did not lead immediately to a breast cancer diagnosis. Thus, for every woman who received a positive diagnosis, many more moved into ambiguous and uncertain positions along the breast cancer continuum. Perhaps their mammograms were not alarming enough to require additional diagnostic procedures but were suggestive enough to require intensified medical and self-surveillance—active watching and anxious waiting.[74]

In addition to the women who were recalled for additional testing but not diagnosed with breast cancer, a rapidly growing number of women entered an even more frightening liminal position. Improvements in the technology of mammography, on the one hand, and the growing utilization of mammographic screening, on the other, led to a dramatic increase in the diagnosis of ductal carcinoma in situ, a symptomless condition that radiologists can identify on mammographic film and digital images but that is otherwise impossible to feel or see. DCIS, which is cancer confined to the milk ducts of the breast, is considered "preinvasive" by some doctors, "noninvasive" by others, and "precancerous" by yet still others.[75]

DCIS presented a challenge to physicians not only because its classification was unsettled but also, and more importantly, because its clinical significance was uncertain. Physicians knew that, left untreated, some cases of DCIS would turn into invasive breast cancer and others would not, but no means existed for distinguishing between them. As a result, women diagnosed with DCIS were typically treated as if they had stage 1 invasive breast cancer. During the 1970s and 1980s, this meant that the majority were treated by mastectomy. Later, as breast-conserving surgeries combined with radiation therapy became an increasingly popular option among women diagnosed with small tumors, women with DCIS often found themselves in the peculiar position of having fewer options than women with invasive breast cancer. Because DCIS often presented as a multifocal disease, women with DCIS were often poor candidates for breast-conserving surgery. Thus, many of the women who received mastectomies were, technically speaking, treated prophylactically for invasive breast cancer.[76]

Between 1973 and 1983, for women aged forty to forty-nine years, the incidence rate of DCIS grew an average of 4 percent a year. Between 1983 and 1992, incidence rates for this group of women grew approximately 17.4 percent a year. For women aged fifty and over, DCIS incidence rates increased approximately 5.2 percent a year between 1973 and 1983, and 18.1 percent a year from 1983 to 1992. Between 1983 and 1989, incidence rates for DCIS increased 213 percent among white women and 153 percent among black women. By the mid-1990s, DCIS accounted for 30–40 percent of mammographically detected breast cancers.[77] Yet because DCIS was counted and classified separately from invasive breast cancer, the skyrocketing rates of DCIS were largely invisible to the lay public. The incidence rates typically reported by the National Institutes of Health, the National Cancer Institute, the Centers for Disease Control and Prevention, and the American Cancer Society included cases of invasive breast cancer only. But even incidence rates for invasive breast cancer, as Paula Lantz and Karen Booth have shown, were increasingly portrayed in women's magazines as evidence of a growing epidemic that called for women's utmost vigilance and adherence to screening guidelines.[78]

## CONCLUSION

The diffusion of breast cancer screening and the movement of the mammographic gaze into asymptomatic populations helped give rise to a new regime of breast cancer. In this new disease regime, the message of early detection shifted from "Do Not Delay" to something more along the lines of "Go in Search." By the end of the 1980s mammographic screening was firmly entrenched in state legislation and in a vast network of interlinked industries, professions, and organizations.

The diffusion of screening technologies—breast self-exam, clinical breast exams, and mammographic screening—reconstituted normal breasts into suspect purveyors of disease and asymptomatic women into risky subjects. Every ambiguous mammogram and every liminal diagnosis with an unclear prognosis resulted in the deeper entanglement of seemingly cancer-free women in the increasingly complicated regime of breast cancer. Screening campaigns thus moved the awareness, fear, and anxiety of being diagnosed with breast cancer onto the horizons and into the psyches of a growing number of women.

The acceptance and practice of breast cancer screening made more permeable and ambiguous the rigid borders that had formerly separated women with breast cancer from other women. It transformed healthy, asymptomatic adult women into risky subjects who took up residence on the breast cancer continuum. Thus, rigid separations were replaced by blurred and shifting positions on a new breast cancer continuum, and the future that every woman sought to avoid was searched for and anticipated within the present.

But this did not happen uniformly. The history of health care and medicine in the United States is a history of countervailing tendencies. On the one hand, medicine has continually expanded its jurisdiction by colonizing new territories and dimensions of experience. On the other hand, it has marginalized and excluded poor people, people without health insurance, immigrants, and racial and ethnic minorities.[79] The expansion of screening that took place during the 1970s and 1980s continued this well-established pattern of unequal access, or what Adele Clarke and her colleagues have referred to as "stratified biomedicalization."[80] Whereas white, middle-class women were successfully interpolated into the new disease regime, less privileged women were marginalized in this regime of practices. Thus, as the discourses and practices of breast cancer screening increasingly penetrated the social spaces, bodies, and psyches of the white middle classes—constructing new subjectivities and sensibilities—they skirted the edges of communities of color and took a detour around poor women and women without health insurance.[81]

During the 1990s the culture of screening activism that emerged in the Bay Area—as was true elsewhere—drew attention to racial and class disparities in the use of mammographic screening and sought to remedy those disparities through privately and publicly funded screening programs for medically marginalized women. Before turning to an analysis of the first of three COAs, however, we need to examine the transformations that took place during the 1970s and 1980s in the anatomo-politics of individual bodies—in the medical diagnosis, treatment, and "rehabilitation" of women with breast cancer. This is the subject of chapter 4.

# Biomedicalization and the Anatomo-Politics of Treatment

Why did the identity of being a woman with breast cancer change from passivity to action? . . . What impelled women with breast cancer to break out of their isolation and assemble under the banner of a new social movement?

—PATRICIA A. KAUFERT, "Women, Resistance, and the Breast Cancer Movement"

The biopolitics of screening, as we saw in chapter 3, changed the popular discourses and public administration of breast cancer. As it did so, it reconstituted ordinary women as risky subjects and repositioned them along the breast cancer continuum. This chapter explores the other half of the transformation in disease regimes: the anatomo-politics of treatment, focusing on key changes in the diagnosis, decision making, treatment, and "rehabilitation" of breast cancer patients. This chapter is not a history of cancer policy, cancer research, or cancer medicine but, rather, a genealogy of the breast cancer patient within the regime of biomedicalization. My analysis focuses on the medical practices and technologies that most directly shaped the embodied experiences and social relations of disease for women with breast cancer—the most important, and least voluntary, subjects of this regime.

## DIAGNOSIS AND DECISION MAKING: THE RISE OF INFORMED CONSENT AND THE DEMISE OF THE ONE-STEP PROCEDURE

During the 1960s and 1970s the norms of disclosure among physicians underwent a dramatic shift. By 1977 a full 98 percent of the physicians surveyed reported that they believed patients had the right to know their diagnoses and that disclosure of cancer diagnoses to cancer patients was their usual policy.[1] Twenty years earlier, 90 percent of the physicians surveyed had believed it was best not to tell cancer patients of their diagnoses, and a majority had claimed that they never or seldom told their patients the truth about their diagnoses.[2]

Beyond the basics of disclosure, however, lay the question of informed consent and decision making. By the mid-1970s it was standard practice for physicians to inform their patients of their breast cancer diagnoses, but the patients were still being informed postoperatively, and there was still a one-size-fits-all approach to treatment. The one-step procedure, as discussed earlier, combined a surgical biopsy with an immediate mastectomy if the frozen-section biopsy—analyzed by a pathologist while the patient was still on the operating table—yielded a positive diagnosis of breast cancer. As long as there were no alternatives to the radical mastectomy, however—or no alternatives that U.S. surgeons were willing to perform—informed decision making was a relatively empty concept. What physicians had, instead, was post hoc informed consent. Meaningful participation in decision making was dependent upon the fulfillment of two preconditions that, in practice, were closely linked: the abandonment of the one-step procedure and the willingness of American surgeons to offer alternatives to the Halsted radical mastectomy.

The movement to abandon the one-step procedure in favor of a two-step process was led by Rose Kushner, the mother of breast cancer activism. Kushner was married, middle-class, and working as a freelance medical journalist when she discovered a lump in her breast in 1974. Kushner complied with the script that she and other women of her racial and socioeconomic background had been taught: She immediately consulted her family physician. Afterward, however, she went off script by driving directly to the public library and locating the one copy of the one book that the library owned on the topic of breast cancer. The title of the book was *What Women Should Know about the Breast Cancer Controversy,* and its author was George Crile Jr., a maverick physician who defied professional norms and the medical establishment by writing, for a lay audience, a book on breast cancer that encouraged breast cancer patients to challenge their physicians. It included a "Patient's Bill of Rights," which was reprinted in *Ms.* magazine. The book was published in 1973, a year before Kushner consulted her family physician about the lump in her breast. As Kushner recounted it, "I hadn't even known, then, that there *was* a breast cancer controversy!"[3]

Based on what she learned from Crile's critique of the one-step procedure, the frozen-section biopsy, and the radical mastectomy, along with additional research that she conducted in the medical library of the National Institutes of Health, Kushner decided that she would not agree to a one-step procedure. As she later recounted in *Breast Cancer: A Personal History and an Investigative Report* (1975), she locked herself in a public phone booth and started calling a list of surgeons that her physician had suggested. "No patient is going to tell me how to do my surgery," was the response of one of the surgeons when she asked for a two-stage operation. "I've never heard of such a thing" was the response of another. A third surgeon exploded with "You're absolutely ridiculous!" And so it went, as Kushner recalled, as she made her way down the list.[4]

Kushner eventually found a surgeon who agreed not to perform the one-step procedure if breast cancer were diagnosed during the operation—but only, he later explained, because he was so sure that the lump would turn out to be benign. Kushner drew up her own consent form, which read: "Under no circumstance is [the doctor] or anyone else in the operating room of [the doctor] to perform the procedure known as mastectomy."[5] Kushner insisted that the document be signed by the surgeon prior to the operation. When the surgeon, working with the pathologist, determined that the tumor was malignant, he was furious that he had signed away his right to perform a radical mastectomy. Kushner encountered a similar battle when she attempted to find a surgeon willing to perform a modified radical mastectomy, an operation that leaves the chest muscles intact.

In publishing *Breast Cancer: A Personal History and an Investigative Report,* Kushner launched a one-woman battle against the one-step procedure, against the Halsted radical mastectomy, and, more than anything, against the exclusion of women from access to the information they needed in order to make informed decisions about their own bodies and treatment.[6] "My ideas may differ from those of other women," Kushner wrote, "but the point of this book is to show that we women should be free, knowledgeable, and completely conscious when the time comes for a decision, so that we can make it for ourselves." "*Our* lives are at stake," she added, "not a surgeon's."[7] Although Kushner's body politics grew out of feminism and the women's health movement, she emphasized that she did not agree with "women's liberationists who see an evil plot to mutilate women by mastectomy." None-theless, her first book did include a chapter entitled "Male Chauvinism, Sex, and Breast Cancer" and pointed out that "the United States' entire breast-cancer Establishment is masculine."

In 1979, prompted by public controversies over the one-step procedure and radical mastectomies, the NIH convened a consensus development conference titled The Treatment of Primary Breast Cancer: Management of Local Disease.[8] By 1979 Kushner had become such a powerful figure in the world of breast cancer that she was named to the NIH consensus development panel of experts. She was one of only two women, and the only member who was not a medical doctor.[9] A consensus statement issued by the NIH panel of experts explicitly encouraged physicians to abandon the one-step procedure.[10] The rationale for this recommendation, according to Kushner, was to allow women diagnosed with breast cancer "to get other opinions and to look into options."[11] Although the consensus statement did not have the force of law behind it, it constituted a symbolically loaded nod toward the growing rights of breast cancer patients.[12]

That same year, Massachusetts became the first state to pass breast can-cer informed consent legislation, and a year later, in 1980, California became the second. By the end of the decade, breast cancer informed consent leg-islation had been proposed in twenty-two states and adopted in fourteen.[13] According to medical sociologist Theresa Montini, breast cancer informed consent campaigns were single-issue campaigns typically launched by a small handful of former breast cancer patients in each state. In most cases, these patient-activists were not connected to the women's health or patients' rights movements, nor did they publicly engage in what Mary Fainsod Katzen-stein has termed the "discursive politics of feminism."[14]

In fact, Montini discovered that although informed consent activists expressed their anger in private interviews, they deliberately avoided its ex-pression in public.[15] These breast cancer activists achieved political success by strategically mobilizing the discourses and practices of normative het-erosexual femininity. In presentations to the media and in public legislative hearings, for example, they displayed the gender-appropriate emotions of fear and grief and downplayed the gender-norm-violating expression of anger. They presented themselves as victims of callous individual surgeons who engaged in willful misconduct. In sum, Montini argued, "The activ-ists did not risk being discredited on the basis of being unfeminine. . . .

they attempted to use gender stereotypes to their advantage, presenting an aggrieved, feminine, emotional self in need of the protection that a breast cancer informed consent law would provide."[16]

Informed consent legislation was resisted by physicians and by the American Cancer Society, which on this issue, as on most others, deferred to the interests of physicians. In fact, it was the American Cancer Society, in conjunction with the American Medical Association, that organized opposition to these laws on a state-by-state basis. The opposition was effective enough to seriously weaken and undermine the efforts of informed consent activists. In some states, the ACS and AMA were successful in defeating the legislation. In others, they succeeded in inserting language that protected physicians from future lawsuits and liability.[17] As a result of the ACS and AMA interventions, in almost every state, the final form of the breast cancer informed consent legislation was written in weak language, lacked enforcement mechanisms, and made no provisions for patient education.[18] Nonetheless, as Montini and Ruzek have argued, "the effectiveness of informed consent laws cannot be assessed entirely by their enforcement through the courts or regulatory agencies. Although these laws [were] highly problematic in many ways, what they [did] most effectively [was] publicly challenge the acceptability of physicians' monopoly over access to scientific information and interpretation of its implications for clinical management."[19] Informed consent legislation, like the 1979 NIH Consensus Conference on Breast Cancer, brought the state into the sacrosanct relationship between surgeons and breast cancer patients. In both cases, the state stepped in to protect breast cancer patients from the sovereign power and authority of surgeons.

The implementation of informed consent legislation and the two-step procedure did not happen overnight, and their practical effects varied tremendously from patient to patient, surgeon to surgeon, state to state, and even region to region. During the 1980s, however, breast cancer patients gradually emerged as biomedical citizens. No longer anesthetized into silent submission to the will of the surgeon, breast cancer patients finally gained the right to "gaze back" at their physicians and participate in their treatment as conscious, speaking, decision-making subjects. The next section explores important changes in the repertoire of treatments available to breast cancer patients.

CHANGES IN TREATMENT: SURGICAL RETRACTION,
ADJUVANT EXPANSION

In their nuanced, feminist history of changes in breast cancer diagnostic
and treatment practices during the 1970s and 1980s, Theresa Montini and
Sheryl Ruzek offered several explanations for the reluctance of U.S. surgeons to abandon the Halsted and incorporate less radical techniques into
their surgical repertoire.[20] They argued, first, that in a fee-for-service system such as existed in the 1970s, there was a strong economic incentive for
surgeons to perform radical mastectomies because this procedure was billed
at approximately three times the cost of a lumpectomy ($1,080, versus $351
in 1976). Second, they argued that a social-psychological element also fed
surgeons' resistance, because the adoption of less radical surgeries required
an acknowledgment that the radical surgeries they had performed in the
past—which undoubtedly caused a great deal of pain and suffering for their
patients—had been unnecessary. Third, most surgeons, as Montini and
Ruzek pointed out, are not scientists or clinical researchers, and they do not
automatically accept the results of clinical trials that appear to contravene
their experientially based knowledge—the evidence of their experience.[21]

Montini and Ruzek argued, further, that surgeons had a professional
interest in maintaining their "ownership" of breast cancer and the prestige
of their specialty. The radical mastectomy, unlike a local excision or lumpectomy, was a technically complex and challenging procedure that demonstrated the special skills of the surgeon. In addition, breast-conserving
surgeries were usually accompanied by radiation therapy, and radiation
therapy moved the treatment of breast cancer beyond the exclusive control
of surgeons. It forced them to share, confer, and work with other specialists, namely, radiologists (later radiation oncologists). Finally, offering more
than one treatment opened the way to the meaningful participation of
patients in treatment decision making, "yet the idea of a patient choosing
her treatment was anathema to most surgeons."[22] Surgeons resented efforts
to redefine the sick role and redistribute power within the surgeon–patient
relationship.

Building on the work of Ruzek and Montini, Barron Lerner also traced
the rise and demise of the Halsted radical mastectomy, underscoring the
"public controversy that erupted during the seventies" when the Halsted radical became a symbol of the "powerless [female] patient" and the "imperious

[male] physician."[23] By the late 1970s, according to Lerner, "dozens of studies had found that it [radical mastectomy] was no more curative than more conservative procedures," but American surgeons, unlike their European counterparts, "were slow to abandon the procedure."[24] Eventually, "as more and more women 'refused to consent to radical mastectomies' and searched for surgeons 'willing to perform more conservative and less disfiguring operations', offering procedures other than radical mastectomy [became] a necessary business decision."[25] When the radical mastectomy began to decline in the late 1970s, much of the impetus, as Montini and Ruzek and Lerner demonstrated, came from breast cancer patients and the women's health movement.

In a famous study of the women's health movement, Sheryl Ruzek quoted a prominent San Francisco surgeon speaking at a public forum in the early 1970s: "The state of the art isn't such that we can do lumpectomies now despite what the *Ladies Home Journal* says, which has caused an enormous amount of mischief. I think this is something that has gone too far. . . . having women tell the doctor what he should do and not do. . . . I've had several patients recently who've said, 'You're not going to take my breast off no matter what,' and I said, 'Well, that's fine. You can go here, there or the other place, but I'm not going to do a lumpectomy.'"[26] In *Cancer*, a journal for clinicians published by the ACS, a group of progressive surgeons argued for careful consideration of less radical breast surgery, but they simultaneously argued "that women have no business making a decision about the extent of surgery for breast cancer on grounds that one cannot make a wise selection when disturbed by tensions and emotions."[27] Thus, even as progressive surgeons moved cautiously toward discussing the scientific merit of less radical surgeries, they resisted sharing decision making with breast cancer patients.

This was not, in many respects, a new battle. As early as 1970, for example, Oliver Cope, emeritus clinical professor of surgery at Harvard Medical School, published a groundbreaking article on the surgical treatment of women with breast cancer in which he called for the adoption of less aggressive and "mutilating" treatments. Cope was a maverick not only in his opinions but also in the media he chose to express them. Instead of circulating his recommendations exclusively within medical and scientific forums, he published an article in the *Radcliffe Quarterly*, a magazine for Radcliffe students and alumnae. Going one step further, in 1974 Cope appeared in a feminist documentary entitled *Taking Our Bodies Back,* which was produced by the Boston Women's Health Book Collective. In it he argued that "local excision, radiation and chemotherapy" were preferable treatments for many women.[28] This statement was reprinted in *Women's Health Care: Resources, Writings, Bibliographies,* an influential women's health publication.[29] Cope's acts of professional whistle-blowing occurred in a fertile environment, already primed by the ascent of the women's health care movement. George Crile joined these efforts, as noted earlier, by publishing *What Women Should Know about the Breast Cancer Controversy.* Two years later Crile published an article in *Harper's* in which he argued that American physicians' reluctance to abandon the radical mastectomy was tied to their financial interests, not to the patient's well-being.[30]

When the Boston Women's Health Book Collective printed the second, revised edition of *Our Bodies, Ourselves* in 1976, it contained ten pages of information on breast problems and breast cancer. The first edition of the book, published in 1970, had contained no mention of breast cancer whatsoever. The new, revised edition included a highlighted box at the end of the section entitled "Key Facts about Breast Cancer for Women Consumers." The "key facts" included the statements that biopsies should be separated from subsequent treatment and that the results of the biopsy should be clearly explained to the patient. The 1976 edition also advised women who received a diagnosis of breast cancer to obtain a second opinion before proceeding with treatment; it warned women that radical mastectomy was not the only surgical possibility and that radical mastectomy had never been proven superior to other options.[31]

The 1979 NIH consensus development conference that led to the abandonment of the one-step procedure also sounded the death knell for the Halsted radical mastectomy.[32] Three broad categories of surgical techniques were evaluated by the panel of experts: radical mastectomy, total mastectomy (which removes the axillary lymph nodes but preserves the chest muscles), and "lesser surgical procedures such as segmental mastectomy with or without radiotherapy." The panel concluded that a total mastectomy with axillary lymph node dissection "provides an equivalent benefit" to women with early-stage breast cancer "and should be recognized as the current treatment standard." The panel also reviewed the early research from clinical trials of "lesser surgeries" and expressed its "enthusiastic support" for this research. Finally, the panel endorsed a clinical protocol developed by the National Surgical Adjuvant Breast Project to measure the effectiveness of total mastectomy against lumpectomy with radiation therapy.[33]

NIH recommendations were not binding on physicians, but they did signify the shifting surgical norms and standards of practice within the medical profession. Even before the 1979 NIH consensus development conference, however, the number of radical mastectomies performed in the United States had declined significantly, from a high of 54,000 in 1968 to 40,000 in 1975; 32,000 in 1976; 24,000 in 1977; and 19,000 in 1978. In 1980, 11,000 radical mastectomies were performed, and by 1983 the number had dropped to 5,000.[34] Thus, although the consensus conference speeded the demise of the Halsted, its decline was in large part the result of the efforts of maverick physicians, women's health activists, and the media.

The demise of the Halsted and the rise of less radical surgeries made more feasible the performance of breast-reconstructive surgeries, which were difficult to perform on women who had undergone a radical mastectomy. Thus, reconstructive surgery expanded rapidly during the 1980s, along with the development of new surgical techniques and implant technologies.[35] With the multiplication of types of breast surgery, the treatment options continued to increase. In the context of new norms of disclosure and informed consent procedures, this expansion made it possible and even necessary for growing numbers of women to weigh options and make choices about their treatment. The demise of the Halsted radical mastectomy thus repositioned women as agents, not just objects, of medical treatment.

Adjuvant Chemotherapy

During the 1980s the standard treatment repertoire expanded to include adjuvant chemotherapy. The first clinical trial to test chemotherapy as an adjuvant treatment for breast cancer was begun in 1957.[36] The trial protocol, which was adopted in standardized form by twenty-three institutions, was designed "to determine the efficacy of administering chemotherapy in conjunction with 'curative' cancer surgery to decrease recurrence and extend survival of patients with cancer of the breast."[37] It is interesting to note that by the time the results of this trial were published in 1968, the term "curative surgery" was surrounded by quotation marks, signifying the growing problematization of the idea of the "surgical cure." A second trial was conducted between 1973 and 1975, and soon thereafter chemotherapy trials were initiated in Britain and Italy. The early results of the Italian trial—

the Bonadonna trial, published in 1976 in the *New England Journal of Medicine*—had a dramatic impact on clinical practice and stimulated a rapid shift toward the use of chemotherapy as an adjuvant treatment for breast cancer.[38] The "adjuvant era" of chemotherapy for women with breast cancer began, as Rose Kushner recalled, "on February 19, 1976, with the first results of Bonadonna et al. from Milan." "I doubt," Kushner added, "that any data have ever had such a rapid and revolutionary impact." "It took almost a century to abandon the Halsted radical," Kushner continued, "but fewer than five years to embrace adjuvant chemotherapy."[39]

In 1976, only 7 percent of breast cancer patients received chemotherapy.[40] In 1985–1986 that figure had climbed to 23.7 percent.[41] This was true despite the fact that the NIH had recommended in 1980 that adjuvant chemotherapy for women with breast cancer should be given only in the setting of a controlled clinical trial.[42] In 1985 the NIH held a second consensus conference to review the results of new clinical trials and recommended multiagent cytotoxic chemotherapy as the standard treatment for all women with lymph node positive, estrogen receptor negative breast cancer.[43] This trend was given a final boost in 1988 when the NCI issued a clinical alert to all physicians urging them to administer chemotherapy to *all* breast cancer patients, regardless of their stage of diagnosis or tumor biology.[44]

Cancer chemotherapy, as historian Ilana Löwy has argued, represented a "new domain of medical intervention."[45] As the use of chemotherapy grew—fed by the infusion of funding for cancer chemotherapy research and clinical trials following the passage of the National Cancer Act of 1971—so too did the number of chemotherapists. The growth of chemotherapy for the treatment of breast and other cancers created a growing need for physicians trained to use these "highly toxic" drugs. The growing specialization of physicians who used drugs to treat cancer patients, as Löwy observed, led to the development of a new subspecialty in internal medicine: medical oncology. The first certifying examinations in medical oncology were administered in 1973.[46] The number of board-certified oncologists grew rapidly thereafter. By 1985 there were more than four thousand board-certified medical oncologists in the United States, and by 1992 there were almost six thousand.[47] In the United States, according to Löwy, the medical oncologist quickly came to be viewed "not as a consulting specialist, but as the primary doctor caring for cancer patients."[48]

But what did the addition of radiation and chemotherapy mean to the women who suffered through it? How did it change their embodied experiences of this disease? In a word: radically. This new domain of medicine and these new repertoires of treatment prolonged, expanded, and deepened the experience of treatment. No longer did women enter the hospital for a single surgical procedure and leave, several days later, as officially rehabilitated ex-patients. Now, in addition to undergoing surgery, breast cancer patients could expect to return over and over again for adjuvant treatments—primarily radiation and chemotherapy—designed to reduce the risk of recurrence.

Patients who received some form of breast-conserving surgery, including many women with partial mastectomies, could expect to undergo several weeks of radiation therapy, delivered on a daily basis. Common side effects of radiation included nausea, lack of appetite, skin changes, radiation burns, and cumulative, sometimes extreme, fatigue. It also, of course, increased their risk of long-term complications, as radiation will tend to do. Following their recovery from radiation therapy, which often left them weak and exhausted, they could look forward to several months—sometimes a full year or more—of cytotoxic chemotherapy.[49]

Chemotherapy, like radiation therapy, in the words of Rose Kushner, "made healthy people sick."[50] Chemotherapy regimens usually included a mixture of toxic drugs, a "chemo cocktail," that was administered intravenously in the hospital. Unlike radiation therapy, chemotherapy was a systemic therapy. Chemotherapy was administered in multiple cycles of varying length. A typical cycle might require three or four weeks to complete and would consist of an infusion followed by a period of recovery. Common side effects of chemotherapy, which patients often experienced as its main effects, included cumulative anemia, often bone-crushing fatigue, nausea and vomiting, diarrhea, weight loss, hair loss, depression, dry skin, disintegrating nails, loss of vaginal lubrication and painful intercourse, premature menopause and loss of fertility, and a weakened immune system that could lead to any number of opportunistic infections, including thrush. Longer-term complications included liver and kidney damage, memory loss, difficulty concentrating, and the development of secondary cancers—cancers caused by chemotherapy.

Adjuvant chemotherapy and radiation therapy, which were designed to reduce the risk of recurrence, prolonged the treatment experience of breast cancer patients, expanded treatment into parts of women's bodies left untouched by the previous regime, and required that women return over and over again for repeated treatments and reenactments of the new risk role of the breast cancer patient. In this way, breast cancer treatment shifted from the one-step procedure of the previous regime to a series of procedures repeated over a prolonged period of time.

As Dee, who was diagnosed with breast cancer in 1993—and whose treatment included a lumpectomy followed by chemotherapy followed by radiation therapy followed by additional chemotherapy—explained in a 1995 interview: "Having breast cancer [is] a lifestyle. . . . It impacts your whole life. . . . the consequences . . . are so broad and so long-rooted . . . All these skin changes, all these stupid yeast infections, the dryness, the lack of lubrication . . . the little things like bleeding hands and disintegrating nails and cracked skin . . . and the big things like early menopause, loss of fertility, toxic chemicals and radiation . . . extreme fatigue . . . changes in muscletone and physical shape and body image . . . So when you say 'breast cancer'—yeah, that's the disease, but that's not really what's going on. What's going on is much more encompassing than just little ol' breast cancer."[51] The rational response to the physical and time demands of treatment, as another woman put it during a support group meeting, was to become a "professional patient."[52]

Another systemic therapy, tamoxifen, was approved by the U.S. Food and Drug Administration (FDA) in 1978 for the treatment of women with metastatic breast cancer. Tamoxifen was a hormone therapy that was self-administered orally, once a day, over a period of years. Compared to cytotoxic chemotherapy, it was relatively well tolerated by most women, but like all drugs, it introduced new risks and, for some women, intolerable side effects. During the 1980s tamoxifen was incorporated into the treatment regimens of a growing number of women diagnosed with breast cancer, often in addition to cytotoxic chemotherapy.[53] In 1985 tamoxifen was given an additional boost when the NIH Consensus Development Conference on Adjuvant Chemotherapy recommended tamoxifen as the treatment of choice for postmenopausal women with positive nodes and positive hormone receptor levels in their excised tumors.[54] Thus, during the 1980s, adjuvant hormone therapy expanded to embrace an increasingly wider band of breast cancer patients.

As the role of the breast cancer patient underwent redefinition, it also underwent a process of repositioning and, in many respects, a process of multipositioning. The incorporation of adjuvant therapies into standard treatment regimens resulted in the multiplication of cancer specialists and health care professionals. As this occurred, breast cancer patients were repositioned at the hub of a much larger circle of activity. Instead of having exclusive relationships with their surgeons, breast cancer patients began to participate in a much larger network of relationships. Increasingly, patients moved from site to site and appointment to appointment, consulting with surgeons, oncologists, and radiation therapists. They also interacted with a wider array of nurses, technicians, and other health care workers. This matrix of relationships was further complicated, in the San Francisco Bay Area, by the popularity of alternative medicine, which added to the mix acupuncturists, herbalists, massage therapists, nutritionists, and other practitioners of alternative medicine.

Between the early 1970s and the early 1990s, the treatment of women with breast cancer shifted from a one-step procedure to months upon months of grueling treatments; the process of recovery often lasted well over a year. For many women, this grueling treatment regimen occurred while they continued to work full-time jobs and, in many cases, raise children. Although treatment eventually ended, being at high risk for breast cancer did not, nor, in many respects, did being a breast cancer patient. The risk role of the regime of biomedicalization was not a temporary role that breast cancer patients simply exited. Instead of exiting, women treated for breast cancer rejoined the breast cancer continuum further along the line, in a permanently higher risk position. They remained risky subjects, but they also became members of the "remission society," a society of people who were "effectively well but could never be considered cured."[55]

### The Rise of Rehabilitation: Individual and Group Support

Once created, the space of patient participation continued to expand and deepen as the medical management of women with breast cancer changed in a third dimension: The isolation of breast cancer patients was replaced by structured opportunities for interaction. This shift was fed by two developments: the institutionalization of the Reach to Recovery program by the ACS and the growth of cancer support groups and organizations.

*Reach to Recovery*

Reach to Recovery was created by Terese Lasser in 1952 when, following her radical mastectomy, neither her doctor nor her nurse was able to tell her where to buy a prosthesis or what exercises to perform to regain strength and range of motion. Between 1952 and 1969 Lasser petitioned the ACS on several occasions to incorporate Reach to Recovery into their programming and develop it on a national basis. In 1969 the ACS decided to do so.[56] The ACS finally moved in the direction of rehabilitation, according to Lester Breslow and Devra Wilner, when it realized that cancer self-help programs were growing successfully without them.

Reach to Recovery was designed as a peer-based, one-on-one, hospital-based visitation program for new mastectomees. Run entirely on volunteer labor and modeled after Alcoholics Anonymous, Reach to Recovery used ex–breast cancer patients to provide newly postoperative breast cancer patients with a breast prosthesis, practical information, social and psychological support, and instruction in therapeutic exercises (physical therapy) designed to restore physical strength and functioning. Reach to Recovery quickly became one of the largest and most successful volunteer programs ever developed by the ACS.[57]

Although the limits of this program were carefully circumscribed and tightly controlled by the sovereign power of physicians, breast cancer patients were luckier than other cancer patients, most of whom were left on their own to navigate their way as ex- and possibly future cancer patients. But women with breast cancer came to be seen as having a unique set of needs, and those special needs were directly connected to the cultural significance of women's breasts in American society and the importance of women's "breasted existence" to their individual and social identities.[58] The loss of a breast came to occupy a place of special significance in the programming of the ACS, and the needs of women with breast cancer were programmatically constituted as different from the needs of other cancer patients.

Reach to Recovery, which many surgeons initially viewed with a mixture of skepticism and suspicion, nonetheless became institutionalized within hospitals and cancer-treatment facilities during the 1970s. The ACS was dependent upon surgeons, however, who controlled access to their patients; and the surgeon's preapproval was required before a breast cancer patient could be visited by a Reach to Recovery volunteer. As a condition of access,

Reach to Recovery volunteers were prohibited from expressing their opinions or offering advice about physicians, treatments, or medical concerns.
The volunteer, in turn, was required to be certified by her physician as psychologically fit before she could begin visiting patients.[59]

The purpose of the program was to provide emotional support to the
breast cancer patient by demonstrating, in the volunteer's attitude and physical appearance, that breast cancer was a survivable disease and that it need
not alter either the mastectomee's self-perception or the way she was perceived by others. To this end, Reach to Recovery volunteers, all ex–breast
cancer patients, were required to be (ostensibly) cancer-free, to behave in
an upbeat and optimistic manner, and to present an attractive, heterofeminine appearance that was wholly indistinguishable from the appearance
of cancer-free women. They were required, in other words, to appear as
"normal" and as "normalized" as could be.[60] In the 1970s Dr. William Mar-
kel, a strong supporter of the program with the ACS, described the effectiveness of Reach to Recovery:

> I think the big bang in Reach to Recovery is when the patient in the bed looks
> up and a woman comes through the door. (And we insist [that she] wear a
> tight fitting gown so that both breasts show and her hair is all combed.) We
> think we've made it then at that point. She looks up. You are a Reach to Recov-
> ery volunteer and you've had a mastectomy. If something clicks here, then all
> the rest of it is not terribly important, because then she wants to get well.[61]

In addition to embodying a model of adjustment and recovery, each
Reach to Recovery volunteer brought a gift for the new mastectomee: a temporary breast prosthesis made out of cotton. The temporary prosthesis
allowed the new breast cancer patient to begin disguising the evidence of
her mastectomy immediately so that she could receive visitors and leave
the hospital without shame or embarrassment. The volunteer also taught
the new mastectomee how to dress in order to hide the evidence of her
surgery. And the volunteer provided the only form of instruction in physical therapy that the patient was likely to receive. She taught her client how
to perform exercises with a handheld rubber ball so that she could regain
full range of motion in her upper body as she rehabilitated from surgery.

By instructing a new mastectomee in the art of concealment, affirming
the temporary nature of her illness, and assisting her transition back to

normality, Reach to Recovery strengthened the dominant spatial, temporal, and visual social relations of disease. At the same time, however, Reach to Recovery laid the groundwork for the construction of new social relationships and nascent group identities. These nascent identities and limited forms of association were originally organized, to be sure, to maintain their invisibility as mastectomees and sustain their identities as "normal women" by helping them pass beneath the public radar. In this sense, Reach to Recovery can be seen as the practice of anti-identity politics and an important supporting structure in the architecture of the closet.

In order to discourage mastectomees from thinking of breast cancer as a disability or an ongoing source of suffering or difficulty, Reach to Recovery volunteers were discouraged from maintaining ongoing contact or building ongoing relationships with their clients.[62] A statement from a Reach to Recovery representative, quoted by Rose Kushner, conveys the sprit of the program and its practices quite effectively:

> We didn't want Reach to Recovery to become a crutch. . . . After all, the whole point of Reach to Recovery is to convince women they do not have a disabling handicap. We talked about having a mastectomy club. . . . But that would have defeated our whole purpose. Having a mastectomy is *not* a permanent handicap, and even the worst of scars can be hidden by a well-fitting prosthesis and the right clothing. So we decided we would help the patient for just a few weeks, and then leave her to her own psychological recovery.[63]

The anti-identity philosophy of Reach to Recovery was not an aberration in the ACS approach to rehabilitation. The ACS also sponsored peer-visiting programs for people with laryngectomies and colostomies. In the latter case, the ACS worked closely with the independent United Ostomy Association (UOA) but had a very different philosophy. According to Lester Breslow and Danile Wilner, the ACS "does not believe in the club principle." An ACS spokesperson explained, "'We don't want colostomates making a social life out of being colostomates. The UOA has membership drives; we don't want membership drives. We want people leaving us.'"[64]

For many women, being visited by a Reach to Recovery volunteer was a welcome experience. It provided them with their only link—perhaps no more than a fleeting contact—with a "mastectomy underground," and it provided visual evidence that breast cancer was neither an automatic death sentence nor an unconcealable disfigurement. The expansion and promotion of the Reach to Recovery program, beginning in the 1970s, signaled the ambivalent, ambiguous beginnings of the transition to a new regime. Reach to Recovery created temporary social supports and social ties to the mastectomy underground while simultaneously teaching women to disidentify with their history of disease, to continue on as if nothing had happened, and to avoid stigmatization by engaging, on a daily basis, in the practice of passing.

Most certainly, Reach to Recovery did not create the stigmas associated with breast cancer, but it did in some ways strengthen the architecture of the closet that enabled these stigmatizing discourses to continue circulating freely, even as it helped women avoid directly encountering them. Ironically, however, the inscription of Reach to Recovery's anti-identity policies and practices on the bodies and psyches of new mastectomees began to change the social relations of disease and opened the door to the formation of more enduring relationships and identities.

### The Institutionalization of Support Groups in the San Francisco Bay Area

The implementation of Reach to Recovery challenged the isolation of women with breast cancer from each other, but it was limited by its programmatic structure to short-term, one-on-one peer support. Some women became Reach to Recovery volunteers, which opened the door to maintaining an ongoing contact with the mastectomy underground, but the degree to which the disease could become a shared experience and collective identity among breast cancer patients was limited by the anti-identity philosophy of Reach to Recovery. It was the proliferation of women's cancer and breast cancer support groups that created the social networks and group solidarities that fed the breast cancer movement.

During the 1970s and 1980s cancer support groups arose at the margins of medicine and the health care industry. Like Reach to Recovery, cancer support groups were (and are) a deeply gendered social technology. Like Reach to Recovery, support groups were initially resisted by surgeons, and for all the same reasons. Like Reach to Recovery, support groups really did represent a challenge to the authority of physicians, to their control over patients, and to their monopolization of information. The very structure of support groups—group support—challenged the sick role script, the social relations of disease, and the isolation of patients.

Two grassroots cancer support communities were founded in the San Francisco Bay Area in the second half of the 1980s—the Cancer Support Community in San Francisco, and the Women's Cancer Resource Center in Berkeley. Both organizations were founded by women with breast cancer and both organizations played an important role in the development of feminist breast/cancer activism in the Bay Area (this is discussed in greater detail in chapter 6). During roughly this same period, the number of support groups in hospitals and cancer centers began to rise.

Breast cancer support groups certainly existed in the Bay Area during the 1970s and early 1980s, but they seem to have been few in number, dependent on word of mouth, lacking in institutional support, and largely invisible. A statewide survey of cancer support groups conducted by the California Division of the ACS in 1981, for example, shows only twelve "mastectomy groups" across the entire state.[65] The survey is interesting for a number of reasons. First, it documents the appearance, for the first time, of "mastectomy groups"—a category that did not exist in an earlier survey conducted in 1976. Second, it suggests that, consistent with the philosophy of Reach to Recovery, "breast cancer patients" and "women with breast cancer" had not yet emerged as social categories. Mastectomy groups, in other words, were organized around an operation, not a disease or an ongoing illness experience.[66]

Four examples from my fieldwork illustrate the relative scarcity and invisibility of support groups for Bay Area women with breast cancer during the 1980s. In 1996 I met a woman named Clara.[67] She had been diagnosed with breast cancer in 1979 and received a mastectomy at a private hospital in Berkeley (I return to Clara's story in chapter 8). Despite her strong desire to connect with other women with breast cancer and her involvement in consciousness-raising groups and the women's liberation movement, Clara was not aware of any local support groups or places where she could go to meet other women with breast cancer.[68] A second woman, Laura, who was diagnosed in 1980, eventually learned about a cancer support group that met at Kaiser Permanente Medical Center in San Francisco. She attended the group twice, she said, but became dissatisfied and stopped going because the group's participants were not allowed to question medical authority or expertise.[69] Later, through feminist networks, Laura heard about another support group led by an activist in the Older Women's League (OWL), and she began attending this support group instead. It met in a private home and was not linked to a wider cancer network. A third Berkeley woman named Marla, who was diagnosed in 1984, recalled learning through word of mouth that a support group for women with breast cancer was meeting in San Francisco. She attended the support group for a short time but decided to form her own group in the East Bay so that she could avoid the commute into the city, which she found too exhausting in her weakened state. The support group that she created, like many others, was not linked to a larger institution, and women who attended her group heard about it through word of mouth. According to a fourth woman, Linda, the first breast cancer support group that was organized by a Berkeley hospital began meeting in the fall of 1988.[70] Laura was one of five women who regularly attended this group. In addition, she remembers hearing about the Cancer Support Community, but the commute across the bay to San Francisco was too daunting in her state of treatment-induced exhaustion. Interestingly enough, although WCRC had been founded in Berkeley two years earlier, its visibility was sufficiently low that Linda, who identified herself as a feminist, did not hear about WCRC until 1989 or 1990. There is no way of knowing if the difficulties these women encountered in locating support groups that met their needs is representative of the experiences of other Bay Area women during this period of time. Their stories do suggest, however, that as a social technology, support groups were not visible, accessible, or institutionalized—were not, in other words, part of the regime of breast cancer—until the late 1980s, at the very earliest.

This conclusion is reinforced by a 1989 cancer resource guide for the San Francisco Bay Area called *Who and Where: A Guide to Cancer Resources.*[71] The guide, which was created by Pamela Priest Naeve of the Northern California Cancer Center (NCCC), was published as a small booklet and distributed to nurses, social workers, physicians, and the media. Naeve indicated that, prior to the guide's publication, medical professionals and patients were "on their own" in terms of learning about services and referring their patients to them.[72] No hospital-sponsored support groups were listed in the guide, although a statement at the beginning hints at their existence: "The social service department of your local hospital may be able to provide information regarding other resources including self-help groups and counseling services." Support groups were becoming part of the landscape, but they had not yet been institutionalized within the health care industry. It is worth noting, as well, that the first edition of this cancer resource guide did not focus on breast cancer but, rather, served as a resource guide for people with cancer of any kind.

The incorporation of breast cancer support groups into the health care delivery system was given a boost in 1989 when David Spiegel, a scientist-physician at Stanford University Medical Center, published the results of a follow-up to a case-control study originally published in 1981. His results showed that women with metastatic breast cancer who had participated in a short-term support group ten years earlier had lived an average of eighteen months longer than those who had not. Spiegel had conducted the follow-up study to disprove what he considered to be exaggerated claims about the survival benefits of support groups. Much to his surprise, however, his findings reinforced this set of claims and propelled forward the institution-alization of support groups in the medical care system.[73]

In 1992 a new Bay Area resource guide was published. The guide was substantially larger even though its focus had narrowed to breast cancer. The 1992 revisions provide evidence that the organizational field of breast cancer support groups had dramatically expanded over the course of three years.[74] In the five counties that make up the San Francisco Bay Area, thirty-three different organizational sponsors of support groups were listed. Five or six of these were independent cancer support centers; the rest were hospitals and medical centers. By 1992 only thirteen hospitals in the Bay Area (approximately one-third of the total number listed in the guide) indicated that they did *not* offer cancer support groups.

An updated edition of the *Bay Area Breast Cancer Resource Guide* was issued in 1994. Between 1992 and 1994 the size of the resource guide grew from thirty-nine to eighty-five pages of breast cancer–specific resources.[75] The growth in the size of this guide serves as a measure of the rapid expansion of resources for women with breast cancer. Thus, although the details of the development of support groups in the Bay Area remain obscure, the general pattern of proliferation and institutionalization during the 1990s is clear.

During the 1990s hospitals in the Bay Area shifted en masse from a cautious, halfhearted, and even resistant stance toward cancer support groups to the enthusiastic provision and promotion of free support groups for women with breast cancer. The fact that hospitals developed breast cancer support groups despite the absence of any remuneration (from patient participants, managed care plans, or health insurance companies) provides strong evidence that support groups had become an industry standard, indispensable for attracting the lucrative business of breast cancer patients. The growing institutionalization of support groups during the 1990s constituted an important change in the practices of patient rehabilitation and in the social relations of disease. Reach to Recovery referrals in the Bay Area increased during the 1980s and then gradually began to decline, as women increasingly turned to support groups and accessed other in-house services supplied by hospitals and cancer centers.[76] First developed outside of and at the margins of biomedicine, support groups were gradually institutionalized within the Bay Area medical care system. Initially resisted by physicians, they were eventually reconceptualized by the health care industry as another form of adjuvant therapy.

Support groups expanded and deepened the space available for the formation of patient subjectivities. For the first time, social spaces were created that reconfigured the structures of patient individualization, isolation, silence, and invisibility. They did so through the simple act of bringing patients together in a common space and time, thus facilitating the creation of multiple, lateral, and ongoing ties among breast cancer patients. Support groups repositioned patients within a larger hub of activity and further transformed the hierarchical gaze of the surgeon into the polyvalent gaze of patients, changing its direction from exclusively up and down to down and up and sideways.

Individually oriented rehabilitation programs like Reach to Recovery encouraged women to adopt the sick role: to disidentify with and distance themselves from their experiences as breast cancer patients. They encouraged women to view their encounter with breast cancer as an isolated event that they could leave behind. And although they partially challenged the isolation of breast cancer patients, programs like Reach to Recovery discouraged the formation of lasting bonds with other patients in favor of a process of normalization and reintegration. Support groups, on the other hand, regardless of their structural location and therapeutic philosophy, challenged the institutionalized barriers that separated women with breast cancer from one another. The proliferation and institutionalization of support groups thus created an ever-widening circle of women with new and more enduring senses of group identity.

By the time I began observing support groups in the mid-1990s, a dense web of connections linked breast cancer patients—especially white, middle-class patients—to support groups in a variety of institutional settings.

Although support groups differed along a number of dimensions, it would be difficult to overestimate the significance of their existence and prolifer-ation—both inside and outside of the health care system—for the develop-ment of a sense of collective identity and solidarity among women with breast cancer. Support groups created new forms of biosociality among women with breast cancer. As one support group participant explained it:

> I had this notion that I couldn't possibly be a cancer patient because I didn't have the external workings of a cancer patient—I kept most of my hair during chemotherapy, I hadn't had a mastectomy. . . . And going off to [the support] group and talking with other women, and finding out that what they thought was important was not the loss of hair, not the scar, but the actual . . . it's the minute by minute, hour by hour struggle to feel good about your life. Women would go off to that group partly because it gave them a chance to feel good about helping somebody else, and you'd go off to that group . . . and you'd leave that group and you'd think: "Well, what did I say? Did I say anything that made somebody laugh?" . . . And that's great. Because what happens . . . two things happen. One is, you stop worrying about the external markers of cancer, and the other is, you redefine it in terms of shared experiences . . . a shared struggle.

In addition to providing emotional support and social solidarity, support groups pooled the knowledge and experience of their members. Participants exchanged information, shared experiences, validated and affirmed one an-other's struggles and successes, and encouraged each other to challenge their physicians, insurance companies, and HMOs. Through support groups breast cancer patients learned how to navigate their way through admin-istrative barriers and mystifying procedures. They learned about clinical tri-als, experimental procedures, alternative therapies, the treatment choices and experiences of different women, and the wide variety of resources available to them. During the second half of the 1990s, these resources increasingly included cancer Web sites and Internet mailing lists. In short, what par-ticipants acquired in these spaces was access to resources and a larger body of experiences, new social networks, new friendships, new skills, new knowl-edge, and a growing sense of shared experience and group identity.

What participants *also* often acquired, however, was an unwelcome aware-ness of the amount of guesswork involved in their treatment, the lack of consensus within the research and medical establishments, the primitive state of knowledge about this disease, and the uncertainty of their futures. As Musa Mayer once observed, "the trade-off for getting information and support from other survivors [was] often a poignant one: isolation for anxiety; innocence for knowledge."[77] The establishment of new friendships and social networks increased the likelihood that even women who maintained their membership in the remission society—the society of people who were "effectively well but could never be considered cured"—would love, comfort, and care for women who suffered recurrences and died from the disease.[78] Thus, social solidarity and group identity were also linked to experiences of loss and mortality.

One woman put it like this: "See here's the thing, if in fact any of us [in the breast cancer support group] metastasize . . . or [have] a recurrence of the primary cancer . . . we think of ourselves more as . . . it's like you're a cancer patient but it's like you're living the high risk lifestyle, and it's not even high risk sex. . . . you don't get anything out of it! You've been put in a category where your life is permanently changed. You think about things that other people don't think about, you've been through experiences that other people have never experienced . . . so when you say 'breast cancer' . . . well, yeah, but what's really going on here is that my life has been redefined. . . . thank God that there are women whose lives have been redefined who I can talk to so that I'm not walking around feeling like the only weirdo." Support groups made members of the breast cancer society visible to each other. The breast/cancer movement, the subject of part II, made regular flesh-and-blood women with breast cancer—not just journalists and celebrities—visible to the rest of us.

# Cultures of Action
# in the Bay Area

# Early Detection
# and Screening Activism

The power to endure is found in making the message mainstream, by engaging
the business, government, and scientific communities.

—SUSAN BRAUN, Susan G. Komen Breast Cancer Foundation

We've been invited to participate in a process by people who do not look like
us, do not talk like us, and do not know our culture. Black women do not
buy into what white women say on TV—they do not see themselves in those
women.

—BEVERLY RHINE, "A Faith Centered Model for Activism and Advocacy"

It is October again: National Breast Cancer Awareness Month. Breast health
is in the air and pink ribbons are everywhere. In the past two weeks I have
been asked to Clean for the Cure with a Eureka vacuum, Cook for the
Cure with a pink KitchenAid mixer, Kiss Cancer Goodbye with Avon lipstick, and Shop for the Cure with an American Express card. I can also race,
walk, dance, swim, climb, golf, bike, hike, and kayak for breast cancer
awareness, and I can attend elegant dinners and fashion shows to raise
awareness. Awareness of what? Awareness of the importance of constant
vigilance, annual mammograms, and early detection to "protect" women
against dying from this disease.

This chapter examines the culture of early detection and screening activism that developed during the 1990s in the San Francisco Bay Area. This
culture of action did not represent an abrupt break with the breast cancer
awareness campaigns of the 1970s and 1980s. Like the earlier generation of

screening campaigns, this COA promoted breast self-examination, clinical breast exams, and mammographic screening as life-saving technologies. Like these earlier campaigns, this COA constructed compliance with screening guidelines as a moral responsibility of individual women—a civic duty, yes, but also a family obligation. What was new to the 1990s was the emergence of a full-bodied, three-dimensional, participatory COA. The emergence of this new COA was tied to three overlapping and mutually reinforcing developments: the interpenetration of the state, private industry, and breast cancer screening advocacy; the rise of mass-participation fund-raising events; and growing pressure to expand mammographic screening to medically marginalized communities.

First, during the 1990s the density and diversity of organizational actors involved in the promotion of breast cancer screening and early detection grew by leaps and bounds. Instead of a hegemonic field dominated by the American Cancer Society, a new organizational field took shape. In California this increasingly fragmented field included public agencies and publicly funded programs that designed and implemented large-scale breast cancer screening programs. The field also included breast cancer organizations like the Susan G. Komen Foundation and its local affiliates, local ACS chapters, local businesses, and hundreds of corporations that sponsored breast cancer awareness activities—some of whom, like Avon, Ralph Lauren, and Estée Lauder, created their own multimillion-dollar breast cancer foundations and launched their own campaigns.

During the 1990s breast cancer awareness became the cause célèbre of corporate America, especially the fitness, fashion, and cosmetics industries. But breast cancer—as Lisa Belkin observed in 1993—"is not hot just because Nancy Brinker, Ralph Lauren, Ronald Perelman, and Evelyn Lauder willed it to be hot. Breast cancer is hot because it resonates."[1] And why did it resonate? It resonated, as we know from part I, because by the early 1990s women in the United States had developed a more intimate relationship with the regime of breast cancer. By the early 1990s, many women had discovered a lump in their breast or received an ambiguous mammogram or undergone a biopsy or received a diagnosis of invasive or preinvasive breast cancer—or at the very least knew someone who had. It resonated, further, because by the early 1990s the white middle classes had been transformed by decades of early detection campaigns into risky subjects.

Second, and relatedly, during the 1990s the Komen Foundation and other breast cancer organizations developed an effective means of mobilizing hundreds and sometimes thousands of individual participants, friendship networks, employee groups, civic organizations, churches, small businesses, and health care organizations to participate in fitness fund-raisers. These mass-participation fund-raisers—Komen's Race for the Cure and Avon's Walk for Breast Cancer are the most famous—were incredibly popular with adult women and their families and were incredibly successful at raising money. In addition, they were fun, healthy, social activities that generated good will, solidarity, awareness, and visibility. Mass-participation fitness fund-raisers literally transformed the public face of breast cancer. Corporate cause-related marketing constituted a second tactical innovation in this COA's repertoire of action. Through cause-related marketing, corporations simultaneously were able to elevate their corporate image and visibility among female consumers while expanding their markets and, often, increasing their profits. The flip side of cause-related marketing, thus, was cause-related consumption. The more products consumers purchased, the more the corporate sponsor donated to various breast cancer initiatives.[2] Neither of these tactical innovations, technically speaking, were invented by this COA, but they were developed and utilized in the domain of breast cancer on a scale and with an impact not previously seen. Across the country, hundreds of thousands of women and men joined in the breast cancer movement via mass-participation fitness fund-raisers and cause-related consumption. In 1991, for example, fourteen Race for the Cure events were held across the country. By 1998, however, there were more than seventy such races—and each race attracted thousands, and sometimes tens of thousands, of participants. Since 2005 alone, the Komen Foundation estimates that more than one million people have participated in Race for the Cure.

Third, unlike in the campaigns of the 1970s and 1980s, access to mammographic screening for medically marginalized women—especially low-income, uninsured women of color—finally became a moral imperative for politicians, public agencies, cancer charities, and corporate philanthropies during the 1990s. Communities of color were the primary targets of this expansion in screening programs. Mainstream discourses of breast cancer screening, in turn, were racially recoded in an effort to counteract decades of campaigning that privileged white women. A third tactical innovation, an offshoot of the growing trend toward public–private partnerships in the delivery of social services, was the use of a strategy called "community mobilization" to implement state-funded breast cancer screening programs on the local level.

One of the things that made this COA so puzzling to me at first, and so intriguing, was the challenge it posed to two popular assumptions among social movements scholars: first, that social movements have clear boundaries and can be easily distinguished from the state, private industry, and philanthropic organizations; and second, that social movements engage in contentious forms of action.

Contrary to the first assumption, the culture of screening activism was a composite of public agencies, private corporations, professional associations, health care organizations, community groups, and breast cancer philanthropies, research foundations, and advocacy organizations, as well as churches, beauty parlors, and work sites, and so on. This COA was a hybrid—an example of what Mark Wolfson has termed an "interpenetrated" social movement.[3] It was not identical to, but it was nonetheless solidly anchored in, the state, private industry, and different sectors of civil society.

Contrary to the second assumption, this COA did not engage in contentious forms of protest, although it did target (and was in some ways part of) the state. This was a *consensus* COA that mobilized hope and solidarity, faith in science and medicine, and respect for health care professionals. It privileged the identity of "breast cancer survivor" and tied this identity to the physical display of heteronormative femininity. It created what could be called a "community of the caring" that included virtually every sector of society. It did not mobilize anger against public agencies, private corporations, the health care system, the pharmaceutical industry, or other nonprofit organizations. Rather, it mobilized a discourse of solidarity in which the only enemies were lack of awareness and other barriers—financial, cultural, physical—to breast cancer screening.

Consensus activism and the culture of optimism resonated with the political styles and sensibilities of many women who had been diagnosed with breast cancer; it resonated with their friends, coworkers, and families; and it resonated with many of the ostensibly healthy risky subjects who occupied shifting positions on the breast cancer continuum. It also resonated with many small businesses and large corporations who wanted to be associated with a popular, bipartisan, "consensus" movement that would appeal to their customers. As a representative of the Komen Foundation explained,

"The power to endure is found in making the message mainstream, by engaging the business, government, and scientific communities."[4]

The culture of breast cancer awareness and screening activism was not unique to the San Francisco Bay Area. Indeed, many of its participants—social movement organizations, corporations, philanthropic foundations—operated within national and international theaters. But the San Francisco Bay Area is nonetheless an interesting site to study, because it offers the opportunity to observe the local development of this COA in a field of contention that included two other cultures of action. The Bay Area is an important site to study for a second reason: California was the first state to make a serious commitment of its own resources—catalyzed by a legislative mandate and funded by a tax on cigarettes—to the promotion and *provision* of breast cancer screening to medically marginalized women, especially low-income, uninsured racial and ethnic minority women.

This chapter is divided into two parts. The first part focuses on the corporatization of the breast cancer awareness movement during the 1990s, highlighting the role of the Komen Foundation and Race for the Cure, the quintessential public event of this COA. The second part explores the expansion of breast cancer screening into medically marginalized communities, highlighting the role of public agencies and local organizations in the racial and sexual diversification of the discourses and practices of early detection.

THE CORPORATIZATION OF BREAST CANCER AWARENESS

Linking brand names and consumer products to a disease associated with death and disfigurement seems "like the prescription for a marketing disaster," as an article in the *Wall Street Journal* once put it, but that is exactly what happened to breast cancer. During the 1990s, the article continues, corporations discovered "that the strong emotions provoked by breast cancer [could] translate to a company's bottom line." As a result, breast cancer was transformed into "a powerful selling tool" that leading corporations in the fitness, fashion, and cosmetics industries "jockey[ed]" to attach their names to.[5] The decoupling of breast cancer from images of death and disfigurement and the construction of powerful new associations with popular images of heterofemininity changed the corporate calculus of charitable giving and cause-related marketing. According to one industry analyst, breast cancer appealed to marketing departments because "it hits that sweet spot in all modern American women where soap-opera fan and feminist meet."[6]

Cause-related marketing emerged in the mid-1980s, as Samantha King has shown, "as a strategic marketing tool for differentiating a brand and adding value to it."[7] Corporations contributed generously to breast cancer foundations and charities during the 1990s because breast cancer had become an important issue to women and women were the consumer market they aimed to please. Research conducted by General Motors (GM), for example, led the company to conclude that 54 percent of its potential consumers were more likely to consider buying a GM vehicle after hearing about its "Cure Campaign."[8] Unlike the pharmaceutical companies and mammography equipment manufacturers that had promoted breast cancer screening during the preceding decade, however, the corporations that sponsored breast cancer fund-raisers and foundations during the 1990s, by and large, were not invested in the business end of cancer. This is an important shift in the corporate sector's involvement in and support of breast cancer initiatives.

Some corporations contributed directly to existing breast cancer organizations. Others created their own breast cancer charities, research foundations, and even medical facilities—the Nina Hyde Center for Breast Cancer Research, for example, was established through the initiative of fashion mogul Ralph Lauren.[9] Still others organized various kinds of breast cancer awareness campaigns that revolved around the purchase of special products and pink ribbons. Numerous corporations sold tickets to special events—fashion shows, elegant dinners, and other public events—and donated the proceeds to their favorite breast cancer organization. Corporations mobilized cause-related marketing, strategic giving, and corporate philanthropy to build name recognition and customer loyalty.

Avon was a particularly generous contributor to the culture of breast cancer awareness and screening activism. In 1993, for example, Avon established its own nonprofit organization, the Avon Breast Health Access Fund. By December 1996 Avon had spent $20 million to finance "community-based programs that make screening mammograms available to medically underserved women."[10] In addition to funding mammographic screening for medically underserved women, Avon used its 450,000 sales representatives to sell pink-ribbon pins, pens, and other products to raise money for the fund and encouraged its sales force to act as breast health educators and outreach workers—selling cosmetics while conducting breast health education. When a sales representative "begins to talk to a customer about something like this," as an Avon executive explained, "suddenly there's a linkage and a bonding between them."[11] Avon's Breast Cancer Awareness Crusade became one of the largest cause-related marketing programs ever created, and Avon estimated that publicity regarding their Breast Cancer Awareness Crusade campaign "created 700 million media impressions— opportunities for people to read, watch or hear about Avon's good works."[12] These "impressions," according to James E. Preston, the chairman and chief executive of Avon, "had a substantial impact on sales."[13]

Cosmetics giant Revlon also established a strong relationship with the breast cancer research, treatment, and advocacy communities. During the 1990s Revlon created fund-raising "runs" modeled after Race for the Cure and an annual fund-raising event called the Fire and Ice Ball. Revlon also founded the Revlon–UCLA Women's Cancer Research Program and sponsored the National Breast Cancer Coalition's petition drive in support of a "national agenda" on breast cancer.[14] And the list goes on and on.

Other companies incorporated breast health messages directly into their merchandise. Nike, for example, created a line of running shoes displaying the pink-ribbon symbol. Kenar sold T-shirts emblazoned with a large pink ribbon. American Airlines added pink ribbons to its luggage tags. Titleist imprinted pink ribbons on two lines of golf balls. The Hanes Hosiery unit of Sara Lee Corporation included plastic BSE shower cards in their stocking packaging. Dozens of companies contributed to the promotion of breast cancer awareness through pink-ribbon add-ons to consumer products marketed to women. In theory, companies donated a percentage of the sales or profits from these products to breast cancer research, treatment, screening, or education. In practice, there was very little transparency in many of these pink-ribbon campaigns.

Regardless of the motivations of corporate marketing departments, however, their participation in this COA was very real and very consequential. First, they provided direct financial support to organizations like the Komen Foundation. Second, in seeking to burnish their own corporate images, they did indeed promote awareness of breast cancer. Corporate involvement in the breast cancer movement, as one study of cause-related marketing revealed, "profoundly changed the public's awareness of the disease and significantly increased the budget of many breast cancer organizations, thereby increasing the impact of their work."[15] And as the vice president of the Komen Foundation acknowledged, the Komen Foundation could never have afforded the sort of advertising that its corporate sponsors provided.[16]

*The Susan G. Komen Breast Cancer Foundation*

The Susan G. Komen Breast Cancer Foundation was founded in 1982 in Dallas, Texas, by Nancy Brinker. It was named in honor of her sister, Suzy, who died from breast cancer in 1980 at the age of thirty-six. Two years after founding the organization, Nancy Brinker was diagnosed with breast cancer. Brinker was luckier than her sister, however. She became a "breast cancer survivor" and remained the driving force behind the Komen Foundation.

Nancy Brinker's husband, Norman Brinker, was a tremendously wealthy and well-connected businessman—a founder of three national restaurant chains—and was active in Republican politics. Through her husband's connections, Brinker became acquainted with Dan and Marilyn Quayle and other powerful Republicans whose support and name recognition she was able to enlist.[17] During the early 1980s, when the ACS was the only organization working to raise breast cancer awareness, Nancy Brinker mobilized her tremendous cultural, economic, social, symbolic, and political capital to raise the visibility of breast cancer as a public issue and mobilize support for access to mammographic screening.

The Komen Foundation deserves a great deal of the credit for reshaping the publicly available meanings and representations of breast cancer. This was not an easy thing to do. Brinker likes to recount the story of her first attempt to enroll a lingerie manufacturer in the body politics of her political agenda. In 1984 she approached a lingerie manufacturer with the following proposition: Why not attach a tag to each bra reminding women to get regular mammograms? The lingerie manufacturer, according to Brinker, responded by throwing her out of his office, exclaiming, "That's negative advertising and I'm in the business to make money!"[18] A decade later, at its annual fund-raising dinner, the "intimate-apparel" industry raised almost $200,000 for the Komen Foundation. By then multinational corporations were competing for the honor of becoming "official sponsors" of the Race for the Cure and other Komen Foundation events.

Not only did the Komen Foundation mobilize hundreds of thousands of individuals across the country to participate in Race for the Cure events during the 1990s, but it also successfully linked the cause of breast cancer to the purse strings of corporate America. It did so in large part by transforming popular discourses of breast cancer from images of death, deformity, and victimization to images of feminine triumph, strength, and beauty.

At the same time, the Komen Foundation maintained a safe distance from feminist and environmental breast cancer activism. Nancy Brinker, for example, was involved in the initial series of meetings that led to the formation of the NBCC in 1991. But Brinker pulled out of the committee that eventually issued the call that resulted in the establishment of the NBCC. One Bay Area activist told a well-known story about one of these early meetings: "The Komen ladies, dripping in diamonds, sat on one side of the table, and across from them were some women from the Mary Helen Mautner Project for Lesbians and Cancer."[19] According to this narrative— a story that was repeated on many occasions in the feminist cancer community—the Komen ladies (and they were always referred to as "ladies") decided to pull out of the NBCC while it was in the process of formation because they did not want to work with feminists and lesbians. True or not, the repetition of this narrative illustrates the cultural and political divide that, from the perspective of the "feminists and lesbians," the Komen Foundation embodied and represented.

The Komen Foundation embraced mainstream, and in some respects conservative, norms of gender and sexuality, and these resonated with corporate America and with ordinary Americans from across the political spectrum. The Komen Foundation also maintained a respectful, uncritical stance toward the medical and research establishments—raising money for them without directly challenging their authority, priorities, and expertise. The foundation, in other words, embraced a traditional division of labor and distribution of power between the lay populace and the institutions of science and medicine. But the foundation was also at the forefront of legislatively focused efforts to force the health insurance industry to cover mammographic screening. In 1987, for example, Komen volunteers successfully lobbied members of the Texas State Legislature for insurance coverage of baseline mammograms, helping set a precedent for legislation in many other states and federally.[20] The Komen Foundation consistently pushed for expanded access to mammographic screening and used its own resources to provide mammograms to low-income women. The Komen Foundation helped transform the *issue* of mammograms for low-income, uninsured, and underserved women, especially women of color, into a *moral imperative*.

During the late 1980s and 1990s the Komen Foundation remained headquartered in Dallas, but a network of volunteers spread out across the country as local chapters formed, often for the purpose of staging Race for the Cure events. It was through these events that the Komen Foundation achieved its greatest success in constructing a new public culture of breast cancer, mobilizing the middle-class masses, and converting corporations to the cause. The first Race for the Cure was held in 1983 in Dallas, Texas, and it was a unique event. Road races had grown popular during the 1970s, but they were seldom associated with charitable causes or social movements.[21] Race for the Cure—a trademarked event—represented an important strategic innovation in the tactical repertoire of social movements. It created a template that was adopted by countless social movement organizations in their efforts to raise money, promote their messages, and recruit participants.

The San Francisco chapter of the Komen Foundation, one of the oldest foundation chapters, was formed in 1987, and in 1991 San Francisco became one of the first fifteen cities to stage a Race for the Cure event. The race raised $232,000. These funds were used to support biomedical research and to launch a local program, administered by the University of California, San Francisco, to provide free mammographic screening to "the medically underserved" through the use of a mobile mammography van.[22] By

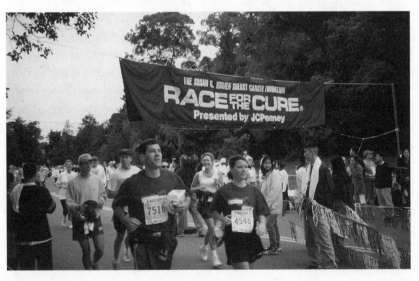

Finish line of the 1996 San Francisco Race for the Cure. Photograph by Maren Klawiter.

1996 the Komen Foundation had raised over $65 million nationally for breast cancer research and early detection, most of it during the previous five years, as a result of Race for the Cure. In 1996 Race for the Cure events were held in sixty-six different cities across the country.

I participated in the San Francisco Race for the Cure in 1994, 1995, 1996, and 1997. The description I give here is of the 1996 event, but the four events were virtually indistinguishable, except that they grew larger every year. The 1996 Race for the Cure was held in Golden Gate Park. The event drew almost nine thousand participants and raised over $400,000.[23] The Komen Foundation required local Race for the Cure organizers to send 25 percent of the proceeds to the national office. The remaining 75 percent could be used to fund local projects.

*Race for the Cure*

On a beautiful October morning in San Francisco's Golden Gate Park, the atmosphere of a carnival prevailed. The sixth annual Race for the Cure was coming to life. The outskirts of Sharon Meadow were lined with corporate booths, from which staffers hawked their wares. Dressed in running attire, thousands of women, children, and men meandered about. The crowd was about 75 percent white and 75 percent women, most of whom were toting clear plastic bags labeled "Vogue" that contained free hair products, cosmetics, lotions, and perfumes. The bags rapidly filled up with more free items—pins of the newly issued breast cancer awareness stamp, pink ribbons, and breast self-exam brochures. Tropicana Orange Juice, one of the national sponsors of the race, offered some encouraging news about how to avoid breast cancer. "Don't gamble with the odds!" their brochure declared. "If you play it smart, you can beat them." Tropicana even provided a convenient set of diet tips and orange juice recipes to that end. The brochure explained that being overweight and not getting enough vitamin C were "risk factors" for the development of breast cancer. The language of risk factors, breast health, and early detection dominated the discourse of the race.

Booths of the corporate sponsors—Chevron, Genentech, JCPenney, American Airlines, Ford, Pacific Bell, Vogue, Nordstrom, Wells Fargo, Bank of America—were prominently positioned. The health care industry was also in attendance—booths for Kaiser Permanente, California Pacific Medical Center, Davies Medical Center, and UCSF–Mount Zion Hospital, and Marin General Hospital lined the perimeter, and the UCSF Mobile

Mammography Van was stationed on the lawn. In the breast cancer capital of the world, breast cancer was a big-ticket item that health care providers could not afford to ignore. During the preceding few years, a whirlwind of sales, closures, and mergers had transformed the health care industry in the San Francisco Bay Area.[24] Many of the health care organizations that survived were reorganized and repackaged, the better to appeal to the concerns and demands of female baby-boomer consumers.[25] Old-fashioned hospitals and general medical centers were replaced by women's health centers, breast health centers, breast cancer centers, and the less specialized, more old-fashioned cancer centers. One of the breast health centers in San Francisco distributed an eleven-page handout listing thirty-four services, groups, and programs for women with breast cancer and "breast health" concerns.

The fitness, nutrition, beauty, and fashion industries were also in attendance. They offered an amazing array of services and top-of-the-line accessories tailored to the special needs of women in treatment for cancer and women who had survived breast cancer treatment. There were nutrition consultants, fitness experts, and hair stylists. There were special lotions and creams. There were special swimsuits, wigs, scarves, makeup, clothing, and vitamins. There were customized breast prostheses, beginning at $2,100, created from a cast made of the customer's breast before she underwent a mastectomy. There were partial prostheses for women with less radical surgeries. For the physically active crowd, there were sports bras, biker pants, and baseball caps, with and without attached ponytails. There was plenty of sexy lingerie. The cover of one catalog featured a quote attributed to Simone de Beauvoir: "One is not born a woman, one becomes one." Inside the catalog were the means of (re)becoming a woman—prostheses, lingerie, ponytails, and fitness wear. This was the style of embodiment given center stage at the race.

Adding to the festive atmosphere were shiny new automobiles adorned with balloons and parked in the middle of the meadow, courtesy of Ford— national sponsors of the race. In every direction one looked, purple and aqua balloons danced in the air. Also bobbing about in the crowds, and easily noticeable from a distance, were women wearing bright pink visors. These visors signaled a special status and were worn with pride. On each visor, below the corporate logos, the following message was stitched: "I'm a survivor." The visors were distributed from a special booth, situated in the center of the meadow—the Breast Cancer Survivors' Station. Here, more than a dozen queues formed with women standing six deep, chatting and socializing while waiting to receive the complimentary pink visor that would mark them—more importantly, that they would use to mark themselves— as breast cancer survivors. As each woman donned her visor and mingled with the crowd, she proudly and publicly marked herself as a breast cancer survivor. In doing so, she visually embodied an identity not otherwise apparent. This was an act of social disobedience—a collective coming out, a rejection of stigma and invisibility, an appropriation of the traditional color of femininity by the survivor identity. Later, after the race had been run and walked, there was an official ceremony during which all the breast cancer survivors who wished to be recognized were asked to ascend the main stage. There they were honored for their courage in fighting breast cancer and for their willingness to demonstrate to other women, through their rejection of the cultural code of silence and invisibility, that breast cancer was not a shameful disease, that it was survivable, and that it was neither disfiguring nor defeminizing.

Another way of publicly remembering and honoring women with breast cancer was provided at the registration tables. Instead of the standard numbered forms pinned to their backs, participants could choose to wear "In Honor of" or "In Memory of" forms displaying the names of women— both living and dead—whom they wished to publicly honor and acknowledge or mourn and remember. Like the visors, these forms were pink and they marked their wearers with a particular status. In choosing to display these forms, the participants identified themselves as part of the expanding circle of those whose lives have been touched by breast cancer. The practice of wearing a sign was a way of enacting community, a way of including oneself in the sea of sympathizers, sufferers, and survivors working together to raise awareness of breast cancer and money for medical research and mammographic screening. The signs and visors were powerful visual reminders of the pervasiveness of this disease. They signified the public display of private losses and personal triumphs. Wearing them was an emotional act at once painful, brave, and hopeful. These moving displays enhanced the intensity of the experience of moving en masse through the park with thousands of strangers united by their relationship to this disease.

Three more displays visually coded and packaged breast cancer. All three were stationed at one end of the meadow, apart from the corporate booths.

The first display was a very large, long cloth banner. The banner was imprinted with thousands of pink ribbons, the symbol of breast cancer awareness. Everyone was invited to write a name on a ribbon, and many of the ribbons were filled in with handwritten names. The second display was the Breast Cancer Quilt. Modeled after the AIDS Quilt but smaller, each quilt—and there were several on display—contained approximately twenty twelve-by-fourteen-inch panels. Each panel was created by a breast cancer survivor or a woman who, at least at the time the quilt was made, was still a survivor. Unlike the AIDS Quilt, which recognized those who had died, the Breast Cancer Quilt recognized survivors. The difference is significant. Not far from the Breast Cancer Quilt was stationed the third display, the Wall of Hope. This display contained a series of panels. Each panel contained fifteen eight-by-ten-inch "glamour photos" of breast cancer survivors. The survivors were photographed in full makeup and adorned in brightly colored evening gowns, sparkling jewelry, and even feather boas. Most of the survivors on display were white women. Women of color, especially dark-skinned women, stood out in a sea of light faces, their visages poorly captured by a photographer seemingly accustomed to working with lighter hues. Each woman was identified by name and by year of diagnosis, or by the number of years of survival postdiagnosis. Frozen in time, all of these women appeared as breast cancer survivors—even those, unknown and unidentified, who had since died.

The core message of the official program, conducted on stage by a woman in a pink visor, was clear and concise. The solution to breast cancer, she made clear, lay in two directions: biomedical research and early detection. The audience learned that the Komen Foundation had contributed more money to breast cancer research, screening, and early detection than any other private organization that was dedicated solely to breast cancer. The audience also learned of the foundation's origin as a memorial to Suzy Komen. "Back then," said the speaker, "there was no follow-up therapy, no radiation, no chemotherapy, no pill [tamoxifen]."[26] In this case, the speaker was mistaken. All three treatments she mentioned—tamoxifen, chemotherapy, and radiation therapy—were used to treat women with breast cancer during the 1980s. The details and accuracy of the speaker's narrative were less important, however, than the trope of medical progress.

The speaker continued with her story of individual control and medical progress. Nancy Brinker, she explained, learned from her sister's experience "that early detection is the key." This knowledge served her well. She was vigilant and proactive in her own "breast health practices" and, soon thereafter, was diagnosed with early-stage breast cancer. Because she practiced breast health and was diagnosed early, she was now a survivor. The speaker concluded, "This is what every woman here needs to know. All women should get a baseline mammogram at age 35, every two years after age 40, and yearly after age 50. And every woman should practice monthly breast self-exam." The message here was clear: Biomedical research had led to advances in the treatment of breast cancer that, in combination with breast self-examination and mammography, were transforming the new generation of breast cancer patients into breast cancer survivors.

This was the archetypal story of Race for the Cure and National Breast Cancer Awareness Month. This was a story of individual triumph and responsibility. It was a story of success and self-determination, not a narrative of failure and victimization. There was nothing sad or tragic about Brinker's encounter with breast cancer. Rather, her story was a narrative of unqualified success. It also, however, served as a cautionary tale. Apparently Suzy, unlike Nancy, did not practice, or perhaps was not aware of, early detection procedures. As a result, or so the logic of the narrative suggests, she died because her breast cancer was diagnosed too late. In this morality tale the unaware and irresponsible died and the proactive survived. In the discourse of the race, survival is a matter of individual choice and responsibility. Regular mammograms never fail to diagnose breast cancer early, and women diagnosed early never die.[27] For those who practice breast health, breast cancer may constitute a momentary setback, but it is not a debilitating, recurring, or chronic disease. In the discourse of the race, breast cancer is part of each survivor's personal history, but it is a finished chapter, not a part of their future. In the discourse of the race, breast cancer is a disease of universal, individual, ahistorical, resilient, reconstructable, heterofeminine, biological females. Thus, the story told by Race for the Cure and enacted by the participants is a story of individual control and survivor pride, a narrative of hope, and a declaration of faith in the steady progress of science and medicine.

In addition to breast cancer survivors, a second category of women were singled out for special attention. These women were constituted as "the medically underserved," and it was for them that the Komen Foundation raised money for free mammograms. The medically underserved were an abstract presence at the race: symbolically evoked by the showcasing of the UCSF Mobile Mammography Van and discursively constituted by speakers at the event and in Race for the Cure publicity. Who these women were, however, and why they were "medically underserved" were questions that went unasked and unanswered. Like the simultaneously individualizing and universalizing category of the breast cancer survivor or the free-floating symbol of the pink ribbon, medically underserved women were discursively disembedded from context and community.

I turn now from an exploration of the ways screening activism blurred the lines between corporate marketing, public health campaigning, and breast cancer activism to an exploration of the equally blurry line between public agencies and social movements.

## The Expansion of the State into and the Mobilization of Medically Marginalized Communities

An equally, perhaps more, significant development that took place during the 1990s was the expansion of the state's role in mammographic screening. For the first time, federal and state agencies were legislatively empowered to organize and fund breast cancer screening services for low-income women who did not have health insurance. Previous expansions, as previously discussed, mandated that health insurance companies and managed care organizations cover mammographic screening but did not address the issue of access for uninsured women.

Furthermore, although the ACS, the Centers for Disease Control and Prevention, and public health departments made efforts during the 1980s to expand mammography screening campaigns to reach racial and ethnic minority women, one result of decades of early detection campaigns that targeted, even if unintentionally, white middle-class women was that breast cancer had been culturally constituted as a "white woman's disease." As the late Beverly Rhine, a California breast cancer activist and "three time survivor" pointedly remarked, reflecting on this history of exclusion, "We've been invited to participate in a process by people who do not look like us, do not talk like us, and do not know our culture. Black women do not buy into what white women say on TV—they do not see themselves in those women."[28]

During the 1990s, publicly funded access to mammography screening for low-income, uninsured, and underserved women in California occurred through the auspices of two major initiatives. The first, the federally funded California Breast and Cervical Cancer Control Program (BCCCP), was authorized by the National Breast and Cervical Cancer Mortality Prevention Act of 1990. The second, the state-funded California Breast Cancer Early Detection Program, was authorized by the Breast Cancer Act of 1993. These were not insignificant programs. The federal program was described by senior officials at the CDC as "one of the largest efforts in chronic disease prevention ever undertaken by an agency of the federal government."[29] Likewise, the state-funded BCEDP was by far the largest cancer-screening program ever undertaken by a state.

Unfortunately, neither program included a mandate to fund treatment services for women diagnosed with cancer under their auspices. The moral imperative to screen that was embraced by elected officials thus did not include a moral imperative to treat. This left low-income or uninsured women diagnosed with breast cancer at the mercy of charity, and it left the staff, community organizations, and volunteers involved with these programs scrambling to find charitable donors of medical treatment.

Both programs were conceptualized as strategies to reduce breast cancer mortality rates among uninsured and underserved low-income women, and both focused their attention on racial and ethnic minority communities. Despite their similarities on paper, however, the federal and state programs were very different in practice. In fact, the California BCEDP dwarfed the federal program in size, impact, and ambition. At its peak, for example, the federally funded BCCCP provided cancer screening at approximately 155 sites across the state. The state-funded BCEDP, on the other hand, grew to include some 2,000 providers statewide. And while the BCCCP left many areas of the state uncovered, the BCEDP was geographically comprehensive. The federally funded BCCCP was budgeted at $4.5 million annually for its first five-year funding cycle, which covered both cervical and breast cancer screening. The California BCEDP, on the other hand, began with an annual budget of $14 million for breast cancer screening alone.[30]

These budget differences had a direct impact on the number of women served by each program. By way of comparison, in fiscal year (FY) 1994/ 1995, the federally financed BCCCP served 24,704 women in California (including both cervical and breast cancer screening). Six years later, in FY 2000/2001, the BCCCP served 28,665 women—an increase of only 4,000 women. In contrast, the California BCEDP served 3,455 women in FY

1994/1995, when it was just getting started. Three years later, in FY 1997/ 1998, the number of women screened by the BCEDP had jumped to 77,260, and in FY 2000/2001, the California BCEDP screened 141,745 women for breast cancer alone—almost five times as many women as the federally financed screening program for breast cancer and cervical cancer combined.[31]

But the differences between the federally funded BCCCP and the state-funded BCEDP extended beyond size and structure. Whereas the BCCCP was a relatively straightforward, top-down program of patient recruitment and service provision, the California BCEDP was an ambitious project of community mobilization, cultural transformation, and political organization. For these reasons, my analysis focuses on the state-funded BCEDP and, in particular, on its implementation by the Bay Area Partnership (not its real name), one of the fourteen regional partnerships that implemented the BCEDP on the local level.

From its point of conception, the California BCEDP was envisioned as a working coalition. The Breast Cancer Act of 1993 specified that the BCEDP would be overseen by an advisory council that would include representatives from voluntary nonprofit health organizations, health care professional organizations, breast cancer survivor groups, and breast cancer– and health care–related advocacy groups. The state was divided into fourteen regions, each of which organized its own breast cancer partnership to administer the BCEDP. The general structure of each partnership was specified by the California Department of Health Services (CDHS), but these requirements left room for local variation and indigenization. The practices through which the BCEDP was administered by each partnership region were shaped by the state, to be sure, but they were also shaped by the fields of contention in which they were embedded.

In a narrow sense, the goal of the BCEDP was to recruit eligible women, especially racial and ethnic minority women, to participate in its screening program. The way in which the BCEDP approached this goal, however, entailed the pursuit of a much broader set of objectives. Rather than adopting the more traditional "If we build it they will come" approach pursued by the federally funded BCCCP, the CDHS and the advisory council required that all regional partnerships adopt a strategy known as "community mobilization."[32] A key element of the community mobilization, according to the CDHS, was the "broad-based participation and collaboration of diverse groups that make up the community."[33]

In the vision of the CDHS, each regional partnership was mandated to include health care providers and other agencies, organizations, and individuals "interested or knowledgeable in breast cancer issues," as well as "high risk underserved groups, breast cancer survivors, health advocates, local businesses, church groups, and low-income women." Furthermore, the regional partnerships were mandated to "include and represent the racial and ethnic populations residing in the region."[34]

The fourteen regional partnerships were thus conceptualized as hybrid social formations that would bring together and bridge different groups, organizations, and communities, creating a complex series of linkages and relationships. According to the CDHS: "Each member of the Partnership is expected to rally around the issue of breast cancer and work towards a common goal." In essence, the BCEDP was envisioned as a state-financed, locally organized, interpenetrated social movement.

As the CDHS noted, the lack of health insurance and the cost of screening services were two of the most important reasons for inequalities in access to mammographic screening. In addition to these economic barriers, however, the CDHS identified a number of cultural barriers to screening, including "the woman's belief that she is not at risk" and "the woman's belief that screening is unnecessary in the absence of symptoms."[35] Whereas the provision of free screening services was designed to mitigate the effects of class- and insurance-based inequalities, the cultural methods and messages used to promote breast cancer screening were designed to change the belief systems of women who did not see themselves as being at risk and who did not routinely search for signs of disease in the absence of symptoms. Like most public health campaigns, this was a project of cultural transformation designed, in this case, to alter the risk perceptions and health practices of low-income, uninsured, and underserved racial and ethnic minority women. The success of the program, according to the CDHS, hinged upon the effectiveness of the community-mobilization approach in changing "community norms."[36]

Instead of directly targeting women eligible for the program, the community-mobilization approach targeted the social networks and organizational environments in which they were embedded. The goal was to transform every social space and social relation into a new site for the diffusion of discourses of early detection—to inspire everyone, as the CDHS put it, to "rally" around the issue of breast cancer early detection. The hallmark of the community-mobilization approach was the recruitment of local businesses, churches, schools, nonprofit organizations, social services, and community leaders, as well as friendship and kinship networks.

A Mother's Day card distributed by the BCEDP provides a simple illustration of the deployment of this strategy. The front of the card looks like a typical Mother's Day card—a bouquet of flowers is accompanied by the salutation "Happy Mother's Day to Someone Very Special." Inside, on the right side, a traditional Mother's Day wish appears: "You've touched my life in many special ways. You've always been there when I needed you. Thank you for all you've done for me. Happy Mother's Day!" On the left-hand side, a rather nontraditional message is accompanied by another bouquet of flowers. It reads, "I'll always need you. That is why I want you to have a long and healthy life. Because I love you, please do something very important for both of us. Get a life-saving check-up. Call today, toll-free. 1-800-511-2300 to get more information about FREE breast examinations and mammograms." The back of the card contains additional information and encouragement to practice breast health, including the claim that "breast cancer can be successfully treated if detected early."

This is just one of many examples of the BCEDP's strategy of mobilizing preexisting relationships, networks, and identities to promote participation in breast cancer screening—in this case, tying the promotion of screening to the expression of filial love and affection and ultimately to successful treatment. Such strategies were by no means unique to the BCEDP, but through the community-mobilization approach, the BCEDP extended this discourse of family responsibility into medically marginalized communities and classes.

In addition, the BCEDP sought to transform the popular perception that breast cancer was a white woman's disease into a shared understanding that breast cancer posed a serious threat to all women. Changing popular understandings of breast cancer required changing the public culture of the disease—the popular images and media representations of "breast cancer survivors" and women at risk. Instead of being shown predominantly white faces and white bodies, the BCEDP visually and verbally recoded the disease through the voices, faces, and bodies of racial and ethnic minority women.

One of the ways the BCEDP did this was through the distribution of posters featuring images of women from the "targeted groups." Similar to the Mother's Day card described above, these posters promoted breast cancer screening by mobilizing preexisting relationships and identities in the service of breast cancer screening and surveillance. One poster produced by the CDHS and the BCEDP, for example, shows six smiling women grouped closely together; two appear to be African American; two, Latina; and two, Asian American. At the top of the poster appears the message "A woman you love needs a life-saving breast check-up." Further down: "Mammograms and breast check-ups every year are the key to a long and healthy life." A toll-free phone number is included, along with instructions to "call and find out if you qualify for a free breast check-up." Another poster includes the same text but shows five African American women spanning three generations, laughing together. Other posters featured three generations of Asian American women or three generations of Latinas.

These posters did not emphasize the eligibility requirements of being low-income and uninsured, nor did they foreground class-based identities. The BCEDP promotional materials foregrounded women's racial, ethnic, and familial identities—visually connecting the exercise and embodiment of these identities to participation in the practices of breast cancer screening. All women who saw themselves in these images and representations were encouraged to call a toll-free number to find out if they qualified for free screening services. In the language of technology studies, it was African American, Latina, and Asian American wives, mothers, and grandmothers who were configured as the primary "users" of these technologies.[37] This is not to say that low-income women and women without insurance were configured out of, or excluded from, this technology. But it was through their racial, ethnic, and familial identities, not their class identities, insurance status, or socioeconomic positions, that women were recruited to participate in this screening program. The discourse of familial duty and responsibility represented by the Mother's Day cards and posters expanded the mechanisms of surveillance from the medical clinic and the media to intimate relationships among women (mothers, daughters, grandmothers, granddaughters, aunts, sisters, and so on) and reinforced the moral imperative of mammography—insisting that mammographic screening not only saves lives, it also saves families.

*The Bay Area Partnership and the Localization of Community Mobilization*
Some elements of the BCEDP's mammography screening campaign were uniform throughout the state—posters, buttons, Mother's Day cards, and

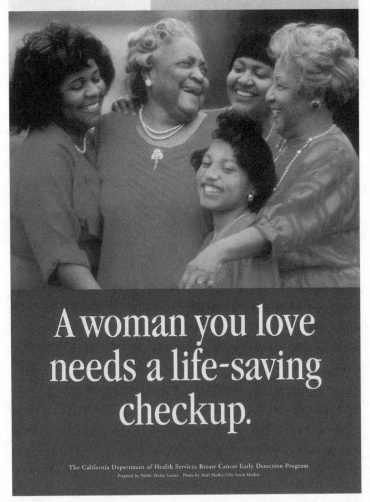

A woman you love needs a life-saving checkup. Poster prepared by
Public Media Center for the California Department of Health Services.
Photograph by Ariel Skelley/The Stock Market.

other educational media—but others varied across the fourteen regional partnerships. Regional partnerships were not, of course, equally adept at operating according to the principles of community mobilization. Each of the fourteen regions hired its own staff, recruited its own partnership members and health care providers, and developed its own leadership style and organizational culture. One of the five partnerships operating in the San Francisco Bay Area, for example, was widely perceived as ineffective, in large part because it was run in an autocratic manner and did not create a participatory culture. The Bay Area Partnership, however, was a model of community mobilization. Its membership meetings were well organized, well attended, productive, and pleasant affairs that generated a high level of good will and participation.

The region served by the Bay Area Partnership was approximately 18 percent Latino, 9 percent African American, 11 percent Asian, and 58 percent white, and the partnership employed a wide variety of social marketing strategies and outreach tactics to recruit eligible women. It placed articles and advertisements in local papers and the newsletters of community groups and local organizations. It placed billboards on buses; distributed posters to local businesses; handed out flyers, pamphlets, and buttons at public events; set up interactive displays at farmers' markets, grocery stores, food banks, and community events; conducted radio interviews; organized free breast health workshops; and placed public service announcements on local radio and television. During a six-month period in 1998, for example, the Bay Area Partnership reported that approximately 2,509,767 women had been reached with "broad-based outreach," including 225,850 African American women, 230,898 Asian or Pacific Islander women, 283,604 Latinas, and 1,749,308 white women.

In addition to broad-based outreach, the partnership created interventions tailored to specific communities. Each year, for example, it distributed small grants to community-based organizations, neighborhood groups, and individual activists who were interested in conducting "culturally appropriate" breast health education. The size of these grants varied from year to year, ranging from $2,500 to $10,000—not a trivial amount for small groups and community organizations. One minigrant, for example, funded outreach activities that included the distribution of twenty-five-dollar food coupons as incentives for women to get screened. In addition to funding small projects initiated by local organizations, the partnership applied for outside funding from local businesses and foundations. External grants of this sort were used to fund a series of culturally sensitive and language-appropriate "breast health workshops." External grants were also used to hire medical interpreters to conduct culturally sensitive and language-appropriate outreach in Latino, Cambodian, Filipino, and Laotian communities, and "patient navigators" to help patients through the complicated, chaotic, and confusing health care system.

The Bay Area Partnership also established special task forces to develop outreach projects tailored to African American, Asian, Latina, and lesbian communities. The African American Task Force, for example, produced a calendar featuring African American breast cancer survivors who were recruited through local church-based and friendship networks. A gala reception was organized to honor the calendar models, and photographs of the models were displayed at the community art center. The calendar was distributed to African American women in the county and was so popular that new editions were produced in subsequent years.

Given that the BCEDP defined its core mission as one of outreach to communities of color, there was nothing surprising about the creation of task forces that focused on the African American, Asian, and Latino communities. The Lesbian Task Group, on the other hand, was a purely local invention, the result of strong ties between partnership members and the lesbian community. The Bay Area Partnership conceptualized lesbians—like racial and ethnic minorities—as an underserved community and organized special activities to improve outreach to women in the lesbian community.[38] In addition, recognizing the low level of awareness of lesbian health issues within the medical community, for example, the Lesbian Task Group organized two public events—a lesbian comedy night and a book reading—to raise money for the production of materials designed to educate local health care providers about lesbian health issues.

A fifth task force was created in response to a controversy that erupted over the broadcast of a video promoting breast health. The video project, which is discussed in the next subsection, illustrates the great extent to which the politics and practices of the Bay Area Partnership were dynamically developed in response to the local political culture and environment. It shows, as well, how the partnership, in responding to this field of contention, influenced its political culture and development.

*The Video Project: (Re)Racializing Risk and Reconfiguring*
*"Normal" Women*

In October 1997 the Bay Area Partnership approached the county public television station and asked them, as part of NBCAM, to air a series of breast cancer educational videos. The TV station agreed, but it pulled the videos after airing them once, claiming that images of women disrobed above the waist were too explicit for public television. The station's refusal to continue airing the BSE videos was ridiculed in the media. The nationally syndicated *Today Show,* for example, made fun of the television station during its morning news commentary, and the *San Francisco Chronicle* printed a political cartoon depicting breast health videos being sold as "triple XXX rated smut" by pornographers.

Outraged by the public television station's refusal to continue airing the videos, representatives from Bay Area Partnership testified before the county board of supervisors. In response, the board of supervisors reversed the decision of the county television station and ordered the videos to be rebroadcast. In addition, they insisted that the county television station work with the partnership to produce a breast cancer awareness video that could be broadcast throughout the year. Over the course of the next year, the eight-member Video Advisory Group established by the partnership worked with the county television station to produce a thirty-minute breast cancer awareness video. The final product was a testimony to the politically engaged, locally controlled, multiracial, multicultural vision of the Bay Area Partnership.

In the opening segment, for example, the core message of the BCEDP, "Every Woman Counts," was repeated by a diverse assortment of women in six different languages. Then, endeavoring to persuade racial and ethnic minority women that breast cancer was not a white woman's disease, the incidence and mortality rates for Latina, African American, and Asian women living in the region served by the Bay Area Partnership were recited. These statistics were framed in order to demonstrate, as dramatically as possible, the breast cancer risks of women of color. The breast cancer incidence rate among Latinas, for example, was described as the highest in the state, while the incidence rate for Asian women was described as the second highest. Mortality figures were chosen and presented in equally dramatic fashion. More Asian women died from breast cancer than in any other county of the state. This shift from rates to absolute numbers dramatized the mortality figures of Asian women, who did not have the highest mortality rate in the state. Because there were fewer African American women in the county than in other parts of the state, however, the narrator once again presented mortality rates rather than absolute numbers. African American women in the region served by the partnership had the third-highest rate of death from breast cancer in the state. The use of dramatic statistics to motivate compliance with screening guidelines was not unique to the partnership, but its video deftly deployed this strategy, shaping the statistical descriptions to fit local concerns and conditions.

In addition to dramatizing the breast cancer risks faced by women of color, the video disrupted the dominant script and visual vocabulary of breast health videos. In one example, a white woman in her fifties with very short salt-and-pepper hair and a "soft butch" lesbian style described how, after being diagnosed with early-stage cancer in one breast and "after listening to and rejecting" every option suggested by her doctors, she decided to have both breasts removed (one of them prophylactically). Instead of breast implants, prostheses, or extensive reconstructive surgery, however, she decided to have her nipples reattached and be done with it. Without even the hint of hyperbole, she explained that she went in for surgery one afternoon and came home the next morning feeling "a little sore, but not too bad." Within two weeks, as she indicated, she was "back on the golf course and pitching for my softball team."[39] At the end of the interview she removed her shirt and proudly displayed a colorful tattoo of a phoenix inscribed on the flat plane of her chest, a celebration of life and beauty on the first anniversary of her surgery. The coded display of lesbian culture and imagery, the representation of breastlessness as an aesthetic choice, and the straightforward rejection of medical advice constituted a threefold departure from the representational practices and conventions of breast cancer educational media.

The video disrupted the dominant script of middle-class, heteronormative corporeal styles along a second axis. Instead of choosing a conventionally attractive woman with firm, youthful breasts to serve as the BSE model, the producers chose an obese middle-aged woman with large, pendulous breasts that were noticeably different in shape and size. In one scene the BSE model, naked from the waist up and wearing pajama-like drawstring bottoms, stood before a full-length mirror scrutinizing her breasts as the narrator explained that "looking at your breasts in the mirror helps you become familiar with the normal appearance of your breasts so that you can be aware of any changes" and that "for many women, it's common for one breast to be larger than the other." In addition to modeling the proper technique for BSE, the model visually demonstrated that it is "normal" for women to have nonidentical, non-gravity-defying breasts and soft, full bodies, and she made it "normal" for women to look as if they spend more time in the kitchen than they do in the gym.

Finally, unlike mainstream educational media, the video closed with an explicitly political message. The final image was that of a young African American woman who explained that she had received two diagnoses of breast cancer within the space of a few years. Early detection was responsible for her survival, she said, but breast cancer activism had also played an important role in her "healing process." In closing, this survivor-activist encouraged viewers not only to get screened but to get active in the breast cancer movement.

The Bay Area Partnership video thus accomplished several things: It challenged the whitewashing of breast cancer and replaced it with multiracial and multicultural representations. It incorporated lesbian-coded images of nontraditional femininity that could fly under the radar of heterosexual audiences yet speak to lesbian viewers. It made "deviant" bodies visible and recoded them as normal variations on a theme. And it served as a tool of recruitment for the breast cancer movement. The Bay Area Partnership enthusiastically embraced the role of serving as a tool of recruitment for the breast cancer movement.

### The Bay Area Partnership as a Social Movement Organization

In many respects, the Bay Area Partnership functioned like a newly established political coalition or social movement organization—recruiting new members, building a sense of collective purpose and identity, publishing a newsletter, creating committees to take on different projects, reaching out to the community through public events and educational activities, working with the media, and organizing support and opposition for legislation.

Beginning with a mailing list of one hundred, the partnership grew, within a couple of years, to include approximately four hundred individuals and organizations, over a third of which were considered active members. Representatives from organizations such as the Older Women's League, the Gray Panthers, Planned Parenthood, Hadassah, The Wellness Community, the Northern California Cancer Center, the Women's Cancer Resource Center, and local chapters of the American Cancer Society were involved with the partnership from its earliest stages—attending meetings and other public events, serving on committees, promoting the partnership's agenda and activities, sharing their mailing lists, and circulating information about the Bay Area Partnership and BCEDP services.

Partnership meetings were pleasant affairs. Coffee, cold drinks, and things to nibble on were provided, and there was time at the beginning to chat and socialize. Conflict and contention were not part of the political culture of these gatherings. Instead, partnership meetings were marked by displays of physical affection, expressions of support and appreciation, laughter, and sometimes tears of compassion. Like any other social movement organization, these meetings served the purpose of building trust, familiarity, commitment, and solidarity.

Partnership meetings also served an educational function. One meeting, for example, featured a panel of speakers who described breast cancer screening outreach projects in local Vietnamese, Korean, and Latina communities. At another partnership meeting a prominent San Francisco activist delivered a talk entitled "The California Breast Cancer Movement: Past, Present, and Future." At another meeting a prominent public health official presented a sharply worded critique of a recently released CDC report, contesting its claim that elevated breast cancer rates in the San Francisco Bay Area could be explained by known risk factors.

The Bay Area Partnership produced a newsletter that grew from a one-page flyer to an eight-page publication. The partnership used the newsletter to communicate with members, but members also used the newsletter to communicate with each other. Members used the newsletter to advertise their upcoming events, for example, and to share information with the wider partnership community. The newsletter also published information on breast cancer risk factors such as exercise, diet, nutrition, smoking, and alcohol consumption and on things individuals could do to improve their health and lower their risk of breast cancer. Every issue included a list of breast cancer resources, including books, Web sites, consumer and breast cancer organizations, government agencies, and the like. On occasion the newsletter reprinted articles from the newsletters of local organizations.

After a while, the newsletter added a feature called the Environmental

Corner. The Environmental Corner was devoted "to sharing information about environmental links to cancer, including what those concerned can do to find out about and fight against the release of potential environmental carcinogens in their communities." The migration of environmental issues into the institutional and discursive space of breast cancer screening was highly unusual. As such, it shows once again that the political culture and commitments of the Bay Area Partnership were not given in advance but, rather, were created over time in response to the local field of contention.

Participation in the Bay Area Partnership offered local organizations an opportunity to help shape its discursive practices and politics. Ever since its founding in 1986, for example, WCRC had positioned itself as a vocal critic of mammographic screening, regularly criticizing the mammography industry and the cancer establishment for overselling what it believed was a deeply flawed technology while ignoring industrial carcinogens. At the same time, WCRC was committed to working in coalition with communities of color. It was this second commitment that prompted WCRC to become an active member of the Bay Area Partnership. Thus, despite its critique of mammographic screening, WCRC displayed BCEDP brochures, videos, and promotional materials in its office space and library and contributed staff time, volunteer labor, and expertise to the Bay Area Partnership.

This does not mean that WCRC abandoned its critical stance or political agenda vis-à-vis mammographic screening and the cancer industry, but it does mean that it turned down the volume, softened the tone, and paid more attention to its audience, recognizing that its critique of mammographic screening was neither welcome nor particularly appropriate in communities where access to basic health care and preventive medicine were top priorities. WCRC sought to influence the political culture of the Bay Area Partnership, but it did so by promoting environmental activism while promoting access to mammographic screening for medically marginalized women.

One of the most important issues confronting the Bay Area Partnership, the BCEDP as a whole, and the federally funded BCCCP was the absence of a permanent source of funding to pay for the treatment of women diagnosed with breast cancer under the auspices of these publicly funded screening programs. This lack was a constant thorn in the side of everyone involved with the screening programs. The breast cancer partnerships fashioned creative stopgap measures to help women diagnosed with breast cancer obtain medical treatment, and no woman diagnosed with breast cancer through either the federally funded BCCCP or the state-funded BCEDP was ever denied treatment, but treatment was arranged on an ad hoc case-by-case basis, and during the early years a large number of patients, in the CDHS's records and words, "refused treatment."[40]

In 1996 Blue Cross of California's Public Benefit Program made a $12.4 million grant to four community foundations to provide treatment services to women identified through the state-funded screening programs.[41] These community foundations selected the California Health Collaborative to administer the program, in cooperation with the California BCEDP. The California Breast Cancer Treatment Fund, as it was called, provided an important, albeit partial and temporary, solution to the "policy gap" between screening and treatment. The solution was temporary because the money was finite. The solution was partial because it necessarily required severe rationing of medical services.[42]

The Bay Area Partnership worked with other regional partnerships, the statewide BCEDP, and other organizations to develop legislation to establish a permanent, state-funded breast cancer treatment program for low-income, uninsured, and underinsured women. This legislation, Assembly Bill 2592, which was sponsored by Assemblyman Howard Wayne, passed the California Assembly and Senate in 1998. The Advocacy Committee of the Bay Area Partnership helped mobilize support for this legislation, sending out alerts, updates, notices of hearings, addresses and phone numbers of key members of the California Senate Health and Human Services Committee, and so on. It operated, in other words, like any other social movement organization. After the legislation passed both arms of the California State Legislature, the Bay Area Partnership helped mobilize support to pressure the governor of California, Pete Wilson, to sign Assembly Bill 2592. In October 1998—during NBCAM—Wilson vetoed the legislation. As Ruth Rosen—a journalist, historian, and breast cancer survivor—wrote in an op-ed published by the *Los Angeles Times,* "Wilson's veto is a disgrace. It reveals a misogynistic indifference to poor women that borders on the pathological."[43] This defeat was not, however, the end of the issue. In 2002, as I discuss in the book's conclusion, California activists succeeded in enacting and the governor, Gray Davis, signed legislation establishing the most inclusive breast cancer treatment fund in the nation.

## CONCLUSION

The culture of early detection and screening activism achieved a remarkably high level of support in the Bay Area. The discourse of hope and salvationist science as well as the construction of the breast cancer survivor identity understandably appealed to the fears and sensitivities of many women who had been diagnosed with breast cancer. It also appealed to their coworkers, friends, and families. Finally, it resonated with the sensibilities of women who had already been transformed into risky subjects by offering them hope and a sense of control over the future.

It also appealed to image-conscious corporations whose philanthropic strategies were increasingly coordinated with their marketing departments. Known as "cause-related marketing," these new forms of corporate giving, as Samantha King has shown, provided strong support for new forms of collective identity that married civic-mindedness to consumption.[44] In addition, mass-participation fund-raisers—often organized around physical activities such as walking, biking, running, climbing, or golfing—provided people with new opportunities to contribute to the cause and express their solidarity while participating in fun, social, and healthy activities. Small businesses and large corporations associated themselves with breast cancer because breast cancer was a popular cause and a consensus issue, as well as an effective strategy for enhancing the company's reputation as a good corporate citizen, strengthening employee and customer loyalty, and expanding into new markets. Investments and involvements in the cause of breast cancer came in different shapes and sizes. Whatever form they took, however, corporate contributors, "via ads and glowing news coverage," promoted the message "that the more of us who participate by buying an object or attending an event, the larger the pot for the charity of choice."[45]

The result of this widespread appeal was a hybrid social phenomenon, an interpenetrated COA that blurred the boundaries between the state, private industry, and social movements. What was most striking about this COA was not its success at reducing breast cancer mortality rates within the communities it targeted but, rather, the cultural and social transformations that it spearheaded. It deepened the expansion of the discourses and practices of breast cancer screening into medically marginalized communities and diversified the public face of breast cancer and survivor identities. It channeled corporate America's passion for profits in the direction of breast cancer–related philanthropic activities. Finally, it mobilized the masses and popularized new practices of good citizenship. Thousands and thousands of ordinary women and men began wearing pink ribbons to honor breast cancer survivors and promote breast cancer awareness, donated money to breast cancer charities, and attended mass-participation breast cancer fund-raising events like Race for the Cure.

But this COA also mobilized the state and local communities to take a more proactive role in the expansion of breast cancer screening to medically marginalized women. The California BCEDP's stated mission was to lower mortality rates among underinsured and uninsured women. For women and men involved in implementing the BCEDP during the 1990s, however, there was no way of knowing if the program was having or ever would have an effect on mortality rates for this group of women. To this day, in fact, the answer to that question is unclear, although a recent study measuring stage of diagnosis among women who participated in the state-funded screening programs provides a basis for cautious optimism.[46] The significance of the BCEDP and its regional partnerships, however, remains wholly invisible if they are evaluated strictly on this basis.

The more immediate effects of these early detection programs lie elsewhere: in their successful mobilization of communities around breast cancer early detection and in their creation of more racially diverse images and representations of breast cancer survivors and women at risk. Their significance lies in their incorporation of medically marginalized women into the screening apparatus and the expansion of the state into a new area of service provision. It lies in the development of new kinds of relationships between the state and at least one strand of the breast cancer movement. Finally, it lies in the creation of new kinds of relationships between organizations that were embedded in, and whose primary allegiances lay with, different cultures of action.

It is important to recognize and remember, however, first, that the culture of early detection and screening activism was cohesive but not monolithic, and coherent but not univocal; second, that it was only one of three COAs in the Bay Area field of contention. We turn now to the culture of patient empowerment and feminist breast/cancer activism.

# Patient Empowerment and Feminist Treatment Activism

If each woman with breast cancer understood medicine's limited ability to control the disease, our reliance on physicians, tests, and medical interventions would be enormously reduced. The power of these institutions over us would dwindle accordingly. Without the Rosy Filter, women with breast cancer would gain the right to map our own future, within the very real constraints imposed by a life-threatening disease.

—SHARON BATT, *Patient No More*

The fact that we as feminists, the fact that we as lesbians, have created these [community cancer] centers as a consumer-feminist movement is so political. . . . If you don't understand why a direct service agency to lesbians is political, you don't really understand anything.

—JACKIE WINNOW, "The Politics of Cancer"

In 1985 Jackie Winnow was diagnosed with breast cancer while serving as the coordinator of the Lesbian/Gay and AIDS Discrimination Unit of the San Francisco Human Rights Commission. Despite her knowledge, position, and experience, Winnow was shocked to discover that even in the Bay Area, the epicenter of health consciousness and health activism, there were very few resources available for women with cancer and no collective consciousness of the political dimensions of the disease. Shortly after her diagnosis, Winnow began attending a women's cancer support group led by Carla Dalton, another Berkeley feminist, who was diagnosed with breast cancer in her thirties. In 1986 Winnow and Dalton, with the help of family and friends, founded the Women's Cancer Resource Center in Berkeley, California. WCRC was the first organization of its kind in the country—a resource center for women with cancer that was animated by a feminist, environmentalist, lesbian-friendly, and anti–cancer establishment political vision.

In 1989, shortly after learning that her breast cancer had metastasized to her lungs and bones, Winnow delivered the keynote address at the Conference for Lesbian Caregivers and the AIDS Epidemic.[1] Keenly aware of the profound gaps and silences that characterized the landscape in which women with cancer lived and struggled to survive, Winnow delivered a provocative speech crafted to galvanize a women's cancer movement.

Winnow began her speech by informing her audience that there were approximately forty thousand women in the San Francisco–Berkeley–Oakland area who were living with cancer, and that approximately four thousand women had died from cancer in 1988. She compared the mortality statistics for breast cancer to those for AIDS and explained that the total number of AIDS-related deaths in the United States since the onset of the epidemic was roughly equivalent to the number of women who would die from breast cancer in 1989 alone. "Cancer," Winnow asserted, "has become an acceptable epidemic. And as someone who has metastatic breast cancer, that is unacceptable to me."[2]

In her speech, Winnow celebrated the inspirational mobilization of the San Francisco lesbian and gay communities around the AIDS crisis:

> From nothing, we created services that educated the gay community and the general community; we housed people with AIDS/ARC, served them meals, provided emotional and practical support, and provided them funds. We created model programs for hospital care, hospice care, and social services. We demanded government responsiveness. We fought for good legislation and endlessly fight against bad legislation and bigotry. We created information services about various treatments and about ways to get them. We honored the dead through building an evolving monument, the AIDS quilt. As need became apparent, we filled the gaps.[3]

Even as she lauded the AIDS activism of the lesbian and gay community, however, Winnow encouraged the audience to examine "the excruciating choices [we make] without even being aware of them."

Referring to a recent newspaper article about women with AIDS in San Francisco, Winnow argued that the forty thousand women living with cancer in San Francisco "don't have the services that the 100 women with AIDS have." "If you have AIDS in San Francisco," Winnow asserted, "you can go to the AIDS Foundation for food and social service advocacy, get emergency funding through the AIDS Emergency Fund, and get excellent meals through Project Open Hand. Your pets are taken care of. . . . We have clinics and alternative centers and organizations fighting for drugs and research and our mental health." But if you have cancer, Winnow explained, "you wait endlessly for a support group, which if you are a lesbian, a woman of color, working class, or believe in alternatives, you don't fit into anyway. No organization shepherds you through the social service maze, no organization brings you luscious meals or sends support people to clean your house or hold your hand. No organization fights for your needs, no one advocates for you."[4]

Having been involved in AIDS work since the beginning of the epidemic, Winnow understood that AIDS organizing in the San Francisco lesbian and gay community was truly exceptional. "In the case of AIDS," Winnow asserted, we "built a model as a community." But the model, Winnow argued, did not serve everyone. Using her own life as an example, Winnow described how, after undergoing surgery and radiation, she was expected to return immediately to her work on the San Francisco AIDS commission. "I felt invisible in our community," she said. "What I found was a community willing to address AIDS, but [nothing else]."[5] Winnow concluded her speech by urging the lesbian and gay community to expand the AIDS model of organizing to serve women with cancer and people with other life-threatening illnesses and to address what she termed "the growing epidemic."

Winnow certainly understood the different contexts and conditions of AIDS among gay men in San Francisco and cancer among Bay Area women. Analyzing the former, Winnow argued that AIDS emerged suddenly and appeared as a "clear, delineated crisis." It "escalated rapidly" and created a deep sense of urgency and a need to respond quickly in order to "help people in our community."[6] Not only was AIDS labeled and perceived as a "gay disease" by both the scientific and gay community, but it was concentrated in a community whose recent history had taught its members how to survive and thrive in the face of powerful forces of stigmatization and normalization by constructing both oppositional and mainstream identities, building their own civic institutions, creating a vibrant public culture, and organizing politically.[7] Thus, when AIDS invaded the San Francisco gay men's community, it attacked an extremely well resourced, well organized, politically savvy, and culturally cohesive social group.

Cancer among women differed along each of these dimensions. First, although breast cancer incidence rates had risen steadily throughout the twentieth century, the omnipresence of breast cancer and the gradualism of its growth made it seem natural, inevitable, and timeless. Second, unlike AIDS, breast cancer was distributed throughout every sector of society, not concentrated among women in an already-cohesive community. Finally, whereas AIDS followed clear lines of person-to-person transmission, breast cancer was almost randomly distributed within populations.

More important than all of these factors combined, however, was the fact that not only was AIDS a new disease, but it was "fresh in terms of who control[led] information about it."[8] Unlike women in their relation to breast cancer, the gay community, as Winnow put it, had been present "at the making" of AIDS. They helped shape the ways AIDS was understood, framed, and represented. They helped shape AIDS-related policies, social services, and public health campaigns. They fought for a role in setting research priorities and designing clinical trials.[9] Furthermore, many organizations within the gay community received federal funding to conduct AIDS-education programs. As a result, at the same time that AIDS devastated the gay community, it also stimulated the flow of public funding, attention, and recognition, which contributed to the organizational and political strength of the community.

There were no parallel developments with regard to breast cancer or other "women's cancers." Although earlier mobilizations around mammographic screening and the right to informed decision making were encoded in state legislation, health insurance regulations, and physician–patient interactions, they had not led to the development of an organized network of women's cancer organizations. Within the women's health movement, issues connected to breast cancer had been used to highlight the misogyny and arrogance of male physicians but not to launch a women's cancer or breast cancer movement. A small handful of breast cancer organizations had been established prior to WCRC, but they were small local organizations (at that time), and they did not articulate a feminist political agenda.[10] Audre

Lorde published *The Cancer Journals* in 1980, but her vision of "an army of one-breasted women descend[ing] upon Congress"[11] and her critique of the "travesty" of breast prostheses did not immediately inspire—nor did it emerge from—a women's cancer movement.

Instead of breast cancer, the women's health movement focused its attention on the politics of reproduction—sexuality, birth control, abortion, pregnancy, childbirth, breast-feeding, unnecessary hysterectomies, forced sterilizations, and the safety of pharmaceutical technologies (for example, the birth control pill, the DES controversy, hormone therapy)—and on violence against women.[12] The women's health movement created an extensive national infrastructure of service agencies, policy, and advocacy organizations that helped institutionalize the women's health movement within multiple domains. Planned Parenthood, for example, created a national network of clinics where women could obtain birth control information and family-planning services. Feminist rape crisis centers were established in almost every major metropolitan area and recruited feminist volunteers to staff the phones and visit hospital emergency rooms. Likewise, shelters and advocacy organizations for battered women mushroomed across the country.[13] But breast cancer was not part of this trend.[14] When Winnow delivered her speech in the late 1980s, ordinary flesh-and-blood women with breast cancer were still invisible to each other and invisible, as embodied speaking subjects, to the public.

In Winnow and the first generation of women who contributed to the founding and functioning of feminist cancer organizations in the San Francisco Bay Area, tributaries from a number of different social movements came together, for the first time, as more than the dreams of individual visionaries. In WCRC and the culture of feminist breast/cancer activism that developed in the San Francisco Bay Area, these streams merged for the first time. Winnow thus represented the dawning of a new era and the rise of a new hybrid culture of action that bore the marks of several preexisting movements. In WCRC the women's health movement, the lesbian and gay movement, the disability rights movement, the AIDS movement, the alternative health movement, and the environmental movement merged with popular critiques of the cancer establishment articulated by whistleblowers like Rachel Carson in *Silent Spring* (1962), Samuel Epstein in *The Politics of Cancer* (1978), Ralph Moss in *The Cancer Syndrome* (1980), and Audre Lorde in *The Cancer Journals* (1980).[15]

Winnow's speech was revised and reprinted in feminist and in lesbian and gay publications and received relatively widespread circulation over the next few years.[16] I remember reading Winnow's speech in the summer of 1989 and feeling stunned by the common sense and the political power of her analysis. If AIDS was a political priority—and I certainly believed that it should be—then shouldn't breast cancer be too? If AIDS warranted a social movement—and I certainly believed that it did—then didn't breast cancer too? Thus, despite vast differences in the history, biology, and social epidemiology of these two diseases, and despite the influence of the women's health movement and feminism, it was the politicization of AIDS that paved the way for the politicization of breast cancer. Using the politics of AIDS as a reference point, Winnow made the politics of breast cancer make sense.[17]

As it turned out, despite the real obstacles to mobilization that Winnow identified, her speech was delivered on the cusp of a remarkable political revolution. This chapter analyzes the emergence and development of the culture of patient empowerment and feminist cancer activism in the San Francisco Bay Area, focusing on the public events, collective actions, and organizational relationships through which feminist cancer activism took shape in the Bay Area, as well as the points of tension, overlap, and inter-action between the culture of patient empowerment and the cultures of screening and environmental activism.

## THE BAY AREA CULTURE OF FEMINIST CANCER ACTIVISM

When I became a volunteer at WCRC in 1994, interactions and collabora-tions among feminist cancer organizations in the Bay Area were relatively few and far between and were a bit ad hoc. By the time my fieldwork ended more than four years later, feminist cancer organizations in the Bay Area routinely interacted with one another and worked together on a wide variety of projects. WCRC, Breast Cancer Action (BCA), Charlotte Maxwell Complementary Clinic (CMCC), the Breast Cancer Fund (BCF), and the Women and Cancer Project formed the backbone of the Bay Area culture of feminist breast/cancer activism. These organizations did not see eye to eye on everything, and there were the usual number of interpersonal con-flicts and defections, but the ongoing development of each organization in this COA was shaped, during the second half of the 1990s, by the devel-opment of the others. Each organization occupied a different niche and filled a different function in the Bay Area field of contention.

What these feminist cancer organizations shared was a commitment to the empowerment of women with breast/cancer and a body politics and emotion culture that challenged the upbeat discourse of survival and the normalizing images of unmarred, unscarred, heterofeminine bodies that were featured prominently in the culture of screening activism and the mainstream media. The culture of feminist activism challenged these normalizing images in part by creating social spaces, cultural events, and public forums that encouraged and supported the expression of alternative images, alternative discourses, and alternative ways of embodying breast cancer.

The culture of feminist breast/cancer activism also fostered an emotion culture that challenged the ban on the expression of difficult and unpleasant emotions such as sorrow, anger, grief, aggression, and accusation. Feminist cancer activists insisted—in their newsletters and body politics—that the hegemonic discourse of survival and the omnipresence of pretty pink ribbons distorted the ugly realities of the disease.[18] They respected the personal and political power of anger directed outward at the cancer industry. At the same time, feminist breast/cancer activism was also founded upon and cultivated a culture of caring and compassion for women diagnosed with cancer. It was this flip side of the coin—the culture of caring and compassion—that fed the development of direct services and support for women with cancer. In place of the iconographic "breast cancer survivors," this COA celebrated the ongoing struggles of women "living with cancer." It was thus a double-edged culture of emotion that emphasized anger, accusation, and contentious protests directed at the cancer culprits while mobilizing public compassion, support, and direct services for women living with cancer.

Although some women's cancer organizations privileged breast cancer over other cancers affecting women, the feminist culture of cancer activism, as a whole, linked the politics of breast cancer to the politics of *cancer in women* and advocated for the needs of all women with cancer. I use the term "breast/cancer" to signify the intermingling of the politics of breast cancer and women's cancer in the Bay Area, but the politics of breast cancer undeniably remained the central focus, and women with breast cancer undeniably received the lion's share of resources and support. Likewise, the term "cancer activism," as I use it, includes but is not necessarily limited to breast cancer activism.

For example, the Women's Cancer Resource Center and Charlotte Maxwell Complementary Clinic were from the beginning explicitly committed to creating social services and community spaces for all women with cancer. Breast Cancer Action and the Breast Cancer Fund, on the other hand, were organized around cancer of the breast in particular. Neither organization, however, hued strictly to these parameters. Both organizations worked on countless projects that extended the parameters of breast cancer activism.

The political culture of these organizations was feminist, lesbian-friendly, antiracist, accommodating toward people with disabilities, and supportive of non-Western healing practices and alternative therapies. All four organizations were founded and staffed primarily by white feminists who had previously worked as professional writers, community activists, businesswomen, lawyers, alternative health practitioners, or graphic artists. The service-oriented organizations—WCRC and CMCC—tried to reach medically marginalized women, especially women of color, low-income women, immigrants, women without insurance, and women with disabilities, though with limited success during the first half of the 1990s. During the second half of the 1990s, outreach to racial and ethnic minority communities became an increasingly important part of their programmatic and grant-writing initiatives. A brief historical overview of each organization follows.

*The Women's Cancer Resource Center*

The Women's Cancer Resource Center was the first agency of its kind in the country. Founded by a small group of women in 1986, its mission then, and its mission when I became a volunteer in 1994, was "to empower women with cancer to be active and informed consumers and survivors; to provide community for women with cancer and their supporters; to educate the general public about cancer; and to be actively involved in the struggle for a life-affirming, cancer-free society."[19] By the end of the decade, the terms "consumers" and "survivors" had been dropped from its mission statement, which was revised to read: "WCRC is committed to empower women with cancer to be active and informed about their disease."[20] The discursive shift from "consumers" and "survivors" to "women with cancer" was part of a larger shift in the discursive politics of feminist cancer activism. As the health care industry shifted to a language of consumerism and as the culture of early detection increasingly promoted the identity of breast cancer survivor, these terms became freighted with new meanings and associations. The consolidation of the discourse of consumerism and the breast cancer survivor identity within one COA made these cultural constructs problematic within the culture of feminist activism and led to the consolidation of the discourse of patient empowerment and the identity of "women living with cancer."

For its first two years, WCRC consisted of an ad hoc clippings library, an answering machine in Winnow's home, and peer-led support groups. A committee of twenty women took turns answering calls, mostly from recently diagnosed women seeking information and support. Word of mouth was the primary means through which women learned of WCRC. Seed money came from the San Francisco Women's Foundation. By the time Winnow died in 1991, WCRC had received a $6,000 grant to expand its library. In addition, the center ran a number of different support groups, including one for lesbian partners of women with cancer—no doubt the first of its kind in the country. The center also offered yoga and *qi gong*, medical information and referrals, and workshops on legal issues. It was also beginning to plan educational forums for the public and had moved into a wheelchair-accessible office.[21] This was during a time when medical articles were not freely available or easy to access, and patients who wanted to conduct research on their treatment options encountered all kinds of professional and institutional barriers. This was before the rise of the World Wide Web and the Internet— if they wanted to read medical articles, they had to go to a medical library, but such libraries were inaccessible and often not open to the public.

After Winnow's cancer metastasized, she handed responsibility for running WCRC to Susan Liroff, another white lesbian who became involved with WCRC when she was diagnosed with breast cancer in 1987. Winnow "kept insisting," as Liroff recalled, "that it didn't take an expert or someone with credentials to respond to callers, it took heart, being willing to listen, and an eagerness to learn and help." It was with that spirit, Liroff recalled, "that I became a cancer activist."[22] It was also in that spirit that Liroff took over leadership of WCRC. Liroff served as the executive director of WCRC for five years. She resigned in the spring of 1993, as the center entered a new phase that required, as she put it, "strategic planning, reporting, personnel issues, budgets, administration" and other things that "are not where my strengths or heart lie." By the time Liroff resigned, WCRC had achieved firm footing and a measure of stability.

I began my fieldwork the following year. By August 1994 WCRC consisted of five paid staff members—an executive director, a librarian, a volunteer coordinator, an office manager, and a program director. By then the center was publishing a twelve-page quarterly newsletter and organizing three to four volunteer-training programs a year (each with ten to fifteen new volunteers), and trained volunteers were providing a number of different services to women with cancer, including research assistance and in-home practical help. They also led support groups, produced the newsletter, and helped with office work and fund-raising.

*Breast Cancer Action*

Breast Cancer Action was founded in San Francisco in 1990 by a small group of women that included Elenore Pred, Susan Claymon, and Belle Shayer, the first president, vice president, and secretary, respectively. Pred, Claymon, and Shayer met in a support group for women with metastatic breast cancer that was organized and sponsored by the Cancer Support Community. The Cancer Support Community had been founded by two other women with cancer, Victoria Wells and Treya Killam Wilber, in 1986 (the same year that Winnow and Dalton founded WCRC). Like WCRC, the Cancer Support Community was an independent organization designed to provide support and community for people with cancer. Unlike WCRC, the Cancer Support Community was not, in principle, a women's organization. Most of the people who used the services of the Cancer Support Community, however, were women, especially women with breast cancer. Although the founders of BCA remained strong supporters of the Cancer Support Community, they were inspired by ACT UP's politicization of AIDS and they wanted to establish an organization that would help politicize the issue of breast cancer. BCA, thus, was founded as an activist, not a support, organization.

Elenore Pred, the charismatic president of Breast Cancer Action, was diagnosed with breast cancer in 1981, at the age of forty-eight. Nearly seven years later she was diagnosed with metastatic disease. She died in 1991. Pred was a veteran of the civil rights and antiwar movements of the 1960s, and she is credited with spearheading BCA's early efforts to incorporate the political insights and strategic innovations pioneered by AIDS activists into the breast cancer movement. Following Pred's initiative, for example, BCA organized tutorials with activists from the AIDS Coalition to Unleash Power (ACT UP). From ACT UP they learned how to make sense of articles in medical journals, how to work with the media, how to apply pressure to pharmaceutical companies and government agencies, and how to chain themselves to the fence if all else failed.[23]

Whereas WCRC focused on direct services and support for women with cancer, BCA focused on research policy and treatment activism. However, the organizations shared a fundamental belief in patient empowerment through access to information. BCA's most direct line to its constituents during the first half of the 1990s was its bimonthly newsletter. An excellent source of updates, information, and critical analyses, the newsletter published critical articles on breast cancer research, clinical trials, and other diagnostic, detection, and treatment issues, as well as information on legislation, the health care and insurance industries, and the inner workings of key federal agencies. During the first half of the 1990s, the bulk of BCA's work was carried out by a small but very active board of directors that included Susan Claymon, Belle Shayer, Nancy Evans, and Marilyn MacGregor.

### Charlotte Maxwell Complementary Clinic

A third feminist cancer organization, Charlotte Maxwell Complementary Clinic, was founded in 1991 by a group of health care providers and women with cancer who were brought together by the vision of Sally Savitz, a licensed acupuncturist and homeopathic doctor.[24] In 1992 CMCC began providing services to medically marginalized women with cancer. CMCC's stated mission was to make complementary forms of care available to women who ordinarily would not know about them or could not afford to pay for them.[25] CMCC's goals were (1) "to address the needs of low income women with cancer," (2) to "improve the physical and psychological health of women living with cancer," and (3) to "enable each woman to make and trust her own treatment choices."[26] CMCC was dedicated to the belief that all women with cancer, not just those who could afford to pay out of pocket, should be able to benefit from complementary therapies, which were rarely covered by insurance.

For the first several years CMCC struggled with funding and was able to offer services only on Saturdays. Proceeds from the Women and Cancer Walk (discussed in the section "Conflict with the Culture of Screening Activism") helped CMCC survive. It provided free massage therapy, acupuncture, visualization, hypnotherapy, and homeopathy. All services were donated by local practitioners. In 1995 CMCC became a state-licensed holistic health clinic and an official 501(c)3 nonprofit agency. At around the same time, CMCC began publishing a modest newsletter that featured the stories, poetry, interviews, and articles of clients and volunteers. CMCC also began distributing bags of freshly baked bread, organic produce, and other groceries—all donated from local suppliers.

## Breast Cancer Fund

A fourth feminist cancer organization, the Breast Cancer Fund, was founded by Andrea Martin in 1992. Martin was diagnosed with breast cancer in 1989, at the age of forty-two, four months after receiving a mammogram that showed no signs of disease. A businesswoman and restaurateur at the time of her diagnosis, Martin underwent a mastectomy and spent a year in chemotherapy. Two years after her original diagnosis she was diagnosed with a new primary cancer in her remaining breast. As Martin put it, "The first time I was diagnosed with breast cancer, I was scared. The second time I was angry."[27] Like the founders of BCA, Martin attended a support group at the Cancer Support Community. In 1991, drawing on her business savvy and passionate desire to do something, Martin held a major fund-raiser to support the Cancer Support Community, which was in dire straits financially. In 1992 she expanded this fund-raising project into a new organization, the Breast Cancer Fund. The mission of the Breast Cancer Fund, as its name suggests, was to raise money to support breast cancer–related projects. "But with a dynamo like Andrea," as Susan Claymon put it, "they were also interested in advocacy."[28]

In its first year of grant-making the BCF awarded $37,015 to the Cancer Support Community to provide direct services to people with cancer and $6,500 to BCA to support its newsletter. In 1993, its second year, the BCF made awards to the Cancer Support Community, six women's cancer organizations in California, two researchers, and two cancer treatment centers in the San Francisco Bay Area. The BCF also supported the continuation of Greenpeace's work on breast cancer and the environment, which led to the publication of the Greenpeace report *Chlorine, Human Health, and the Environment: The Breast Cancer Warning.*[29]

### CONFLICT WITH THE CULTURE OF SCREENING ACTIVISM

There were aspects of the culture of feminist cancer activism that brought it into direct conflict with the culture of screening activism. Feminist breast/cancer activism aggressively challenged what Nancy Evans, an influential

Bay Area activist, termed the "cheery deary" stories promoted by pink-ribbon activists. Feminist cancer activists, for example, supported universal access to mammographic screening for all women, but their relentless critique of the effectiveness and dependability of this technology threatened the efforts of screening activists to portray mammographic screening as a life-saving technology. Feminist breast/cancer activists attempted to replace screening activists' "cheery deary" stories with narratives that drew attention to the false promises and misrepresentations of the cancer establishment, to the ineffectiveness of mammographic screening, the unreliability and toxicity of treatments, the chronic nature of the disease for many women, the inadequacy of research, the lack of scientific understanding and medical progress on the disease, the emphasis on individual risk factors, and the low priority given to cancer prevention.

One example of the difference between these two COAs was the "Cancer Sucks" buttons and stickers that BCA began distributing in 1997. The button was designed by BCA board member Lucy Sherak, who was diagnosed with breast cancer at the age of forty-three and died two years later, leaving a husband and two young children. BCA explained, in response to a member who commented that she found the button "quite offensive," that they "wanted a symbol that would tell it like it is: Breast cancer isn't pretty." BCA used the "Cancer Sucks" button to counter the pleasant, reassuring message symbolized by the pink ribbon. Although they acknowledged that many people found the button offensive, BCA claimed that the message "resonate[d] with many people who have gone through treatment and live with the realities of the disease every day."[30] They were right. Time and time again I was approached by strangers who laughed or smiled in recognition when they saw my "Cancer Sucks" button and asked where they could get one.

A glance at BCA's award-winning Web site reveals an extraordinarily large number of articles and position papers that complicate the rosy picture of mammographic screening promoted by the culture of early detection. For feminist cancer organizations, publicizing the risks associated with mammographic screening and the contradictory evidence regarding its effectiveness was a matter of respect for the principles of informed consent and the right of every woman to "be aware" of the tremendous uncertainty and lack of consensus regarding the costs, benefits, and effectiveness of mammographic screening. This was a very different discourse of breast cancer awareness than that promoted by the culture of early detection.

The culture of patient empowerment and feminist breast/cancer activism thus took shape, in part, through conflict with the culture of screening activism. The Komen Foundation and its signature event, Race for the Cure, served as a central foil and target of the feminist COA. In fact, Race for the Cure offered numerous opportunities for feminist cancer activists to promote their alternative, oppositional message. At the 1993 Race for the Cure, for example, Polly Strand, a volunteer at WCRC, distributed a flyer criticizing the Komen Foundation for its narrow focus on early detection and its track record of refusing to fund local women's cancer organizations. The following year, just a few days before Race for the Cure, Nancy Evans, the president of BCA, wrote a formal letter to the president of the San Francisco chapter of the Komen Foundation. The letter was cosigned by seven feminist health and breast/cancer organizations in the Bay Area.[31] Quoted at length below, the letter vividly illustrates the tense relationship between these two COAs and the efforts of feminist activists to gain access to a greater share of the resources and revenue controlled by the Komen Foundation:

> The powerful effect of women with breast cancer networking with each other cannot be overestimated. Volunteers in breast cancer support and advocacy groups labor long and hard and deserve support for their efforts from money raised in their communities. This proposal asks you to change the priorities for Race funding to include the non-profit groups that have done so much to create the Breast Cancer Movement. Of course, there is much more to be done.
>
> Access to mammography services for underserved and low-income women is a valuable service and Race funds have made a difference in this area. Race funding can help advocacy organizations to work as partners with the research community, government agencies such as the NCI and legislators, to increase research funding and reassess research priorities. Our real goal must be the prevention of breast cancer BEFORE it starts. Toward this end, it is essential that breast cancer groups form alliances with other organizations working to remove dangerous toxins from our environment.
>
> We are deeply concerned that many issues of critical importance to the health of all women are not being presented to the public, and that breast cancer myths and misinformation are being promoted.

The letter went on to say,

we propose that you allocate half of the funds raised to support non-profit women's cancer organizations in the Bay Area. We propose that a review panel that includes at least five activists from breast cancer advocacy groups solicit proposals from area organizations. . . . It would be very appropriate for the Komen Foundation to begin this change in allocation of Race for the Cure proceeds in the Bay Area since we have the highest rate of breast cancer in the world. However, we propose that this sharing extend to every city in which a Race for the Cure is held.

Although the Komen Foundation did not implement the ideas put forward by the leaders of the local women's cancer movement, the San Francisco chapter of the Komen Foundation did begin funding more local projects that provided direct services to women with cancer. In 1995, for example, the Komen Foundation made a grant of $30,000 to the Cancer Support Community for its Ethnic Minority Outreach Program. Komen donated an additional $20,000 to this program in 1996.[32] In 1998 and 1999 the Komen Foundation awarded grants to WCRC to fund its information and referral program. And in 1999 the San Francisco chapter of the Komen Foundation awarded the first of several grants to CMCC.

Feminist Collaborations: The Women and Cancer Project

The culture of feminist cancer activism also took shape through collaborative projects. During the first half of the 1990s a fifth organization, the Women and Cancer Project, created one of the most important opportunities for collaboration. The project lasted less than six years and never grew into an organization with paid staff and permanent office space. Nevertheless, it served an important function in this COA because it provided both a forum in which feminist cancer organizations could work together and opportunities to develop ties to other community organizations serving medically marginalized communities.

The Women and Cancer Project was created in the summer of 1991, when Joanne Connelly, Nancy Levin, and Abby Zimberg—white lesbians in their thirties who had recently immigrated to the Bay Area—organized the group's first meeting. The inspiration for this meeting came from several places: the organizers' histories of involvement in the feminist lesbian community, Zimberg's personal experience of cancer, and the inspiring model of AIDS activism in the Bay Area lesbian and gay community. In

333333333

3333333

fact, it was Connelly's and Levin's participation in an AIDS bike-a-thon that led them to question the absence of a parallel mobilization around women's health issues. They saw that breast cancer was becoming a bigger issue in the media, but at the same time, nothing seemed to be happening in the lesbian and gay community—no fund-raising, no activism, no attention.[33]

The first meeting of the project included representatives from an array of women's health organizations: BCA, WCRC, the National Latina Health Organization, the Bay Area Black Women's Health Project, and the Vietnamese Community Health Promotion Project. Representatives from all the agencies attended the meeting; some of them were meeting each other for the first time.[34] From the beginning, as this assortment of organizations indicates, a multicultural vision guided the development of the Women and Cancer Project. Equally significant was the fact that although breast cancer was the starting point, breast cancer was linked, both discursively and organizationally, to concerns about women's health, broadly conceived.

The first public event that the Women and Cancer Project participated in was a fund-raiser called the Human Race. The Human Race, which was held in Oakland, California, in 1992, was organized cooperatively by local nonprofit organizations. Beginning in 1993, the Women and Cancer Project began organizing its own fund-raising event, which it named the Women and Cancer Walk. The walk was held from 1993 until 1996.

Proceeds from the walk were divided evenly among the participating organizations. In 1993 the proceeds of the Women and Cancer Walk funded eight grassroots health organizations serving women in the San Francisco Bay Area: Breast Cancer Action, Charlotte Maxwell Complementary Clinic, Native American Health Centers, National Black Leadership Initiatives against Cancer, National Latina Health Organizations, Older Women's League, Vietnamese Community Health Promotion Project, and the Women's Cancer Resource Center. By 1995 five additional organizations had joined the Walk: Bay Area Black Women's Health Project, Cancer Support Community, Lyon Martin Women's Health Services, Mission Neighborhood Health Center, and Mujeres Unidas y Activas.

Proceeds from the walk ranged from a high of $7,000 per organization in 1995 to a low of $2,500 per organization in 1996, the last year the walk was held.[35] For some beneficiaries, money from the Women and Cancer Walk constituted a significant portion of their operating budget. CMCC, for example, depended on the walk for basic operating expenses during its

first few years. For other organizations, money received from the walk constituted only a small portion of their budget. The Gray Panthers, for example, donated their portion of the walk's proceeds in 1995 to two local
filmmakers, Irving Saraf and Allie Light, who were raising money to film
*Rachel's Daughters,* a documentary about the linkages between breast cancer
and the environment (which I discuss in greater detail at the end of this
chapter).

In theory, the steering committee of the walk was made up of one representative from each beneficiary organization. In practice, the steering
committee consisted of whoever showed up to the meetings and was willing to work on the event. Most of the volunteer labor and leadership were
performed by a handful of white women connected to local cancer organizations rather than by volunteers or paid staff of the health centers and
organizations with broader mandates, serving racially and ethnically marginalized communities. By the time I became a volunteer with the walk in
the spring of 1995, the project was hovering on the edge of collapse, suffering from the kinds of problems that are endemic to small, underfunded,
grassroots organizations: no paid staff, no permanent office space, rotating
fiscal sponsors, low levels of institutionalization, and burnout among the
handful of volunteers, who organized the walk while working full-time jobs
elsewhere. There was a great deal of discussion at the organizing meetings
about tapping into the resources of the gay men's community in San Francisco, but it never happened. Unlike Race for the Cure, which was organized
by professional event planners hired and paid for by the Komen Foundation, the Women and Cancer Walk never developed a workable template.
Thus, every year the wheel, to a great extent, had to be reinvented.

The stated purpose of the Women and Cancer Walk was to raise money
for Bay Area community-based health organizations and raise awareness
about women's cancer issues. The awareness that the walk sought to raise,
however, and the projects it funded were quite different from the awareness that Race for the Cure sought to raise and the projects it funded, as
the following ethnographic analysis makes clear. Unlike the Komen Foundation, for example, which cultivated corporate relationships—the bigger
the better and the more the merrier—the Women and Cancer Project was
conflicted about corporate donations. It actively solicited sponsorship and
donations in kind (food, beverages, T-shirts, and so on) from local shops
and business owners, but it struggled to define where to draw the line. The

poster from the 1995 Women and Cancer Walk, for example, included a small Chevron logo indicating that Chevron was a "major sponsor." "Major sponsor" in the case of the Women and Cancer Project, however, meant hundreds of dollars, not hundreds of thousands. Even so, Chevron's sponsorship was controversial among participants in the Women and Cancer Walk, and it was discontinued the following year.

### The 1996 Women and Cancer Walk

On a crisp fall morning in San Francisco in 1996 a crowd of between six hundred and eight hundred gradually assembled in front of a temporary stage in Golden Gate Park. This was the fifth annual Women and Cancer Walk. The walk took place in the same meadow as Race for the Cure, and like the race, it sought to create a festive atmosphere. But the same meadow that held nine thousand participants and scores of booths and displays for the race seemed almost empty with fewer than eight hundred participants, a modest stage, a few folding tables, and colorful splashes of artwork here and there. Neither pink ribbons nor balloons were in abundance. There was no sign of pink visors.

Like the race, the walk symbolically constructed and celebrated a community of people concerned about cancer. But the community constructed by the walk was quite different from that of the race. The beauty, fashion, and fitness industries were absent. So too, for the most part, was the health care industry. Instead, the community was made up of the thirteen beneficiary organizations and dozens of volunteers, performers, speakers, and walkers. The beneficiaries included three feminist cancer organizations and six women's health advocacy organizations—two Latina, two African American, one Vietnamese, and one older women's. The beneficiaries also included three community health clinics—one lesbian, one Native American, and one serving a cross section of poor people in San Francisco's Mission neighborhood. The walk sought to construct a multicultural and multiracial community, but the links within this community were visibly weak. Several of the beneficiary organizations were present in name only, with no one there to represent the organization or distribute literature.

As in Race for the Cure, the majority of participants were white women. Many of the women at the walk, however, hailed from a different social location. Certainly there were women here who would have blended in easily at the race, but they were neither the most visible nor the majority. At the walk there was a broad range of nonnormative "corporeal styles" on display that, taken together, created a different kind of body politic.[36] Fit, athletic-looking women in exercise attire were present, but they were not the norm. Soft bodies in comfortable shoes were in greater abundance than hard bodies in running shoes. There was a strong lesbian, feminist, and countercultural presence that was signaled by styles of dress, hair, and adornment, and by the decentering of normative heterofemininity and the visibility of lesbian relationships and queer sexualities. There were women with body piercings and tattoos. There were women with dreadlocks, short hair, and no hair at all. There were women with visible physical disabilities, large women, women for whom walking a mile would be difficult, and women for whom running a race would have been out of the question. The walk, unlike the race, was not certified as an official 5K event by the USA Track and Field Association.

Hair provided an interesting twist on standards of deviance and normality. Whereas at the race corporations marketed feminine wigs, scarves, and

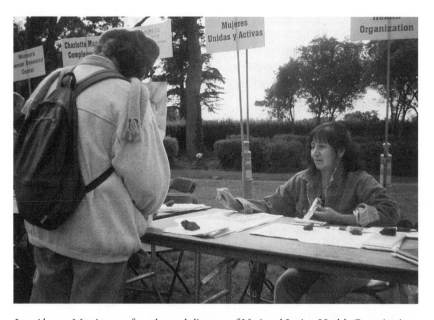

Luz Alvarez Martinez, cofounder and director of National Latina Health Organization, "tabling" at the 1996 Women and Cancer Walk. She is surrounded by empty seats where the other organizations should be. Photograph by Maren Klawiter.

hats to women who wanted to disguise the effects of chemotherapy, at the walk women who had lost their hair from chemotherapy blended in with women who had buzzed their hair and shaved their heads deliberately. The line between women living with cancer and ostensibly cancer-free women was more difficult to discern. At the walk, bald women and women with very short hair moved from the margins to the center, and women with corporate styles and carefully coifed hair looked a bit out of place and weird.

At the same time, many women at the walk had breast cancer histories that distinguished them from cancer-free women in ways visible to the discerning eye. Whereas at Race for the Cure the identities of breast cancer survivors were stitched on the bills of their pink visors, the breast cancer histories of some women at the walk were inscribed upon their bodies in ways that were more subtle than pink visors yet more disquieting for some observers. These women did not wear breast prostheses, and they had not undergone reconstructive surgery. Beneath the shirts of these women it was possible to discern the outline of one breast, but not two. Theirs was a doubly loaded act of defiance. Not only did they challenge the code of invisibility—as did the pink-visor-wearing survivors at Race for the Cure—but the way they did so challenged the tight linkages between the discourse of survival, the display of unmarred bodies, and practices of heteronormative femininity. This form of body politics was carried still further by Raven-Light, who wore a skintight black-and-white dress, black hose, and high heels. Hardly the picture of normative femininity, however, she wore one half of her dress pulled downward and secured in back, revealing the smooth, pale surface of the space where her breast had been.

As I accompanied RavenLight on the one-mile walk through the park, a woman in her late fifties approached us from behind. She pulled up beside us, glanced sideways at RavenLight, and exclaimed, "Oh good! That's what I thought! Well then—I'm going to take my shirt off too!" That said, she proceeded to remove the two shirts she was wearing, which covered a sleeveless, skintight, gray unitard that showed off the asymmetry of her chest and made it clear that she, too, had had a mastectomy. Here, in the context of the walk and in the company of a fellow traveler, this woman was moved to publicly reveal her breast cancer history, to display an otherwise hidden form of embodiment and celebrate an alternative corporeal style, an alternative femininity. She later explained that she lived in the Castro neighborhood of San Francisco and saw gay men with AIDS all the time.

She found them inspiring, and she wanted to be able to walk down the street like they did, without shame. She wanted to be able to walk down the street without wearing extra layers or a breast prosthesis. For this woman, RavenLight made that journey possible, at least within the space and time of the walk.

For the preceding couple of years, "Walkers of Courage" had been named and honored at the Women and Cancer Walk. Women at the walk were singled out for their service and activism, but not for their survival. Sometimes the honorees were women who had faced breast cancer years earlier, but just as often they were women living with metastatic disease—a problematic subject position and identity within the celebratory discourse of the more mainstream culture of early detection and screening activism. In 1995, for example, Gracia Buffleben, an activist with BCA who was living with metastatic disease, was honored as a Walker of Courage. Following in the footsteps of Elenore Pred (one of the founders of BCA), Buffleben and other breast cancer activists worked with ACT UP to organize a protest against the powerful Bay Area biotech company Genentech. In December 1995 they organized an act of civil disobedience against Genentech in order to win "compassionate use" access to Herceptin, a promising new drug available exclusively to women who qualified for the clinical trial.[37] When Buffleben ascended the Women and Cancer Walk stage to accept her award, ACT UP activists, dressed in black, stood behind her holding signs depicting rows of gravestones in a cemetery. The signs read, "DON'T GO QUIETLY TO THE GRAVE! SCREAM FOR COMPASSIONATE USE!" In form and structure, this ceremony was no different from Race for the Cure's onstage recognition of breast cancer survivors. The contrast in images and meanings, however, was telling: pink versus black; survival versus death; gratitude versus anger.

As in previous years, the 1996 walk's program was deliberately multicultural and multiracial—much more so, in fact, than the audience. The prewalk warm-up was led by an Afro-Brazilian dancer and masseuse. The disk jockey was well known within the lesbian club scene. Sign-language interpretation was provided onstage. Live music was performed by a biracial couple—an African American woman and a white man—who were local jazz musicians. The invited speakers were similarly diverse.

The first speaker, one of the main organizers of the walk, began by noting that women's health concerns had been "systematically ignored and

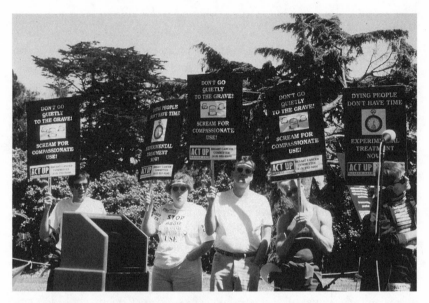

ACT UP and breast cancer activists at the 1995 Women and Cancer Walk. Photograph by Abby Zimberg. Courtesy of the Women and Cancer Walk.

underfunded" and that "health care and social services [were] least accessible to the women who need[ed] them most." At the same time, the speaker noted, cancer rates had risen to epidemic proportions and "one in three women [would] be diagnosed with cancer in her lifetime." This discourse, which was reproduced on the pledge sheets and event programs, broadened the focus of the movement to include all cancer that affected women. Likewise, it bridged from the popular issue of access to mammographic screening to the issue of access to basic health care and social services.

The next speaker was San Francisco's mayor, Willie Brown, who gave a brief speech. This was the first time that a politician of such stature had addressed the Women and Cancer Walk, and it was not entirely clear how the audience would respond to his presence. The mayor affirmed his commitment to solving the problem of breast cancer, and he promoted the upcoming San Francisco Summit on Breast Cancer. Then, however, misjudging at least part of his audience, he reminded the audience that men get cancer too, segued into a sound bite on prostate cancer, and promoted a new prostate cancer initiative that he intended to pursue. Some women in the audience applauded, but others hissed and shook their heads. The woman I was standing next to, for example, turned to me, rolled her eyes and asked, "Does he have any clue about the issues? Does he have any idea who he's talking to? Does he realize that this is the *Women* and Cancer Walk!?"

The next speaker was the director of the Native American Health Center in Oakland. She spoke about the devastation of the environment and its impact on the well-being of the earth and all of its inhabitants. Preaching to the choir, she averred that "this isn't just some little old thing that's attacking us. This is part of a bigger picture. What are we doing to this earth that we walk on?" She spoke about the large Native American community in Oakland and described their lack of access to basic health care services and cancer support programs. "I never wanted to get into this work," she said. "This is painful. But we need to be here for each other. . . . This is a political issue. The highest form of our activity is political . . . and it is spiritual."

The leader of the Native American Health Center then described the ways her health center had used the money donated by the Women and Cancer Walk. Women and Cancer Walk funds paid for cab fare to the hospital for a woman receiving chemotherapy who was too sick to take the bus across town. It paid for phone service for a woman dying of cancer so that she could talk to her family, who lived far away, during her final weeks. It bought Christmas toys for the children of a third woman with cancer. It paid for therapy for a fourth woman, who was dying, and helped pay her burial expenses.

These were stories of physical desperation, emotional devastation, economic hardship, and profound loss. Although the subjects of these stories did not speak for themselves, they were spoken of, and discursively constituted, as women with complicated commitments and biographies. These were women with their own needs, histories, priorities, and desires. They were individuals, but individuals embedded within particular cultures and communities. These women were not passive, but certainly they were victims—victims of multiple institutionalized inequalities. Cancer was just one of many obstacles that they were up against. Perhaps some would become long-term survivors, but this was not where the logic of the narrative led. This was a narrative of suffering, poverty, and dislocation, not a discourse of individual choice and responsibility, not a story of triumph and survival.

The 1996 walk was by far the largest, in terms of participation. There were more individual walkers and more walking teams, and, for the first time, the mayor's office was involved in the event, and the mayor's Commission on the Status of Women helped promote the event among city employees. But the amount of money that was actually distributed to the beneficiary organizations plummeted from a high of $7,000 in 1995 to a low of $2,500 in 1996. In part this was because participants raised less money through pledges, though more people actually participated. In part it was because more money was spent staging the event.

The 1996 walk marked a transitional moment. In order to continue, the walk needed more direction, a permanent home, an event template, a stronger public identity, and paid staff. But it failed to develop any of these structures and disappeared. There were a number of reasons for this. First, for many of the beneficiary organizations, cancer was only one of a broad range of community health concerns, and it was not the most pressing. For these groups, the commitment of limited time and resources to the Women and Cancer Walk was understandably not a high priority. Second, the Women and Cancer Project enforced a strict policy on corporate donations. This policy was a principled stance designed to maintain the organization's independence from corporate interests, but it nonetheless limited the walk's fund-raising potential and access to resources. Third, like many grassroots organizations, the Women and Cancer Project was ambivalent about the process of professionalization. This ambivalence was reflected in the lack of consensus about the direction it should take in the future. One group of volunteers saw promising opportunities in developing closer ties to the mayor's office and public agencies such as the Commission on the Status of Women. This, they believed, could give the walk greater exposure and generate the media attention it needed. Another group wanted the walk to focus on more extensive outreach and alliance building in the environmental justice community. Fourth, there were certain difficulties structured into the "universe of political discourse" that the Women and Cancer Project was unable to navigate.[38] Corporate cause-related marketing and organizations like the Komen Foundation and the American Cancer Society had successfully framed breast cancer as a problem best addressed by medical research and mammographic screening. The Women and Cancer Project was committed to broadening the terms of the debate beyond breast cancer, beyond screening, and beyond research. Such a goal was all well and good, but it was difficult to come up with a compelling frame that tied these larger issues together. Fifth, by 1996 two of the key contributors to the Women and Cancer Walk—BCA and WCRC—had developed their own fund-raising events and strategies. And last, by 1996 the Women and Cancer Project no longer functioned as the only collaborative space within the women's cancer movement.

The Women and Cancer Walk never became a huge event, but during the first half of the 1990s, the Women and Cancer Project was one of the only structures—albeit a temporary and fragile one—that created opportunities for small local organizations to build relationships and work together on issues connected to women and cancer. For this reason, it was more important than either its size or its success at fund-raising suggest. The Women and Cancer Project created a public, participatory event where feminist cancer activists could develop a distinct COA. The Women and Cancer Walk helped build solidarity and a sense of community within the Bay Area culture of patient empowerment and feminist activism. As the next section makes clear, however, the walk's demise signaled not the decline of this COA but, rather, its growing dynamism and strength.

GROWTH OF FEMINIST BREAST/CANCER ACTIVISM, 1996–1998

The growth of WCRC during the second half of the 1990s illustrates the heightened pace of growth and activity within the culture of feminist cancer activism. In 1994 WCRC sponsored support groups for lesbians with cancer and African American women with cancer. It also sponsored a grief group, a post-treatment support group, a group for women choosing alternative treatments, a drop-in group for women with cancer, and a multiple myeloma support group. Within the next few years, additional groups were added to the lineup. WCRC created a support group for lesbian partners of women with cancer; a group for parenting with cancer; a friends and family group; a group about living, dying, and spirituality; and a stress reduction/relaxation group. In 1997 Grupo de Apoyo para Latinas con Cancer was added—a group for Spanish-speaking Latinas. This group, which began as a cancer-education program, met at a Latino church in Richmond and grew to include more than twenty participants.

WCRC also ran an all-volunteer in-home practical support program called the Betts Program and, in 1997, received a grant of $40,000 from the San Francisco Foundation to expand this program. A free therapy program was added to WCRC's lineup of services so that low-income women with cancer would have access to one-on-one counseling with licensed therapists, who were also volunteers and donated their services. WCRC expanded its library by adding video and print materials in Spanish and some Asian languages. The library also added medical databases covering mainstream, alternative, and complementary therapies. WCRC expanded its information and referral hotline to include Spanish speakers, and a TTY line was added to provide greater access for the deaf community. During the mid-1990s the circulation of WCRC's quarterly newsletter—a hodgepodge of announcements, political analyses, updates on programmatic developments, and stories by and about the lives of local women with cancer—grew to nine thousand. WCRC also created a small, informal art gallery in its offices that served as another forum where women with cancer could express themselves, produce new discourses of disease, and share these with the women who visited WCRC's library or attended its support groups.

WCRC also deepened its involvement in environmental activism. In 1998 it organized a series of events called Cancer and the Environment. These events featured writers, community activists, scientists, and practitioners of alternative medicine. Seminars focused on a wide variety of environmental health issues and were held in different locations around the community. WCRC joined a number of environmental coalitions and campaigns and helped found the Toxic Links Coalition (TLC). The TLC, which figures prominently in chapter seven, was an alliance of feminist cancer organizations, women's health organizations, environmental justice organizations, and community groups in the Bay Area that focused on direct action and education about the links between environmental toxins and public health.

BCA also entered a period of tremendous growth and change during the second half of the decade. BCA had always functioned well in its role as critic and gadfly of the pharmaceutical industry and the cancer establishment. During the first half of the 1990s, however, it managed to do so in large part through the Herculean efforts of a small handful of very active board members. In 1995 Barbara Brenner was hired as BCA's executive director. Brenner, who joined the board of directors of BCA in 1994, had been diagnosed with breast cancer in 1993, at the age of forty-one, and again in 1996. Like many other one-breasted women in the feminist COA, Brenner did not wear a breast prosthesis following her mastectomy in 1996. She gravitated toward a confrontational style of political engagement and steered

BCA through an important transition. Under Brenner BCA achieved financial stability and became more powerful and professional without compromising its vision of "speaking truth to power."

Although lesbians were an important BCA constituency, lesbian identities were rarely foregrounded within the public culture of feminist cancer activism.[39] Brenner, who was a Jewish lesbian, strengthened BCA's ties to the lesbian community and made lesbian identities more visible within the Bay Area breast/cancer movement. In 1997, for example, when the San Francisco Lesbian-Gay-Bisexual-Transgender Pride Parade was dedicated to "Our Sisters with Cancer," Brenner gave the keynote address at the postparade rally. In this speech she foregrounded her lesbian identity and the important contributions of the lesbian community to the breast/cancer movement.

Between 1995 and the end of the decade, BCA's staff and budget tripled and its board of directors, which began as a small group of white, mostly middle-class women, expanded to include twelve board members, more than half of whom were women of color. During the second half of the 1990s, BCA attempted, largely successfully, to integrate a wider circle of activists and volunteers into its political activities, and it developed stronger ties to the Bay Area women's cancer community. One of the ways it did so was initiated in 1997, when BCA organized the first of what became an annual town meeting. At the end of the town meeting in 1997, BCA announced the formation of five new task forces—on media, legislation, treatment, community outreach, and street activism—and recruited women from the meeting to sign up for them. These task forces and town meetings created new recruitment opportunities and new opportunities for local supporters of BCA to get more deeply involved in the organization's activities. During this same period of time, BCA, like WCRC, became more deeply involved in the culture of cancer prevention and environmental activism. BCA participated in Californians for Pesticide Reform, was a founding member of both the TLC and Health Care without Harm, and provided crucial support for a number of local projects, including the film *Rachel's Daughters.*

One of BCA's core political commitments was to "follow the money" and see where it led. Over the years BCA's "Follow the Money" campaign translated into a remarkable level of transparency in its own operations and a commitment to ethical fund-raising. In 1998, for example, BCA returned a $1,000 donation from Genentech and adopted a rigorous policy that explicitly prohibited the organization from accepting financial support from corporate entities whose products, profits, or services were based on the diagnosis or treatment of women with breast cancer. BCA also refused to accept funding "from corporate entities whose products or manufacturing processes directly endanger environmental and/or occupational health."[40] The BCA thus expressly prohibited itself from accepting funding from pharmaceutical companies, chemical manufacturers, oil companies, tobacco companies, health insurance companies, and cancer treatment facilities. This policy became part of BCA's public identity. "We cannot be bought" BCA declared, and in making this declaration it implicitly called into question the practices and policies of other organizations that accepted funding from these industries.

In 1998 the Richard and Rhoda Goldman Fund and BCA initiated a new collaborative project, funded with a $221,000 planning grant, called the Practical Support Services Initiative for Women Living with Cancer. The reference point and inspiration for this initiative—as in so many other things—was the AIDS community in San Francisco and its elaborate network of community-based programs and practical support services for people with AIDS. The initiative was originally envisioned as practical support services for women with breast cancer, but the women involved in the planning grant expanded it to include women with any type of cancer. The practical support services they envisioned included money for food, housing, utilities, and transportation and for interpreters in hospitals, in-home support, day-time shelter for homeless women, and holistic services.

The planning grant did not, at that time, lead to the creation of a new program of practical support services for women with cancer. A few years later, however, the Breast Cancer Fund, in partnership with Shanti, an organization best known for providing practical support services for people living with HIV/AIDS, created Lifelines, a new program to provide practical support services to medically marginalized women living with *breast* cancer in San Francisco. This example shows that the tension between privileging the position of women with breast cancer and extending the political focus to include women living with cancer of any kind was a persistent feature of the culture of feminist breast/cancer activism and patient empowerment. It also shows, however, that the commitment to provide services to women living with cancer, or breast cancer, was a persistent part of the vision of this feminist COA.

During the second half of the 1990s the BCF became an increasingly powerful force in the Bay Area field of contention. It became an organizer of major fund-raising events that served the dual purpose of raising the political profile of breast cancer and building a local base of loyal supporters. Second, like other feminist cancer organizations in the Bay Area field of contention, the BCF increasingly defined its priorities in terms of environmental research, regulation, education, and activism. Third, not only did it fund the proposals of other organizations, but it also worked with a wide variety of politicians, philanthropists, scientists, and nonprofit organizations to develop new services, programs, and policies to support women with breast cancer. Finally, although the BCF provided grant money for projects across the country, it was particularly generous to the Bay Area, funding everything from art exhibits to support services to epidemiological research.

In the spring of 1996 the BCF teamed up with the San Francisco Bay Area chapter of the ACS and the San Francisco chapter of the Susan G. Komen Foundation to organize Art.Rage.Us, a juried show of drawings, paintings, sculpture, poetry, essays, and journal entries by women with breast cancer. The show opened two years later at the San Francisco main library with a packed calendar of exhibitions and performances. Art.Rage.Us included visual and verbal images designed to move, inspire, engage, and enrage the viewing audience. The exhibit and performances included stories of healing, recovery, laughter, and redemption, but also of loss, fear, anguish, anger, and amputation. A high-quality book of images from Art.Rage.Us was produced in conjunction with the show, along with posters, postcards, bookmarks, and other publicity paraphernalia.[41]

Although Art.Rage.Us was merely one project among many that grew out of this COA, a closer examination of this project provides insight into the culture of feminist breast/cancer activism. As noted, the project was sponsored by the BCF, the Komen Foundation, and the ACS—an unusual collaboration between two different COAs. The organizer and curator of the project, Susan Claymon, was a well-loved and respected matriarch within the Bay Area breast cancer movement—she cofounded BCA; she helped write the California Breast Cancer Act of 1993; she chaired the Advisory Council of the California Breast Cancer Research Program; she served as a peer reviewer for the Department of Defense's breast cancer research program; she played a role in virtually every major project that was conceived by feminist cancer activists in the Bay Area. The point is that Claymon was in a position to pick and choose her projects, and at this point in her life, she made very deliberate choices about where she invested her time and energy. She worked on projects that she believed would make the biggest difference for women living with cancer. Yet Claymon dedicated two of the final years of her life to producing Art.Rage.Us, and she did so while suffering from bone metastases, enduring multiple rounds of chemotherapy, and undergoing an operation to have pins inserted in her body to hold her bones together. Why did Claymon care so much about this art exhibit?

Claymon believed that carrying the artistically raw and uncensored voices and images of women with breast cancer to a mainstream audience could transform women's experiences of the disease by transforming the way it was popularly understood and publicly represented by mainstream cancer and breast cancer organizations. She believed that challenging the hegemony of pretty pink stories of survival and redemption was one of the most important tasks of feminist breast cancer activism. She viewed Art.Rage.Us as "a unique, landmark thing" because, as she said, "we're broadening their horizons and pushing Komen to do some things that they've never done before." And she believed that the willingness of the ACS and the Komen Foundation to think beyond mammography indicated a growing willingness on their part—or at least on the part of the Bay Area chapters of these organizations—to deal with "the difficult feelings and emotional content of this disease."[42]

These "difficult feelings" and the "emotional content" of breast cancer were vividly depicted in the visual artwork, poetry, and performances of Art.Rage.Us, which included images of one-breasted and bald women, images of surgical procedures, scenes of radiation and chemotherapy, scenes of psychic and physical suffering, and scenes of loss and grief and dying. The public acknowledgment and portrayal of these "difficult feelings" was, for Claymon and many other activists, a politically important statement. Thus, their success in "getting" the American Cancer Society and the Komen Foundation to join them in this public acknowledgment and artistic portrayal was, for Claymon, an important political accomplishment.[43]

In the next section I describe the making of *Rachel's Daughters,* a film that the feminist breast/cancer community threw its support behind. The film, which examines the relationship between breast cancer and the environment, provides another illustration of the important role that artwork—

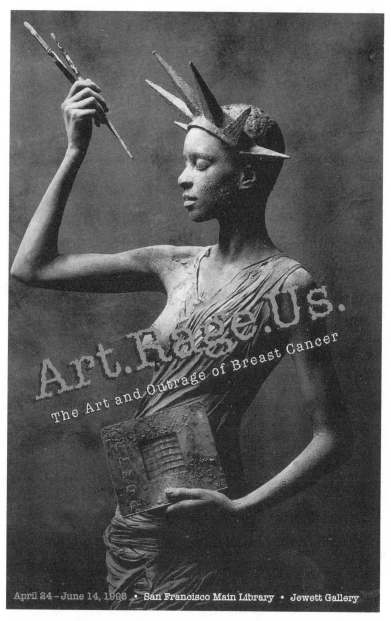

Cover image for Andy Coghlan, *Art.Rage.Us.: Art and Writing by Women with Breast Cancer* (San Francisco: Chronicle Books, 1998). Sperling Sampson West (concept)/Sander Nicholson (photograph).

or what can more broadly be termed the production of culture—played in this feminist COA. My analysis of *Rachel's Daughters* also serves as a segue to chapter 7, which examines the culture of cancer prevention and environmental activism.

### *Rachel's Daughters:* SEARCHING FOR THE CAUSES OF BREAST CANCER

*Rachel's Daughters* was the brainchild of filmmakers Allie Light and Irving Saraf, a wife–husband team from the Bay Area who were inspired to make the film by their thirty-nine-year-old daughter's diagnosis of breast cancer.[44] Filmed between 1995 and 1997, it premiered at San Francisco's Castro Theatre in September 1997 and was subsequently broadcast on HBO. *Rachel's Daughters* is a film about the "known and suspected" environmental causes of breast cancer. However, it was not just a tribute to the vision and persistence of the filmmakers, but a film whose history was deeply intertwined with the cultures of feminist and environmental cancer activism in the San Francisco Bay Area. Tracing the film's pre- and postproduction history provides a window onto the inner workings of one segment of the women's cancer community.

The film was named after Rachel Carson, the environmental scientist and author of *Silent Spring* (1962), the book that launched the American environmental movement. Carson was diagnosed with breast cancer while she was writing *Silent Spring,* but the doctor who removed the tumor from her breast lied to Carson about its malignancy, telling her instead that the tumor was benign. Carson was diagnosed with metastatic breast cancer nine months later. Writing during an earlier regime of breast cancer, Carson concealed her disease from the public, fearing that she would be accused of bias and that her work would be discredited if her cancer diagnosis were made known. She died of breast cancer in 1964.[45] *Rachel's Daughters* thus sought to honor Rachel Carson's contributions to the environmental movement and extend her legacy into the domain of breast cancer, which Carson had been politically unable to acknowledge and address.

Light and Saraf spent several years trying to raise the approximately $250,000 they estimated they would need to make *Rachel's Daughters.* In the mid-1990s they began making contacts and attending events in the Bay Area women's cancer community. By the summer of 1995, for example, bright pink buttons emblazoned with "I Support Rachel's Daughters" began to appear at breast cancer events—purchased from Light and Saraf Productions for a small donation. During the next couple of years, house parties to raise money for *Rachel's Daughters* were hosted by numerous individuals who wanted to support the film. A significant portion of the funding for the film came from individuals within the women's cancer community and from local foundations committed to funding women's cancer projects. The BCF contributed $20,000, the Richard and Rhoda Goldman Fund (a San Francisco foundation) contributed $50,000, and the San Francisco chapter of OWL contributed $5,000 (their portion of the proceeds from the Women and Cancer Walk). The resource guide produced in conjunction with the film was funded by the Jennifer Altman Foundation, a local foundation with a track record of contributing to feminist and environmental cancer activism.[46]

Light and Saraf teamed up with Nancy Evans, then the president of BCA, to select a team of investigators for the film. Most of the women chosen were active within the Bay Area women's cancer community. Jenny Mendoza, for example, was a thirty-one-year-old volunteer with WCRC who was recruited for the film while staffing a WCRC information table at the 1995 Women and Cancer Walk. Others were similarly recruited through word of mouth and at public events. Since Light and Saraf were strangers to the world of breast cancer until their daughter's diagnosis, the film's point of view, as well as their choice of interview subjects, were developed in collaboration with local activists.

*Rachel's Daughters* was organized around the narratives of eight women "living with breast cancer" (not "breast cancer survivors") who played the role of investigators in the film. The main goal of the film was "to shift the focus of public attention from the detection and treatment of breast cancer to environmental toxins and suspected causes of the disease and the possible ways to prevent it or at least reduce the risk."[47] This involved a shift away from "single-cause" theories and individual risk factors to a paradigm of multicausality, synergistic effects, and the "vulnerabilities" created by complex and often low-level exposures to a variety of carcinogens.

Perhaps the most dramatic example of the participation of the women's cancer community in *Rachel's Daughters* was the production of the film's final scene. The social networks of the feminist cancer movement were mobilized in order to recruit women to participate as extras. Approximately 130 women were needed for the final scene, though many more volunteered.

In order to film the final scene, known as the "women in black" scene, all 130 women were loaded onto chartered buses and driven to a grassy, hilly terrain near Half Moon Bay (about an hour outside the city). There, the women, dressed all in black, spent the day waiting, chatting, soaking up the sun, eating the picnic lunches they had brought along, and waiting for the cameras to roll. When the lighting was right, we donned our black veils (donated by a local fabric store) and, with the cameras rolling, slowly descended from the top of the hill. Within a few minutes the entire hillside was dotted with women in black. It was a tremendously moving scene to participate in, and an eerily beautiful scene to capture on film.

In the final scene of *Rachel's Daughters* the main characters of the film, the women with breast cancer who served as the environmental detectives, were seated in the foreground in a semicircle at the bottom of the hill. Susan Claymon, who by then had been living with metastatic disease for almost a decade, spoke the film's final words. Quoting Gracia Buffleben, who had died during the previous year, Claymon solemnly intoned, "I am

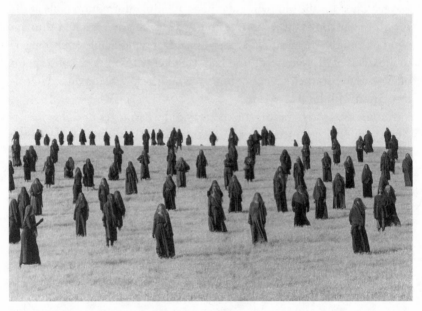

Publicity photograph for *Rachel's Daughters: Searching for the Causes of Breast Cancer* (1997), a film by Allie Light, Irving Saraf, and Nancy Evans. Photograph by Rosalind Delligatti.

still alive, but behind me are four women who have died, and behind each of those women are four women."[48] As she uttered these final words, the camera panned upward, where wave after wave of women in black descended the hill behind her.

Almost four months before the public premiere of the film at the Castro Theatre in San Francisco, the work in progress was screened before an audience drawn from the women's cancer community. A questionnaire was distributed to audience members. Our comments and feedback were then taken into consideration by the filmmakers during the final editing process. The film premiere in September 1997 was hosted and sponsored by the BCF in alliance with ten local cancer organizations, eight of which were active in the culture of environmental cancer activism in the Bay Area. During the months following its San Francisco premiere, the film was shown at various venues and forums around the Bay Area—usually by local women's cancer organizations, often as a fund-raiser for the organization. Copies of the film, taped when it aired on HBO, circulated freely in the Bay Area women's cancer community.

## CONCLUSION

What most distinguished the culture of patient empowerment and feminist cancer activism in the San Francisco Bay Area from the culture of early detection and screening activism was its critique of early detection campaigns, its rejection of the "cheery deary" stories that dominated the media, its adoption of a watchdog role vis-à-vis the medical research establishment, and its emphasis on patient empowerment and direct services for women with cancer. In addition, although breast cancer was certainly the central concern of feminist cancer organizations, only two of these organizations were organized exclusively around breast cancer, and even these organizations often expanded their focus, depending on the context, to include other women with cancer.

What distinguished the culture of feminist cancer activism from the environmental COA, the focus of chapter 7, was its commitment to patient empowerment and the primacy of gender in its analytic framework. Because of its foundation in patient communities, feminist cancer activism was committed to providing direct services and medical information for women with breast cancer, and it was committed to pushing science to develop effective, innovative, nontoxic forms of screening, detection, and treatment.

In these respects, then, feminist cancer activism diverged from the environmental COA by maintaining a broader focus and agenda. At the same time, however, as chapter 7 demonstrates, feminist breast/cancer activism contributed to the creation of a distinct culture of cancer prevention and environmental activism.

# Cancer Prevention and Environmental Risk

To get rid of slavery, abolitionists not only changed their consumer and lifestyle habits—by choosing not to buy slaves themselves—but they also organized underground railroads, demanded legislative change, and, finally, took up arms. In short, they got political and insisted on changing the system. . . . The abolitionists did not settle for reforming slavery, regulating slavery emission rates, conducting cost-benefit risk analyses on slave holding, or attaining state-of-the-art slavery. . . . If we can get rid of slavery—which was at least a two centuries–old institution at the time of the Civil War—we can get radiation and chemical carcinogens out of our air, food, and water.

—SANDRA STEINGRABER[1]

What would happen if an army of one-breasted women descended upon Congress and demanded that the use of carcinogenic, fat-stored hormones in beef-feed be outlawed?

—AUDRE LORDE, *The Cancer Journals*

Chapter 6 examined the culture of feminist cancer activism in the San Francisco Bay Area. It traced that culture's development from a handful of separate organizations with few interactions to a relatively cohesive and co-herent culture of action and highlighted its relationship to, and differences from, the culture of screening activism. It also revealed that from their earliest days feminist breast/cancer organizations framed cancer as an environmental issue. This chapter continues that thread, tracing the growing ties between feminist breast/cancer and environmental organizations during the mid-1990s and analyzing the internally fragmented but dynamic COA that emerged.

The culture of environmental activism used the widespread appeal and familiarity of the dominant discourse of early detection to fashion an oppositional message of cancer prevention. It mobilized the dominant discourse of risk but reshaped it in ways that pointed in new directions. It used the popularity of National Breast Cancer Awareness Month to promote its oppositional educational campaign, National Cancer Industry Awareness Month. Like the two cultures of action already discussed, this COA chose multiple targets for its actions: private industry, local and state government, other cultures of action, and public attitudes and perceptions. Confrontational politics and public protests were part of the political strategy and tactical repertoire that the environmental movement brought to breast cancer activism. This chapter thus explores the synthesis between the breast cancer and environmental movements in the San Francisco Bay Area, emphasizing its relationship to and differences from the cultures of screening and feminist activism.

This chapter also, however, explores diversity within this COA. There were few serious disagreements on policy goals or analyses of environmental causes and culprits, but there were significant stylistic and strategic differences within this COA. These differences and the tensions they provoked illustrate the importance of shared strategies and styles in creating coherence within COAs. Thus, although I trace the dominant strand of this COA through an examination of one organization, the Toxic Links Coalition, (TLC) in the chapter's final section I also explore some of these internal differences and their significance.

## The Toxic Links Coalition: It's Time for Prevention

Late in the summer of 1994, a handful of Bay Area activists convened an informal meeting to network, learn about each other's work, identify areas of overlap, and explore the possibility of working together on issues of mutual interest. These activists came from four organizations: Breast Cancer Action, Greenpeace, West County Toxics Coalition, and the Women's Cancer Resource Center. At their second meeting, they decided to formalize the collaboration and christened themselves the Toxic Links Coalition.[2] The formation of the TLC thus represented a local synthesis of the feminist cancer and environmental health movement. During the next few months, the coalition grew to include a handful of unaffiliated individuals and more than twenty organizations, most of which were drawn from the environmental health movement.

At the suggestion of Henry Clark, director of West County Toxics Coalition—an environmental justice group with a predominantly African American membership whose primary focus was organizing against the toxic output of the Chevron refinery in Richmond—the TLC decided to focus its energies on challenging the pristine image and hegemonic discourse produced and circulated by National Breast Cancer Awareness Month. Invented in 1985 by the London-based Imperial Chemical Industries and taken over in 1993 by its subsidiary, Zeneca Pharmaceuticals, NBCAM was created "to promote the importance of the three-step approach to early detection: mammography, clinical breast examination and breast self-examination."[3]

By the mid-1990s NBCAM had been officially endorsed by more than seventeen governmental, professional, and medical organizations, including the American Cancer Society, the National Cancer Institute, the American College of Radiology, and the Susan G. Komen Breast Cancer Foundation. Working in concert with these agencies, industries, professional groups, and foundations, NBCAM designed and produced the promotional materials used in breast cancer early detection campaigns and disseminated them via a wide variety of means—public service advertising, speaker's programs, and brochures, flyers, and posters placed in churches, beauty parlors, retail stores, physicians' offices, pharmacies, fitness centers, and so forth.[4] NBCAM, in other words, was an extremely popular and successful public health campaign.

NBCAM was viewed by TLC activists, however, as a public relations campaign that practiced deliberate obfuscation in three ways: First, NBCAM legitimized early detection programs as the only conceivable public health approach to breast cancer. Second, it concealed from the public the fact that multinational corporations and their allies were causing cancer through the production of toxic products such as pesticides and plastics (and their industrial by-products, such as dioxin). Third, it concealed from the public the fact that some of the same corporations that contributed to the rising rates of cancer also profited from its diagnosis and treatment. In other words, as TLC activists liked to say, "They getcha coming and going." From their perspective, NBCAM was a wolf in sheep's clothing.

The basis of these claims was simple. Zeneca Pharmaceuticals not only bankrolled and controlled the publicity for NBCAM's breast cancer early detection campaigns, but it also, through its parent company ICI, was one of the world's largest manufacturers of the pesticides that, according to TLC activists, contributed to causing breast cancer. Adding more fuel to the fire, Zeneca was also the manufacturer of tamoxifen, under the brand name Nolvadex. Tamoxifen was the best-selling drug in the world for the treatment of breast cancer. And just to complicate the story still further, it was later categorized as a known human carcinogen by the World Health Organization, among others. NBCAM thus represented a textbook case of vertical integration.[5] Of course, neither the word "carcinogen" nor the word "cause" had ever appeared in NBCAM publicity.[6] The TLC thus declared that October was National Cancer Industry Awareness Month and initiated its own public education campaign.[7]

The TLC's first public action took place at the 1994 San Francisco Race for the Cure, where they set up an "educational picket." The TLC targeted the race because the Komen Foundation was a leading sponsor and promoter of NBCAM and because the Komen Foundation, like NBCAM, studiously avoided any mention of causality, carcinogens, or the environment in its publicity. The TLC's goal in targeting the race, however, was not just to attack the Komen Foundation but also to use the Komen Foundation's success at mobilizing support—evident in the thousands of people who participated in Race for the Cure events across the country—to get a captive audience for its alternative, oppositional message. The educational picket, described below, illustrates the stark contrast between these two COAs.

*TLC's Educational Picket at the 1994 Race for the Cure.*

Long before the race got under way, activists from the TLC lined the walkway between the starting line and Sharon Meadow, the open space where Race for the Cure participants gathered to warm up, cool down, socialize, listen to music, and browse the booths. The atmosphere in Sharon Meadow was very upbeat, positively buzzing with energy. The atmosphere changed dramatically, however, as the race participants (myself included) encountered the TLC activists on their way to the starting line. The activists wore sandwich boards, each with a photograph of Matuschka, her torso cast in plaster, with an alarm clock embedded in the space where her second, now missing, breast had been. "It's TIME for prevention" was the not-so-subtle message.[8]

The demonstrators chanted in unison, "Cancer is murder. Stop cancer where it starts." Whereas the mood had been upbeat and happy in Sharon Meadow—with people enjoying a beautiful Sunday morning in the park and participating in a "feel good" cause—all conversation died out as we passed through this double-sided picket line. It did not feel like an educational picket. It felt like walking the gauntlet. It felt as if we, the runners, were the enemy, the target. Once we were safely past the demonstration, runners around me made comments reflecting this sentiment: "*Scary* looking bunch of women!" (from a man). "Well *that* was a real downer" (from a woman). "Nice range of voices" (said sarcastically, in reference to the chant's remarkably dirgelike, monotonic sound). In short, the TLC's message came across as accusatory and aggressive, and there was no sign of enlightenment on the part of race participants. The educational picket was followed a couple of weeks later by the first Toxic Tour of the Cancer Industry, the highlight of the newly declared National Cancer Industry Awareness Month. The Toxic Tour quickly became the signature event of the TLC and has been performed on an annual basis ever since, and the race continued to serve as an attractive site for disseminating the TLC's political message about breast cancer and the environment.

In the following ethnographic description of the 1996 Toxic Tour, I highlight the distinctiveness of this particular COA and conclude with a brief comparison of the Toxic Tour and the events highlighted in the preceding chapters: Race for the Cure and the Women and Cancer Walk.

### The 1996 Toxic Tour of the Cancer Industry

At noon on a Wednesday in downtown San Francisco a crowd gathered on Market Street in front of Chevron's corporate headquarters. Metal barriers and uniformed police lined the sidewalk for about a hundred feet, separating the pedestrian and street traffic from the protesters assembled inside the barriers. A large banner identified the organizers of the event: "Toxic Links Coalition—United for Health and Environmental Justice." Another large banner read, "Stop Cancer Where It Starts!" The demonstrators walked in an oval, carrying signs aloft and loudly chanting, "Stop cancer where it starts! Stop corporate pollution!" "Toxins outside! Cancer inside! Industry profits! People suffer!" "People before profits!"

The 1996 Cancer Industry Tour was the third of these annual events, and it drew approximately 150–200 participants. As in previous years, the Toxic

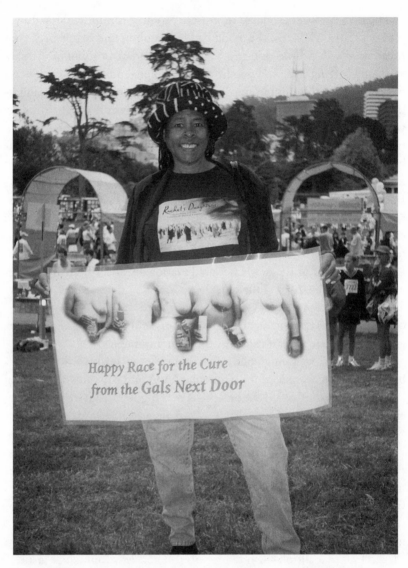

San Francisco environmental breast cancer activist Essie Mormen demonstrating at the 1996 San Francisco Race for the Cure. Her poster contains images of African American women holding plastic containers of toxic chemicals (for clearing clogged drains and for killing insects and weeds). Their naked torsos display various scars and deformities from breast cancer surgery. Beneath the images, the text reads, "Happy Race for the Cure from the Gals Next Door." Photograph by Maren Klawiter.

Tour was designed as a two-hour tour de force that snaked through down-town San Francisco, stopping at specific targets along the way. The 1996 targets were Chevron, Pacific Gas and Electric, Senator Dianne Feinstein, Burson Marsteller (a public relations firm), Bechtel (a builder of nuclear power plants), and the ACS. The Toxic Tour was similar to the Women and Cancer Walk in that many of the speakers identified themselves as members of particular organizations and communities, but the Toxic Tour shifted the focus of political discourse *away* from organizational and com-munity identities in order to discursively construct and physically identify the local outposts of the global cancer industry.

The theme of the tour was "Make the Link!" and the tour was choreo-graphed so that each stop along the way represented a link in the chain of the cancer industry. TLC publicity materials asserted that "the cancer industry consists of the polluting industries, public relations firms, [and] government agencies that fail to protect our health, and everyone that makes cancer possible by blaming the victims and not addressing the real sources." This was a smear campaign, a strategy of public shaming, an attack on corpo-rate images. At each stop the name of a cancer culprit was bellowed over a bullhorn, followed by a description of the practices it pursued that were destructive to human health and the environment. Literally and figuratively, the cancer industry was mapped through the delivery of speeches, the dis-play of props and signs, and the movement of protesters and police from site to site. The speakers called for a politics of cancer prevention and an end to environmental racism.

There were clear lines separating "them" from "us," and those lines were reinforced by the uniformed police escort and barricade. This was street theater. It was ritualized confrontation and condemnation that mobilized the expression of oppositional identities. As in Race for the Cure and the Women and Cancer Walk, about three-quarters of the participants were white and three-quarters were women, but many—about one-half—of the scheduled speakers were people of color, both women and men. They spoke not as individuals, however, but as members and representatives of envi-ronmental justice organizations, feminist cancer organizations, and indi-viduals living with cancer. All of the speakers expressed anger, outrage, and a sense of injustice, and these emotions were mirrored and affirmed by the Toxic Tour participants. Although some speakers identified themselves as women living with cancer and as breast cancer survivors, many did not.

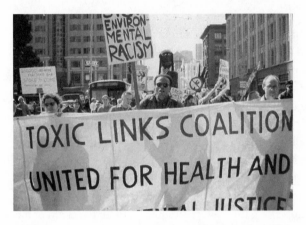

Toxic Links Coalition activists marching in the 1996 Toxic Tour of the Cancer Industry. Photograph by Maren Klawiter.

Cancer was not the only salient identity. As at the race and the walk, men were in the minority at the tour. But unlike at the race and the walk, men spoke from positions of entitlement to justice equal to those of the women speakers. There were no men, however, who identified themselves as cancer survivors or as men living with cancer. If they were present, they did not speak from that subject position.

This demonstration was not primarily an expression of solidarity with or sympathy for people with cancer. It was a collective expression of rage at the cancer industry's destruction of the health of all people, particularly those living in communities victimized by environmental racism. As at Race for the Cure and the Women and Cancer Walk, breast cancer occupied a privileged position in speakers' narratives and in the visual signs and signifiers. But just as the Women and Cancer Walk decentered breast cancer by connecting it to other forms of cancer that affected women, the Toxic Tour decentered breast cancer by linking it to cancers that affected men, women, and children and, further still, to a host of environment-related health conditions such as reproductive, respiratory, and autoimmune diseases. In this context, everyone was part of the inner circle of the aggrieved. But it was not grief that was mobilized, it was rage.

The neon orange flyers distributed along the way announced that one-third of U.S. women and one-half of U.S. men would be diagnosed with cancer during their lifetimes. It stated that the lifetime risk for breast cancer in the Bay Area was one in eight and rising, that the Bay Area had the highest rate of breast cancer in the world, and that African American women living in Bayview–Hunters Point—a low-income and predominantly African American community—had a breast cancer rate double that of the rest of San Francisco. The flyer also stated that "we are all exposed in increasing doses to industrial chemicals and radioactive waste *known* to cause cancer, reproductive, and developmental disorders" and, furthermore, that "big profits are made from the continued production of cancer-causing chemicals."

In the 1995 tour the sixty or so protesters had carried handmade signs painted with slogans, miniature coffins, and gravestones emblazoned with a handwritten name, a lifespan, and the letters "R.I.P." In 1996 there were more than twice as many participants, but the coffins and gravestones were

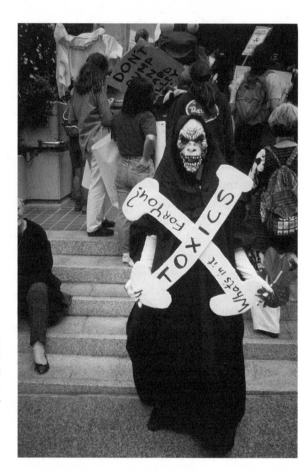

Toxic Links Coalition activist at the 1996 Toxic Tour of the Cancer Industry. Photograph by Maren Klawiter.

nowhere to be seen. Instead, two show-stealing props appeared. The first prop was a gigantic puppet with moving arms, deftly operated by a team of three. The twenty-foot puppet was a papier-mâché woman with blue skin and a mastectomy scar dripping blood where one of her breasts should have been. In each of her gigantic movable hands she held a container of toxic substances, painted with a skull and crossbones. The second prop was a tall, narrow wooden float on wheels, one side of which was painted to resemble a headless man in a business suit. The other side of the float was painted as a skyscraper with an assortment of corporate insignias: Chevron, Pacific Gas and Electric, Dow Chemical, Dow Corning, Monsanto, UNOCAL, and US Ecology. This float was named the Tower of Evil.

Images of death, deformity, and destruction abounded at the Toxic Tour. One woman held high an exhibit of photographs of women's nude torsos. The photographs included many startling images of disfigured women with double mastectomies. Some of these photographs featured the concave chests characteristic of the Halsted radical mastectomy—images from an earlier regime of breast cancer whose effects were still inscribed on the bodies of thousands of women. Other women, members of an organization representing women suffering from implant-related health problems, distributed vivid color photographs of ruptured implants and mutilated chests that were identified as the result of negligence on the part of Dow Corning, the manufacturer of silicone implants. These were exactly the sorts of images that Race for the Cure and the culture of screening activism sought to banish from the public culture of breast cancer. The Toxic Tour, on the other hand, adopted the opposite approach, resurrecting these banished images and pasting them onto sandwich boards worn by angry women marching through the streets of downtown San Francisco in a gruesome example of the return of the repressed.

There were no freebies distributed at this event—none of the beauty products, pink ribbons, or breast health brochures that abounded at Race for the Cure. There were no corporate sponsors. Although Chevron and the ACS were present at both Race for the Cure and the Toxic Tour, they were participants and sponsors of the race whereas they were targets of the tour. At the ACS stop along the tour, for example, Judy Brady—an environmental breast cancer activist and self-described "cancer victim"—delivered a series of withering accusations against the ACS that she substantiated by distributing copies of a recent internal ACS memo marked "Confidential."

The memo, which appeared to have originated in the national office of the organization, instructed local offices to ignore and suppress a brochure on cancer and pesticides that had been created and distributed by a small office in the Great Lakes region. Brady charged the ACS with miseducating the public, ignoring cancer prevention, refusing to take a stand against industrial and agricultural pollution, and colluding with the corporation's stakeholders to hide evidence of carcinogens resulting from the company's products and processes.

Brady's assertion that she was a "cancer victim" was loaded with significance. The identity of breast cancer survivor that was celebrated by the culture of screening activism was constructed in direct opposition to the stigmatizing label "cancer victim." The word "victim" in this instance brought to mind a certain passivity in the face of a cancer diagnosis that would be followed by a slow, painful death. The culture of screening activism worked diligently to dispel these fatalistic assumptions about the meaning of a cancer diagnosis by replacing them with images of women who were surviving and thriving after having been diagnosed and treated for breast cancer.

"Cancer victim" was a label from an earlier era, resurrected and recoded to signify a different kind of victimization. In earlier times, people were *called* cancer victims, but not usually to their faces; and people with cancer did not publicly identify themselves in this way. Brady, on the other hand, publicly identified herself as a cancer victim in order to draw attention to the existence of injustice. Brady claimed the identity of cancer victim not because she was passive and fatalistic but because she was positioning herself, and all people with cancer, as victims of the brutal and unjust cancer industry. Interestingly enough, as I discuss later in this chapter, the media consistently ignored the political content of Brady's assertion of victimhood and referred to her, instead, as a "breast cancer survivor," reflecting the political and cultural gains that had already been made by the culture of early detection.

At the Toxic Tour there was no call for more research to uncover the mysteries of tumor biology or to discern the patterns of cancer epidemiology. There were no visions of more or better science or of more or better social and medical services. There was no call for women to be vigilant or to practice breast self-exam and get mammograms. Mammography *was* invoked, but as an example of false promises and corporate profiteering rather than as a life-saving technology. These activists did not promote the ideology of early detection. They did not promote the notion that disease growing within community bodies could be mapped onto the genetic structures and risk factors of individual lifestyles. Cancer, they stressed, was not a lifestyle choice. Instead of mapping the biomedical geography of individual women's bodies and behaviors, as in Race for the Cure, or mapping the social geography of communities and health services, as in the Women and Cancer Walk, the Toxic Tour mapped the political economy and geography of the cancer industry—the hidden maze of linkages and networks connecting the bodies of state agencies, politicians, charities, and profit-driven corporations to the unhealthy bodies of people involuntarily exposed to toxins and living in contaminated communities. The Toxic Tour mapped the sickness and disease of toxic bodies and the body politic onto the corporate corpus. Cancer prevention, they made clear, required a different kind of cartography.

Comparing the Toxic Tour to Race for the Cure and the Women and Cancer Walk illustrates key differences between the COAs embodied by each event. First, whereas Race for the Cure singled out breast cancer, the Women and Cancer Walk expanded their focus to include all cancers affecting women, and the Toxic Tour of the Cancer Industry expanded the category still further, to include cancer in general and other environment-related diseases. Second, whereas Race for the Cure drew upon biomedicine and represented breast cancer as a universal, ahistorical disease of biologically female bodies that could be controlled through scientific research, medical technology, and individual vigilance, the Women and Cancer Walk drew upon multicultural feminism and represented cancer as a body-altering, life-threatening source of suffering that was compounded by institutionalized inequalities in access to health care and social services. The Toxic Tour, on the other hand, drew upon the environmental justice movement and discourses of environmental racism to represent breast cancer as the product and source of profit of a predatory cancer industry.

In Race for the Cure, the most privileged and honored identity was that of the breast cancer survivor. The Women and Cancer Walk, on the other hand, created more space for the identities of women living with cancer and women dying from the disease. The Toxic Tour decentered women as a category, gender as a lens of analysis, and even, to some extent, the individual identities of participants altogether and instead shifted the focus to victimized communities, on the one hand, and the identities of specific organizations and industries, on the other. Finally, the Race for the Cure called for more biomedical research and early detection and supported the provision of mammograms to the medically underserved; the Women and Cancer Walk called for better health care and social services and supported the work of community clinics and women's health advocacy and activism; the Toxic Tour called for cancer prevention instead of early detection and for more corporate regulation instead of more research, and it supported the work of coalition members on behalf of environmental health and justice. One thing the race, walk, and tour shared, however, was a common language, or vocabulary, of risk. The next section examines the strategic mobilization of risky discourses by a conference on women's health organized by the culture of environmental activism.

### The Women, Health, and the Environment Conference and the Politicization of Risk

The synthesis between feminist cancer activism and environmental health activism was facilitated by the release of a 1994 report by the Northern California Cancer Center entitled "Breast Cancer in the Greater Bay Area: Highest Incidence Rates in the World." The report stated, "Given the available data, white women in the San Francisco/Oakland Area have the highest rate in the world. The rate is about 50% higher than in most European countries and 5 times higher than in Japan."[9] This article was published in the *Greater Bay Area Cancer Registry Report,* a professional publication mailed primarily to cancer researchers, clinicians, and other health care professionals.

The issue of high cancer rates was not a new one, but when the NCCC released its report in the fall of 1994, it was seized upon by breast cancer and environmental organizations in the Bay Area and used to great political effect. The Breast Cancer Fund, for example, called a press conference to publicize the report, and the media started referring to the Bay Area as the "breast cancer capital of the world." In the summer of 1995 the Women, Health and the Environment Conference further publicized and politicized this Bay Area discourse of risk.

The Women, Health, and the Environment Conference was a two-day affair co-organized by the TLC and the Women's Environment and Development Organization (WEDO). WEDO provided funding for the event, as part of its new Action for Cancer Prevention Campaign.[10]

Although the words "breast cancer" and "risk" were absent from the conference title, they were the conference's primary focus, signifying the growing political salience of breast cancer in the environmental health movement. The press release, for example, framed the conference like this: "Seventeen women's health and environmental justice organizations calling themselves the Toxic Links Coalition (TLC) have formed an unprecedented local campaign to demand answers to the question raised by the NCCC's report on breast cancer in the Bay Area: 'Why does the environmentally conscious Bay Area have some of the highest rates of cancer in the nation and perhaps the world?'" At the conference the NCCC's report was copied onto neon green paper and distributed to the media and all attendees. The subtitle of the report, "Highest Incidence Rates in the World," was circled in thick black marker and an arrow was drawn pointing to the top of the page, to a big fat "Why?"

The first day of the conference, which was held in San Francisco's City Hall, was staged as a public hearing. During the first day, nineteen activists representing nineteen organizations provided "expert testimony" to a group of seventeen panelists who were attending the conference as representatives of state agencies, public health departments, political offices, and research organizations. Bella Abzug, the executive director of WEDO, presided over the "public hearing."

The NCCC was accused of sitting on data that had been available since 1992. What was *not* a part of the attack on the center, however, but nonetheless made this sudden "discovery" even more fascinating, was the fact (evident in the report) that the Bay Area had been the site of the highest documented rates of breast cancer since 1947. Only when breast cancer became a politically charged issue, however, did these statistics migrate out of professional circles and galvanize action.

The level of animosity toward the scientific research establishment and the political tendentiousness of breast cancer incidence rates were never more apparent than during the question-and-answer period at the end of the first day's testimony, when a heated debate erupted over the NCCC's report. The executive director of the NCCC was one of the panelists, and he responded to questions about the high rates of breast cancer in the Bay Area in a way that appeared to the audience to minimize, medicalize, and depoliticize their significance. He stated that the higher rates of breast cancer were due to Bay Area women's greater utilization of mammography. The audience hissed and booed at this interpretation of the risk data. Abzug, for example, publicly chastised the NCCC representative, arguing that "we should be able to expect more from public agencies than cast-off remarks like that." Abzug then called for a thorough examination of the environmental implications of the Bay Area's high incidence rates.

The next day, the conference moved across the bay to Richmond, a predominantly African American community just north of Berkeley, located next to a major Chevron refinery. The eight workshops that day once again emphasized cancer and chemicals: (1) Chlorine, Zenoestrogens, and Breast Cancer; (2) Pesticides: The Circle of Poison; (3) Radiation and Cancer; (4) Toxins, Multiple Health Effects, and Toxic Free Life Style Changes; (5) Cancer in the Workplace—Petrochemicals, Solvents; (6) From Richmond to Bayview–Hunters Point: Chevron, Incineration, Toxins, and Power Plants; (7) The Politics of Breast Cancer; (8) Women's Bodies as a Cancer Battlefield. The community-action day concluded with a public demonstration staged at the nearby Chevron plant, where protesters gathered outside the gated facility and demanded that Chevron close an on-site hazardous-waste incinerator that was releasing dioxin and other hazardous compounds into the community.

Several environmental justice organizations that were based in communities of color were represented at the conference, and environmental racism was a strong theme in the presentations of the conference participants. Nonetheless, the vast majority of conference participants were white women and organizations with predominantly white middle-class constituencies. Even on the second day of the conference, when the location shifted to a community center in a predominantly African American community, the racial mix of the participants barely changed. The feminist cancer and environmental health networks did not extend very broadly or deeply into local communities of color.

The conference was nonetheless an important event in the development of this new COA. It brought together activists from all over the Bay Area and strengthened the linkages between feminist breast/cancer activism and environmental health activism. It strengthened the politically charged identity of the Bay Area as the "breast cancer capital of the world"—an identity that proved compelling to local politicians and the media and simultaneously served as an effective mobilizing discourse for the culture of environmental cancer activism.

In addition, the conference galvanized the foundation of one environmental cancer organization and gave a boost to another. The first, the Marin Breast Cancer Watch (MBCW), was founded in the fall of 1995 by Francine Levien and Wendy Tanowitz, who had attended the conference shortly after Levien was diagnosed with breast cancer.[11] It was at the conference that Levien and Tanowitz learned that not only did the Bay Area have the highest breast cancer incidence rates in the world, but Marin County had the highest incidence in the Bay Area. Levien had been active in the antiwar and civil rights movements during the 1960s and was now part of the diffuse alternative health movement in the Bay Area. Tanowitz was active in a variety of environmental and social justice issues. Both lived in Marin County. MBCW started out as a small group of women meeting in Levien's living room, almost like a book group—sharing materials, ideas, and information. Their goal, from the very beginning, was to discover and eliminate the reasons for Marin's high breast cancer rates. The reasons, they assumed, were environmental in origin.[12]

The second organization infused with new energy, support, and visibility by the conference was the Southeast Alliance for Environmental Justice, which was campaigning to prevent the siting of another power plant in its already heavily industrialized neighborhood.

## Politicizing the Discourse of Breast Cancer Risk in Bayview–Hunters Point

Several months before the Women, Health, and the Environment Conference, a small environmental justice organization called the Southeast Alliance for Environmental Justice (SAEJ) had formed in Bayview–Hunters Point (BVHP), a highly industrialized, low-income, primarily African American neighborhood in San Francisco. SAEJ was founded to mobilize community opposition against the proposed siting of a new power plant in the neighborhood, which already had two such plants. In response to community concerns regarding the potential impact of the plant's emissions on the health of residents of Bayview–Hunters Point, the San Francisco Department of Public Health (DPH) conducted a community environmental and health assessment. In conducting this assessment, they discovered that breast cancer rates for African American women under the age of fifty were 50 percent higher than what they expected. In fact, the breast cancer rate for this group of women was the highest in the city.

Although the San Francisco DPH did not release its report until after the Women, Health, and the Environment Conference, word of the report leaked out and the information contained within it was circulated at the conference. The high rate of breast cancer among African American women in Bayview–Hunters Point was widely publicized and debated at the conference. A petition requesting a moratorium on polluting facilities in Bayview–Hunters Point was drawn up, signed, and circulated at the conference and delivered to the San Francisco Board of Supervisors.

The discourse of disproportionate health risks and higher breast cancer incidence was extremely powerful. Although breast cancer was only one of many health problems in Bayview–Hunters Point and certainly one of the rarest, it carried a great deal of political weight. The release of this Bayview– Hunters Point health assessment report set a number of wheels in motion. It resulted, first, in the decision of the San Francisco Board of Supervisors to overrule the California Energy Commission by approving a moratorium on new polluting facilities in BVHP. It resulted, second, in the establishment of the Health and Environmental Task Force for Bayview–Hunter's Point, a collaborative project between BVHP residents and the San Francisco DPH. The task force, in turn, became a lightning rod for a series of controversies involving community representation, the conflict between "lay" and "expert" knowledges, the politics of epidemiological research and risk-assessment science, and the tension between *studying* the problems of pollution and ill health and *doing* something about them.

When, for example, additional studies conducted by the DPH failed to confirm BVHP residents' beliefs that they were being made sick by their toxic environment, they became increasingly angry and distrustful of the DPH's motives and the legitimacy of the science behind the studies. Frustrated by the disjuncture between the experientially based knowledge of local residents and the epidemiologically based knowledge generated by the DPH, community activists in Bayview–Hunters Point argued for solutions that did not depend upon unimpeachable scientific proof that the toxic environment was causing ill health. Community activists demanded instead that toxic sites be cleaned up, that toxic emissions from power plants be better regulated, and that community access to health care be expanded.[13]

Battles over the political meaning of breast cancer took place on multiple fronts, and organizations that were active in the culture of environmental cancer activism played a number of different roles in these struggles. The next section examines the strategic multipositioning in which environmental activists engaged in the planning and execution of the San Francisco Breast Cancer Summit.

*Strategic Multipositioning and Dueling Discourses at the San Francisco Breast Cancer Summit*

In November 1997, San Francisco's mayor Willie Brown fulfilled his campaign promise to host a summit on breast cancer in San Francisco. An article in the *San Francisco Chronicle* promoting the event said, "Alarmed by the city's abnormally high rate of breast cancer, San Francisco Mayor Willie Brown announced plans yesterday for a summit to focus on ways to curb the disease. . . . The goal of the summit is to develop strategies similar to those devised in the early 1980s to battle the AIDS epidemic, said city health director Sandra Hernandez."[14] Clearly, as this framing suggests, the San Francisco Summit on Breast Cancer was a response to what had by then become common knowledge regarding the city's "abnormally high" rate of breast cancer. It was a response, in other words, to the strategic politicization of risk by the culture of environmental cancer activism.

Like any event that brings together representatives from diverse communities, a great deal of the conflict within the summit's planning committees concerned the politics of framing. How would breast cancer be framed? Would it be discussed in terms of individual risk factors, biomedical treatments, and promising new research developments? Would it be framed as an environmental issue? Was it possible to bridge between these two conceptualizations? Because of the centrality of environmental issues to feminist cancer organizations in the Bay Area and the circulation of activists from the environmental justice movement in these networks, environmental issues won a prominent position in the summit's program.

Environmental activists from the TLC were also able to ensure that the panels of women living with breast cancer included women whose personal narratives—their "illness narratives," in the language of medical sociology—explicitly linked breast cancer to issues of environmental health and justice. One of the featured speakers in the Living with Cancer Plenary, for example—and note that it was *not* called the Breast Cancer Survivors Plenary—was Essie Mormen. Mormen was an environmental breast cancer activist, a retired nurse, and a member of the San Francisco African American community. Mormen gave moving testimony about the stigma of breast cancer, about her initial desire to tell only her closest friends, and about her subsequent decision to "come out of the closet" because "keeping quiet would mean betrayal." Mormen also, however, linked her personal narrative to an explicitly political narrative about the relationship between breast cancer and environmental carcinogens. She closed by discussing her involvement in the film *Rachel's Daughters.*

Organizations active in the TLC were nonetheless dissatisfied with the final form of the conference program. Their dissatisfaction stemmed from a series of last-minute changes that, they felt, weakened the environmental component of the summit. These changes included the prerelease and presentation of a new study conducted by the San Francisco DPH showing that, upon further analysis, breast cancer rates among women in Bayview–Hunters Point—the area formerly shown to have exceptionally high rates of breast cancer—had dropped from highest to fourth-highest in the city.

Following the study's prerelease at the summit, for example, the headline of the lead article in the *San Francisco Examiner* read, "Summit on Breast Cancer: No Greater Risk Here." Out of the twenty-eight speakers on the program—twenty-five of whom were women—the newspaper article quoted three male scientists, the only three men who spoke at the summit. The expertise and experience of the twenty-five women speakers—scientists, doctors, health practitioners, activists, and women living with breast cancer—were written out of the newspaper script entirely. Instead, the newspaper article reported that "alarm at local clusters of breast cancers" was unwarranted because breast cancer was "a false epidemic."

Although many of its member organizations were influencing the shape of the summit from the inside, the TLC decided, after learning of the study's prerelease and of the spin it was likely to receive, that they would stage a separate protest from the outside. Knowing that the television media would be covering the summit, they seized the opportunity to broadcast their message of environmental cancer prevention. The television coverage showed TLC activists outside the summit holding a "Stop Cancer Where It Starts! Clean Up the Environment!" banner and moved from there to a close-up of the giant hands of the papier-mâché woman with the blood-dripping mastectomy scar and toxic barrels painted on her palms. The television news story that was aired that evening, November 9, 1996, on the KTVU Channel 2 ten o'clock news demonstrated that the terms of discourse established by the culture of environmental cancer activism had migrated into the local media. It also illustrated the ongoing battle over the right to "frame" the meaning of the Bay Area's breast cancer incidence rates:

> ANCHOR: In San Francisco today, medical experts and breast cancer sur-
> vivors met to share new information on cancer research. The Bay Area is
> an appropriate place to hold such a meeting—Marin County and San
> Francisco have the highest rate of breast cancer in the world and nobody
> seems to know exactly why. John Sasaki reports.
> JOHN SASAKI: Inside San Francisco's Yerba Buena Center for the Arts, ex-
> perts, officials, and cancer survivors gathered for a breast cancer summit.
> Their goal was to bring to light the latest evidence on that devastating
> disease. Outside the summit gathered another group of people known as
> the Toxic Links Coalition who said the experts were missing the point.
> They argue the main focus should be on how the environment is play-
> ing a major role in causing breast cancer.

Next, Judy Brady, who was identified on-screen as a "breast cancer survivor," although she asked to be identified as a "breast cancer victim," added:
"This conference is denying that link. And in so doing, they are contributing to the cover-up of what is going on, and they are helping to guar-
antee that the body count of women will go up."

> JOHN SASAKI: Many of these people also attended the summit. And they
> argued that the Bay Area—San Francisco in particular—is littered with
> old toxic waste dumps. And they say many women have contracted breast
> cancer directly because of all that toxic material. Several speakers from
> the summit say the research just doesn't support that theory and pointed
> to other explanations such as genetics and nutrition for the Bay Area's
> high breast cancer rate.

Then the show quoted two scientists, invited speakers in the plenary sessions on Epidemiology and on Treatment Issues and Options; they were
identified on-screen as "breast cancer experts":

> CRAIG HENDERSON, "BREAST CANCER EXPERT": A lot of the evidence is
> lacking, even though studies have been done, the evidence linking the
> environment to breast cancer specifically . . . ah . . . it just isn't there.

DR. ROBERT HIATT, "BREAST CANCER EXPERT": Right now, we don't have any evidence that links toxins to breast cancer, and I think we have to work on more research in this area to support it . . . before we can expect action on a societal level.

The news story cut to Lorraine Pace, an environmental breast cancer activist from Long Island with strong ties to the Bay Area culture of environmental cancer activism:

LORRAINE PACE, "BREAST CANCER SURVIVOR": I did not have a mother with breast cancer, but now my daughter and my granddaughter have a mother and grandmother with breast cancer. How come so many women in San Francisco have breast cancer? [voice rising in volume] You can't tell me that so many women with a genetic predisposition to breast cancer all got together and moved to San Francisco or Long Island! No way!

JOHN SASAKI: One doctor who says the environment is a major cause of breast cancer offered to debate any of his colleagues who disagrees with that hypothesis.

DR. LEWELL BRENNERMAN, "BREAST CANCER EXPERT": I will show these people numerous studies that show that volatile organic chemicals can cause hormonal problems, can cause neurological problems, cancer problems, and a whole host of other problems.

JOHN SASAKI: Experts on both sides of the issue agree. The Bay Area has one of the highest rates of breast cancer in the world. In fact, this year alone, they say 4,500 women will be diagnosed with this disease and another 1,000 will die. Maybe the questions now are, Does the environment actually play a role in this disease and other diseases like it? And if so, what can be done about it? [end of broadcast].

Environmental breast cancer activists were thus able to position themselves within different terrains, simultaneously working from the inside out and from the outside in. In the newspaper coverage, the environmental framing of breast cancer was challenged and the voices of female speakers at the summit were dismissed. Nonetheless, it was the environmental discourse that set the terms of the debate. The television coverage of the summit, on the other hand, provided an entirely different spin on the event. In this case it was the recognized "breast cancer experts" who were put on the defensive and forced to respond to the claims of environmental activists. The mere fact that leading scientists were forced to address the challenges articulated by environmental activists positioned the environmentalists' claims as a legitimate challenge to the biomedical discourse of individualized risk.

## New Campaigns and Coalitions

In addition to these local struggles, statewide and national coalitions were created by environmental cancer activists and organizations in the Bay Area. California Zero Dioxin Exposure Alliance formed in 1997 to broaden the struggle for a dioxin-free environment. As a result of its efforts and the growing recognition of the dangers of dioxin, three city councils in the Bay Area approved resolutions to create dioxin-free environments: Berkeley, Oakland, and San Francisco. Californians for Pesticide Reform worked toward banning the use of the worst pesticides, reducing the use of the rest, and improving access to information on pesticides through public right-to-know legislation. Almost all the organizations involved in the cancer prevention movement also participated in these two coalitions.

Health Care without Harm was created in September 1996 when Commonweal brought together representatives from organizations around the country to develop a new project to promote environmentally responsible health care. Commonweal was a highly respected organization within the environmental health movement, and it was famous, as well, for the holistic healing and education programs it organized and hosted at its beautiful retreat center in Bolinas, California, for people with cancer. Commonweal had deep ties to the Bay Area culture of cancer prevention and environmental activism. It was, for example, a founding member of the Toxic Links Coalition. In turn, a number of feminist cancer organizations in the Bay Area were charter members of Health Care without Harm.

Health Care without Harm built upon the foundation laid by local coalitions and community-based environmental justice campaigns that sought to create dioxin-free environments, but Health Care without Harm was conceived on a national scale and sought to work with hospitals to eliminate the production of dioxins and mercury at the source. Health Care without Harm's campaign targeted the health care industry because that industry was one of the major sources of dioxin and other toxic by-products of medical care and medical waste management processes. The campaign's goals were to provide expert assistance to hospitals to help them redesign their waste-management systems so that they could minimize the production of PVC waste and, at the same time, help hospitals cut costs. The Bay Area was a center of activity around this campaign and was able to make quick inroads into the local health care system.

*Differences in Style and Strategy*

Unlike in the cultures of feminist and screening activism, however, there were significant differences within the culture of environmental cancer activism. These differences surfaced at the interface of breast cancer and environmental activism, but there were differences, as well, in the ways that breast cancer organizations positioned themselves within this COA. These were differences in style and strategy more than in policy goals and analyses. They included differences in the preferred style of interaction, willingness to work with private industry, and approaches to scientific research. An example of each is highlighted below.

First, as should by now be clear, confrontational politics and public protests were an important part of the political strategy and tactical repertoire employed by the culture of cancer prevention. Not all participants in the culture of cancer prevention, however, were equally comfortable with this approach. Andrea Martin, for example, the founder and executive director of the Breast Cancer Fund, viewed the contentious politics and street protests of the TLC as an "old-fashioned" and "1960s-style" approach whose time had come and gone.[15] Martin and the BCF preferred to negotiate and dialogue with powerful politicians and institutions, and as a successful businesswoman Martin had the skills, inclination, and connections to succeed at it. Breast Cancer Action and the Women's Cancer Resource Center, on the other hand, were founding members and active participants in the TLC. These organizations were much more comfortable with public demonstrations and confrontational politics.

Marin Breast Cancer Watch fell somewhere in between, or rather, on both sides of the issue. On the one hand, it was a product of the confrontational politics of the Women, Health, and the Environment Conference. On the other hand, many of the women who contributed the most to MBCW's development remained deeply ambivalent about this more contentious style of activism and did not participate in it. Women who became involved with MBCW through the environmental health movement tended to be more comfortable with confrontational politics. Women who found their way to MBCW through a diagnosis of breast cancer usually preferred the more collaborative style that, over time, became the dominant organizational culture of MBCW. Although MBCW was the progeny of the TLC, it developed an emotion culture at odds with the confrontational style of the environmental health movement.[16]

These differences in style and strategy were in part differences in the emotion cultures that prevailed in different organizations. There were also, however, differences in the boundaries that organizations established and maintained, and these boundaries mapped onto differences in their relationships to scientific research. Environmental health organizations in the Bay Area were relatively unified on these issues. Scientific discourses were strategically wielded by environmental organizations, but, generally speaking, demands for more scientific research were viewed as delaying tactics by industry, not solutions to the problem. Instead, the environmental health movement demanded the regulation, elimination, and remediation of industrially produced toxins and carcinogens.

Although breast cancer organizations supported demands for the elimination of industrially produced carcinogens, their relationship to the institution of science was more complicated, varied, and ambivalent. While they tended to be very critical of scientific research, Bay Area breast cancer organizations were not willing to abandon science altogether. MBCW, for example, during its first two years of existence maintained a steady focus on developing an environmental mapping project (modeled along the lines of mapping projects in Long Island) that, it believed, could help solve the puzzle of Marin's elevated rates by mapping the relationship between environmental risk factors and breast cancer incidence. MBCW eventually abandoned the mapping project, but it did not abandon its commitment to community-based research.

Other organizations, however, were much less enthusiastic about community-based collaborations with research scientists. In 1997, for example, the Breast Cancer Fund created a loosely organized group of what policy analysts would call stakeholders to begin discussing what could be done about the high breast cancer rates in the Bay Area. The idea behind the Bay Area Study Group, which brought together research scientists, clinicians, public health officials, breast cancer activists, and representatives of community organizations, was to use the Bay Area as a "laboratory" in which to study the causes of breast cancer, with a special interest in examining environmental risk factors. As part of its planning, the BCF solicited feedback from a wide variety of organizations and constituencies in the Bay Area. As part of this process, I agreed to solicit input from the TLC.

When I explained the BCF's plans at a TLC meeting, however, my enthusiastic solicitation of input was greeted with silence. Confused, I tried again to explain that this was an attractive proposal, that we could get in on the ground floor and help design a study that would address environmental issues and questions. "So do you have any ideas? Any requests? Any demands?" I asked again. But still, much to my surprise, no one was interested in brainstorming ideas for a new study or contributing in any way to its design. The goal, from their perspective, was not to figure out why breast cancer incidence rates were higher in the Bay Area than elsewhere, but to eliminate known carcinogens from the environment. The goal was not to reduce breast cancer in the Bay Area to "normal" levels but to reduce the incidence of cancer everywhere, for everyone.

More to the point, there was very little to be gained, they believed, and much to lose by putting their eggs in the basket of cancer epidemiology. Cancer epidemiology, they rightly argued, did not have the technical or analytical tools to identify, measure, or assess the multiple chemical exposures that people were subjected to on a daily basis, nor was it capable of measuring the synergistic effects of different chemical combinations or of uncovering multiple pathways and causal mechanisms. Given the limitations of cancer epidemiology, there seemed no benefit to participating in the design of a study that would further legitimize epidemiological knowledge as a basis for public policy or as an excuse for doing nothing. The more sound approach, they believed, was a political, not a scientific one: eliminate communities' exposures to known carcinogens and toxic substances, even in the absence of definitive proof that they were responsible for the rising rates of breast cancer. Within the next two years, this approach was revised, formalized, and institutionalized within the environmental health movement—locally, nationally, and globally—as the precautionary principle, to wit: "When an activity raises threats of harm to human health or the environment, precautionary measures should be taken even if some cause and effect relationships are not fully established scientifically. In this context the proponent of an activity, rather than the public, should bear the burden of proof."[17]

The TLC's cautionary approach to participating in cancer research, it turned out, was well founded. Later that year, results from a small, preliminary study funded by the BCF and conducted by Bay Area epidemiologists were widely interpreted as showing that known individual risk factors could account for the higher incidence of breast cancer among Bay Area women. Once again, the newspaper headline declared—although this was not the interpretation of the study's senior epidemiologist—that breast cancer in the Bay Area was not an environmental disease. The BCF was furious at the media's coverage, but what could they do? How could they object to a study they had funded? The study was published in the *Journal of the National Cancer Institute,* where the BCF's financial support was gratefully acknowledged.[18]

## CONCLUSION

Within the next few years the Breast Cancer Fund gradually moved out of the business of funding and commissioning scientific studies and threw its weight behind the precautionary principle, as did Breast Cancer Action, the Women's Cancer Resource Center, Marin Breast Cancer Watch, the Toxic Links Coalition, and dozens of environmental health and environmental justice organizations in the Bay Area and beyond. The synthesis between feminist breast/cancer activism and the environmental health movement, however, remained partial and incomplete. In the final analysis, it was more of an alliance than a shared COA. The partial synthesis of the environmental health movement and feminist breast/cancer activism, however, created a powerful synergy that led to the development of numerous innovative campaigns and coalitions. The tensions within this alliance/ COA were productive tensions.

In a very different way, and for very different reasons, the culture of cancer prevention and environmental activism also benefited from its direct and explicit conflicts with the culture of early detection. Without National Breast Cancer Awareness Month there would have been no National Cancer Industry Awareness Month. It was NBCAM that provided National Cancer Industry Awareness Month with an audience that was already primed to notice—even if it did not fully embrace—the alternative message that it promoted. It was the strength and predictability of the original script that generated the power of radical divergence. It was, in other words, the popularity of campaigns for early detection that provided campaigns for cancer prevention with their punchline and their logic—a logic with a real potential for a reversal of fortunes. Thus, in the final analysis, it was the complex and shifting relationships of conflict and cooperation *within* and *between* different COAs that best explained the dynamism of the Bay Area field of contention.

# PART III

# From Private Stigma to Public Actions

*c h a p t e r   8*

# The Impact of Disease Regimes and Social Movements on Illness Experience

And the visibility which makes us most vulnerable is that which also is the
source of our greatest strength.

—AUDRE LORDE, *The Cancer Journals*

This chapter uses the narrative of one woman, Clara Larson, to examine
the impact of disease regimes and social movements on illness experience,
paying particular attention to the ways gender and sexuality shape and are
shaped by disease regimes, social movements, and illness experiences.

Clara Larson was recuperating from a stem-cell transplant with high-dose
chemotherapy when I interviewed her in January 1998. A white, middle-
class, fifty-six-year-old lesbian, a former social worker, and the mother of
four adult children (one of whom introduced us), Clara had undergone
the risky experimental procedure, preceded by six months of conventional
chemotherapy and radiation therapy, in November 1997.[1] Although she
was feeling quite well by the time we met, Clara's immune system had not
yet fully recovered, and she was still at high risk of contracting opportunistic infections. Thus, although she remained relatively housebound, she
was looking forward to returning to work in the near future.

Clara was diagnosed with breast cancer first in 1979 and then again in
1997. While there is nothing about Clara that is ordinary or average, her
experiences nonetheless open a window onto a disease regime at two different moments in time. Her lesbian identity and feminist sensibilities
provide a particularly insightful view of the ways gender and sexuality were
embedded, embodied, exercised, and enacted within the first and second

regimes of breast cancer in the social milieu that she inhabited in the San Francisco Bay Area. In like fashion, although the Bay Area terrain of social movements is not "representative" of the rest of the country (nothing is), the depth and dynamism of the Bay Area field of contention reveals the remarkable extent to which disease regimes and illness experiences can, under certain conditions, be transformed by social movements.

Divided into two parts—the late 1970s and the late 1990s—Clara's narrative helps illuminate key changes over time in the regime of breast cancer, the field of social movements, and the range of experiences available to the involuntary subjects of each regime. Certainly, these changes were not experienced in the same way or to the same degree by every woman. Subject positions and social locations—age, race, class, gender, sexuality, family, culture, ethnicity, physical location, religion, and political convictions—also shaped women's relationships to the regime(s) of breast cancer. Nonetheless, Bay Area women diagnosed with breast cancer during the late 1990s encountered a different set of conditions—a different regime of practices—than had the generations that preceded them. This chapter explores those changes, refracted through the eyes of one extraordinary woman.

The first part of Clara's narrative illuminates some of the defining qualities of the first regime of breast cancer, even as it was beginning to change. These include the sovereign power of physicians (surgeons in particular); the isolation, normalization, and disempowerment of patients; the hegemony of gender-normative and heteronormative assumptions about female embodiment, attractiveness, and sexuality; the invisibility of women with breast cancer and mastectomees in the public domain (despite the public disclosures of a handful of celebrities); and the absence of a group identity. This earlier regime was indeed rather totalizing, but Clara's narrative reveals how her lesbian identity and feminist experiences and sensibilities provided her with the intellectual tools and the social and emotional resources to maintain a critical distance—a self-protective barrier of sorts—from the gendered technologies of control and normalization that she encountered. Although a partial outline of the second regime of practices can be discerned in Clara's narrative, her experience of breast cancer was shaped primarily by key practices of the first regime and the temporal, spatial, visual, and social dimensions of disease that resulted.

The second part of Clara's narrative illuminates some of the defining qualities of the second regime of breast cancer. These include the dethroning of surgeons, the limitations on physicians' authority, and the replacement of the surgeon–patient dyad with a web of relationships; the expansion of patients' access to medical information and their participation in decision making; the creation of new social spaces, services, and resources for women with breast cancer; the growing visibility of breast cancer patients and ex-patients in the public domain; the emergence of new collective identities; and the development of a multistranded and multidimensional breast cancer movement.

## CLARA LARSON IN 1979: DOMINATION, ISOLATION, AND THE LIMITS OF RESISTANCE

In the early 1970s, when she was in her early thirties, Clara Larson followed the advice of her obstetrician/gynecologist and scheduled her first mammogram. Mammograms had been used as a diagnostic tool since the 1950s, but it was not until the 1970s that the National Cancer Institute and the American Cancer Society began to heavily promote the use of mammography as a breast cancer screening technology. Clara was part of the first wave of healthy, asymptomatic women to undergo routine mammographic screening, and she did so before the age and safety guidelines for mammographic screening were first challenged and changed. According to Clara's recollection, "My doctor said 'this is something you need to do now, so go here and do this.' And so that's what I did."

In 1979, when Clara was thirty-seven, a routine mammogram revealed a suspicious lump in her breast. Six weeks later she went into the hospital to have the lump biopsied. She entered the hospital expecting to emerge a few hours later with a clean bill of health. But things did not go as planned:

> I had the biopsy and I was in the recovery room because I had general anesthesia, that's what they did then, and this giant person loomed over me in his green outfit and he said, "Well it's cancer! Do you want me to cut it off now or in a couple of days?"

Recalling this experience in vivid detail almost twenty years later, Clara said, "So I allowed as how I would like to wait a couple of days." Shaking her head and laughing in outrage and disbelief, she continued,

> But he was just gonna do it!! Right then and there!! And me explaining things to my kids, or making arrangements for them and my dog and cat—or

whatever! It was totally unimportant [to him]. He just wanted to wheel me back in and cut my breast off! What an idiot! [pause] He's actually still around. But I'll bet he can't get away with *that* anymore.

At the time of Clara's diagnosis, neither professional norms nor legal regulations required surgeons either to separate the diagnosis of breast cancer from its surgical treatment or to inform their patients of alternatives. It was later that same year that the National Institutes of Health held a second consensus development conference on breast cancer that resulted in, among other things, a nonbinding recommendation that surgeons discuss treatment alternatives with their patients and abandon the one-step procedure.[2] In 1980 California became the second state to pass breast cancer informed consent legislation. This legislation did not criminalize the one-step procedure, but it did characterize as "unprofessional conduct" the failure of a physician "to inform a patient being treated for any form of breast cancer of alternative, efficacious methods of treatment."[3] Thus, Clara was more fortunate than many others: Instead of awakening to the voice of her surgeon informing her that she had breast cancer and asking whether she wanted him to "cut it off" now or later, Clara could easily have awoken to the voice of her surgeon telling her that while she was unconscious, he had diagnosed and treated her for breast cancer by removing her breast, her chest muscles, and her lymph nodes. As callous as Clara's surgeon surely proved himself to be, he was actually on the progressive end of the spectrum on this issue.

Clara went home to make hasty arrangements for the care of her four children; she then returned to the hospital for surgery and underwent a mastectomy. After spending three or four days recovering in the hospital, she returned home in time to take her final exams and finish up her first semester of graduate school. As she recalled,

There was no process. No sensitivity to any feelings I might have about this. Or anything! It was very mechanical. . . . The medical establishment was horrible. Horrible. Horrible. Horrible. . . . It was just kind of like you were having your tonsils out. . . . I just don't remember any supportive medical personnel at all.

In addition to surgery Clara had one appointment with a medical oncologist, who determined that adjuvant therapy was unnecessary. At her follow-up appointment with her surgeon, on the other hand, Clara was advised to undergo an additional, elective procedure:

This was a time when I was visiting him myself [without her lover/partner Regina]. And he said, "You know, you really need to have reconstructive surgery." And I said, "Why?" And he said, "I have seen many a marriage founder on the shoals of a mastectomy." And I thought, "Okay. I'm gay. Now how do I explain this to a guy in a way that doesn't make it sound like my body's not important in this relationship?" . . . and I got so confused trying to figure out how I should respond to him . . . that I lost the opportunity. And I never did explain that to him.

Asked what it was that she had wanted to communicate to her surgeon almost twenty years earlier, Clara responded,

I wanted him to know that I was gay, and that he shouldn't talk to me about heterosexual marriage. But I couldn't figure out how to do it without making it sound . . . I couldn't figure out how to give him the right message. I don't think he could have heard it anyway. . . . If I were to explain it to him today I would say, "This is my body and I see no reason to try to protect people from the fact that I have cancer. Had cancer. Whatever. That is their problem if they can't deal with it." But at the time it did not occur to me [how] to explain that to him.

Reflecting later, she said,

I can imagine if I had been straight that that really would have affected me. But I just thought it was weird! And I didn't know how to verbally respond to make myself understood by this goon. So I think it would have affected me. It would have hurt my feelings. It would have worried me. It would have scared me. If I had not been a lesbian . . . I probably would have killed myself or started drinking.

She added,

My body was my body. And certainly I went through all the consciousness-raising groups in the seventies and . . . certainly, the women's movement and all that stuff that we were going through in the seventies gave me words and concepts to be able to understand how I felt about this stuff. . . . And certainly if I hadn't been through all that stuff, I don't know that I would have been a lesbian. I'd probably still be married to Sally's [her daughter's] father. And I would have taken the stuff that that doctor said to me very seriously. And I would have been worried about it, because it certainly echoed the messages about femininity and womanhood that I'd learned growing up. . . . And if I hadn't been freed from it by the women's movement, then I just would have . . . I wouldn't have questioned it. . . . If you don't have the words to express how you feel, you're really kind of stuck with the feeling. And that's what I got out of those early years and it definitely . . . definitely created my response to the whole cancer experience.

Instead of internalizing the sexism and heterosexism of her surgeon, Clara's feminism and her lesbian identity provided her with the emotional, experiential, and intellectual resources to reject these male-centric and heterocentric assumptions about women's breasts, bodies, desires, pains, pleasures, preferences, and priorities.

From the health care system's point of view, Clara's rehabilitation was simple and speedy. In the 1970s the only institutionalized form of rehabilitation and support available to women with breast cancer was Reach to Recovery, which was adopted by the ACS in 1969 to provide support and practical advice to postsurgical mastectomy patients. The goal of the program was for the postsurgery patient to reenter her former life and become again the person she was before she was diagnosed and treated for breast cancer. The goal, in essence, was to facilitate a quick transition back to normality.

For many women, being visited by a Reach to Recovery volunteer was a welcome experience. It provided them with their only link to the mastectomy underground. For Clara, however, this experience was one of alienation instead of sisterhood:

I felt sorry for her. I mean, she meant well. She really meant well. But, you know, she wanted to tell me all about prostheses and how you could dress to minimize looking like you'd had a mastectomy and . . . it was not what I needed. I got rid of her as soon as I could.

Later, looking back on her first brush with breast cancer, Clara shared an interesting insight about the impact of breast cancer on her relationship to heteronormative standards of beauty. She explained that although being diagnosed with a life-threatening disease had been terrifying, and losing her breast had been traumatic, not everything about the experience was negative:

> One of the interesting things about having cancer is that it's not all bad. In some ways it's very freeing. . . . One of the epiphanies the first time was that, like all young American girls, I mean, I grew up in the forties and fifties . . . I was oppressed by the idea that I had to be beautiful and I had to look like a Playboy centerfold, which I never did. I was never beautiful. I never looked like that. I never *could* have looked like that! It would have been impossible. And it tortured me. And having cancer really liberated me from that. It was like, "Okay, I only have one breast now so I can't possibly compete!" And it was extremely freeing! I didn't have to try anymore! I didn't have to worry about it. I was out of the running. . . . That part was really cool. I loved that.

Clara never opted for reconstructive surgery, and she neither acquired nor wore a prosthesis. She continued wearing the same clothing she had before, tight tank tops and T-shirts. She continued taking her children to the public swimming pool wearing her old bikini. "I was very exhibitionist about it," she said, "especially at the beginning . . . and people were shocked!"

Clara "went on" with her life, as she put it, without hiding the visible signs of her cancer history. But she was forced to come to terms with this history and to make sense of it without the benefit of other women who shared her experience:

> In 1979 people just wanted you to have surgery and they didn't want to talk about it. . . . You were in and out of the hospital and that was that! There was no social workers, no support groups. . . . the closest thing to that was the Reach to Recovery lady and that was awful . . . and that was all there was. There wasn't anybody! I didn't know a single soul! And . . . um . . . that would have been nice, if I'd known other people. Yup. That would have been nice. Because . . . my partner certainly didn't understand it. I mean, nobody understands this experience unless they've gone through it. They just really don't. . . . But I had no idea how to get ahold of people. And the

Women's Cancer Resource Center didn't exist. It wasn't there. And there were no resources that I knew of.

Thus, except for follow-up appointments, Clara was officially "done" with breast cancer when she recovered from surgery. Summarizing the environment for women with breast cancer in the late seventies, she said,

People didn't talk about it then. And I think that's probably the most global thing that I can say about having breast cancer in 1979. People. Didn't. Talk. About it. Period.

Although she was part of the first wave of women who were mammographically screened for breast cancer, Clara knew almost nothing about the disease either before or after her diagnosis. Scientific studies and medical information were not readily available, and breast cancer patients, even middle-class graduate students, had not yet become lay experts. In theory, Clara could have gone to a medical library and conducted her own research, but it did not occur to her to do that. It was not something patients typically did. And this was true despite the fact that Clara was active in the women's movement, despite the fact that she possessed a healthy distrust of the medical establishment, and despite the fact that her lover/partner, Regina, was a physician. Even if medical information had been accessible, the treatment options available to her were negligible. The space for patient agency and the room for maneuvering were minimal.

Clara was unusual in that she forced open the space of participation and created an alternative path. She chose not to hide the evidence of her mastectomy. She refused, as she put it "to protect people from seeing this." Her visibility to others, however, did not make other women with histories of breast cancer visible to her. Clara remembers that after she learned, much to her surprise, that one in thirteen women (now one in eight) could expect to meet a similar fate, she used to walk down the street looking in vain for those invisible one-in-thirteen women and wondering who and where they were. She thought of her friends and all the women she knew. She wondered how many of them would get breast cancer, and she wondered, as she said, "how many of them already had."

In 1979 Clara's act of refusal was a symbolic gesture without a language, disembedded from either the context or the community that could recognize and respond to it. Although Clara struggled against the limits of that disease regime, those limits were finite and rigid. Feminism, women's liberation, and a lesbian identity could take her only so far. They could change her relationship to the regime of breast cancer and they could buffer her against its sharper edges, but they could not, or rather, they had not yet, thoroughly transformed its practices.

CLARA LARSON IN 1997: NEW SOCIAL RELATIONS, SOLIDARITIES, AND SUBJECTIVITIES

In 1997 Clara was diagnosed with metastatic breast cancer when she sought medical treatment for a painful back injury. In the end, rumors of a cure proved to be greatly exaggerated, as they did for so many women who were optimistically pronounced "cured" and, after five years, counted as survivors in the official survival rate statistics. Prognostically speaking, Clara's second diagnosis was much worse than her first. By 1997 her original breast cancer had metastasized to her vertebrae, her hip, and her lungs.

This time around, Clara turned to a variety of sources of information and was gratified by what she found:

The Internet was really helpful. And then you've got the 1-800-4CANCER [the NCI cancer information number]. And I know a lot more people who've had cancer. And . . . there's the cancer center, and the cancer center is just so full of people who are helpful and tell you things, and my doctor is incredibly helpful and supportive. I mean, everybody's just really nice.

Clara used the Internet to research the chemotherapeutic drugs she was given, and she checked out the breast cancer chat rooms and bulletin boards. She received gifts of books from family and friends. Her son, for example, presented her with a copy of *Cancer in Two Voices* (1991) an illness narrative written by a lesbian couple, Sandra Butler and Barbara Rosenblum, chronicling their life together, and Rosenblum's illness and death from breast cancer.[4] Another friend gave her a copy of *Dr. Susan Love's Breast Book* (1995), a book written by a well-known breast cancer surgeon, feminist, lesbian, and breast cancer activist that was wildly popular among women diagnosed with breast cancer.

But it was not just access to information that had expanded; the whole environment of health care delivery had changed. Contrasting the breast cancer regime of 1997 with that of 1979, Clara said,

> I just don't remember any supportive medical personnel at all [in 1979]. In contrast to what I'm going through now, where, you know, I'm in an HMO, and health care is [supposed to be] so terrible and so seemingly unavailable . . . but the medical people have just been fabulous this time around. They're just wonderful. And that just didn't happen before.

Not only were the hospital staff and health care professionals helpful and supportive, but the sexism and heterosexism that infused her first encounter with the regime of breast cancer had been replaced (at least in the Berkeley hospital where Clara was treated) by a lesbian- and feminist-friendly staff whose own views of breast cancer had been influenced by the breast cancer movement. As Clara said,

> A lot of these women are feminists, a lot of these women are lesbians. And people have a political consciousness about the whole cancer thing. . . . I mean, in Berkeley it is so okay to be gay—it's just totally okay. [It's] totally accepted. Now. Not before. And people have been fabulous with Susan [her new partner]. They treat her as my partner. They give her all the respect that they would give a heterosexual partner. . . . One woman, she wasn't a nurse, she was a pharmacist or something, and she came into my room to ask me about something and she said, "Well you're a lesbian aren't you?" and I thought, "Whoa! What an assumption! What a turn around!" And gradually they all [the lesbian health care workers] came out to me. It was great. . . . It was fabulous. I loved it.

What a contrast to Clara's first experience of breast cancer! In 1979 her lesbian identity and her lover's identity were either invisible to or ignored by her surgeon, who did not appear to think twice about his assumptions. Now the presuppositions ran in the opposite direction, but in a way that delighted Clara and her lover and made them feel seen, recognized, and accepted.

Not only had the social and cultural environment of cancer care changed, but so too had the organization and delivery of services. Instead of feeling isolated and powerless, as she had in 1979, Clara felt like the captain of a well-functioning team dedicated to aiding and assisting her treatment and recovery. She gave a long list of the individuals whom she viewed as members of her team:

> Well certainly there's my oncologist. Then there's my regular general practitioner. There's my acupuncturist. There's my chiropractor. Also, my acupuncturist is an herbalist. And then there's other people that have been helpful in this process. . . . A couples counselor . . . and I would also put on the list my hair cutter [who shaved her head when she started losing her hair and continued shaving it during chemotherapy] . . . and I would also put my housecleaner on that list because I'm not supposed to get anywhere near dust [due to her compromised immune system]. And so the list just goes on and on and on and I feel like all those people have really contributed to solving the problem.

In addition to revealing the tremendous impact of alternative health movements on the Bay Area regime of breast cancer, this passage reveals one of the ways the experiences of illness available to women diagnosed with breast cancer were increasingly being shaped by class distinctions. In the earlier regime of breast cancer there was more of a one-size-fits-all approach to the diagnosis and treatment of the disease, and treatment itself, especially for women diagnosed with early-stage breast cancer, was fairly simple (albeit radical) and straightforward—amputation of the breast. With minimal options, alternatives, or amenities available to women diagnosed with breast cancer, the social, cultural, and economic capital possessed by individual patients was less consequential. There were simply fewer investment opportunities—fewer ways of converting these various forms of capital into better treatment outcomes and illness experiences.

In contrast, between April 1997 (her second diagnosis) and January 1998 (when I interviewed her), Clara estimated that she spent $6,000 of her own money on alternative and complementary treatments and services not covered by her health insurance. Beyond that, the treatment she received, high-dose chemotherapy with stem-cell transplant, was an expensive and experimental procedure. Without evidence from clinical trials demonstrating its superiority over standard chemotherapy for the treatment of women with breast cancer, health insurance and managed care companies proved reluctant to cover the procedure, which carried a price tag ranging from

$80,000 to $150,000.[5] This reluctance led, during the 1990s, to proliferating lawsuits, arbitration hearings, testimony before Congress, and attempts at legislation in many states.[6] "These legal and political pressures," according to Michelle Mello and Troyen Brennan, "led most health plans to capitulate and pay for the treatment by the mid-1990s."[7] Despite the absence of any evidence of effectiveness, breast cancer patients underwent more stem-cell transplants combined with high-dose chemotherapy during the 1990s than did any other group of patients. It was within this larger context that Clara underwent this particularly dangerous and grueling procedure in 1997. Ironically, despite the popular backlash against a health care system increasingly organized around the logic of market mechanisms, certain dimensions of the regime of breast cancer had improved for middle-class patients with good health insurance.[8] By 1997 middle-class breast cancer patients with health insurance in the San Francisco Bay Area had become savvy consumers, forcing medical facilities to compete for this ever-expanding market. The number of "women's health" and "breast health" centers grew during the 1990s, along with special resources, support groups, and other amenities. These improvements did not benefit all patients equally, however, and almost certainly exacerbated existing inequalities, but they did contribute in positive ways to the illness experiences of many middle-class, medically empowered patients.[9]

The cancer center where Clara received her treatment offered free patient-education workshops and cancer support groups. These were organized according to various criteria: type of cancer, stage of cancer, age, sex, and so on. There were drop-in groups, ongoing groups, and coed groups for people with metastatic disease. If Clara had wanted to avoid medical settings (as many cancer patients do), there were free support groups and educational forums in alternative settings. Just down the street, the Women's Cancer Resource Center offered a series of support groups, including one for lesbians with cancer. It also offered a variety of practical services to women with cancer, including a medical library, research assistance, patients' evaluations of local physicians, phone access to women willing to share their treatment experiences, and one-on-one assistance with transportation, shopping, cleaning, and other errands and activities.

Clara attended a series of workshops for cancer patients who were contemplating undergoing a stem-cell transplant. These workshops provided her with an opportunity to establish relationships with other, similarly positioned patients and put her in touch with additional resources, support, and information. Certainly, Clara did not access all, or even a significant portion, of the resources available to her, but their existence, and her awareness of their existence, nonetheless shaped her illness experience by changing what had been (in 1979) an individualized experience of isolation and alienation into a shared experience of social support and solidarity.

Even Clara's son benefited from the new openness about breast cancer. Clara related a story about her son, who ran into an old friend of his from high school. Her son's friend asked, innocently enough, "How's your mother?"—and her son responded that his mother had cancer. His friend replied "Mine too! What kind of cancer does your mom have?" "Breast cancer," her son explained, and his friend once again responded "Mine too!" Clara smiled and said, "This never would have happened when I was growing up! We never would have had a conversation like that about our mothers in the 1950s." Instead of hiding their mothers' stigmatizing illnesses and suffering alone and in silence, these two young men were able to bond over their shared experience, support one another, and renew their friendship.

But even for a white, middle-class, lesbian feminist living in Berkeley, the new regime of breast cancer was not a disease utopia. Clara, for example, did not particularly like WCRC:

> They reminded me of . . . in the seventies all the lesbians that I knew . . . were downwardly mobile . . . and there was a certain way that you were supposed to be . . . and I had way too many kids to be politically correct, and I also lived a very middle-class lifestyle . . . and there were a lot of people that were very critical of me because I wasn't the right kind of lesbian. And that's the same feeling that I had when I walked into WCRC. And I'm sure that this is not everybody's experience, but it was my experience . . . and that probably had a lot to do with my resentment with all the people who basically just discounted me in the seventies because I wasn't a politically correct lesbian. I guess it [her negative reaction] probably just hooked into that.

Although WCRC was a feminist- and lesbian-friendly organization, Clara did not respond positively to its organizational culture because it evoked painful memories of rejection, which in turn inspired feelings of anger and resentment. She felt rejected not by WCRC per se but by the lesbian feminist community with which she associated it, a community that twenty years earlier had rejected her, she believed, for being too mainstream, too middle-class, and too motherly.

This aspect of Clara's illness experience is a powerful reminder of two things. First, it reminds us of the importance of cultural differences, even within groups we assume are relatively homogeneous. In this case, differences in class culture and political culture separated Clara from an organization for which one might reasonably have expected her to feel a fair amount of enthusiasm. Further, giving an ironic twist to sociological assumptions about class-based exclusions, Clara felt rejected not for being too poor but for being too middle-class.

Second, it reminds us that disease regimes shape rather than determine illness experiences. The development of lesbian and feminist cancer organizations created new social spaces, solidarities, and subjectivities, thus expanding the kinds of illness experiences available within the second regime of breast cancer. But individual experiences, memories, personalities, and perspectives also shape the illness experience. Just as Clara's feminist politics and lesbian identity served as resources during her first encounter with the regime of breast cancer, painful memories of rejection by the lesbian community created barriers that prevented Clara from fully accessing the resources offered, twenty years later, by a grassroots organization serving the lesbian community.

Social movements in the Bay Area also changed the way the issue of breast cancer was publicly framed and understood. Environmental activism was a key focus of the breast cancer movement in the San Francisco Bay Area, and by 1998 this particular orientation had crept into Clara's own cognitive framework and political sensibilities. No longer did she view breast cancer solely through the lens of gender and sexuality. She now viewed breast cancer as an environmental disease and an issue of corporate profits and pollution:

> In those days, I thought it [wearing breast prostheses] was to protect men from seeing that there were women walking around with one tit. And now I think it's because . . . the increase in cancer, I believe, is environmental. And people need to be protected from us so that they don't realize what an epidemic this is, especially here in the Bay Area, and start questioning some of the people who are polluting the environment, polluting the bay. Because

that's big corporate money. And they don't want people to think about it. That's also why they focus on detection instead of prevention.

Clara indicated that she had arrived at this analysis "probably in the last five years, when I started hearing the statistics that breast cancer is so much more prevalent in the Bay Area than anywhere else in the country." The wide circulation and politicization of these statistics, framed as evidence of environmental influences, was the handiwork of the feminist cancer and environmental justice movements. Clara's understanding of breast cancer was thus shaped by environmental breast cancer activism even though she was not active in this, or any other, social movement.

In fact, her lack of involvement in breast cancer activism was a source of real consternation and guilt. She explained that when the Bay Area women's cancer community and breast cancer activism gained a measure of visibility in the early 1990s, a number of her friends assumed that she would want to get involved. But, Clara said, "I just didn't want to." She explained, "For me . . . my cancer experience was really . . . awful and it was something that I wanted to leave behind. I didn't feel like going up there and being part of all that. I would have rather volunteered at the SPCA [Society for the Prevention of Cruelty to Animals] or something." Since her second diagnosis, Clara had been feeling a growing sense of moral obligation to get involved in the breast cancer movement. "I think I should get involved," she said, "but I bet that I won't." She continued,

I think that something has to be done about it and it's important to push for more money for research, and it's important to be part of the movement to expose the environmental hazards and all that kind of stuff. That's important work to be done . . . but I probably won't do it, because when this is over, I'm gonna want to shut it out of my life again.

Clara's desire to avoid involvements with disease-based activism was not in the least bit unusual or difficult to comprehend. After all, most people, given the choice, would prefer to put the experience of cancer behind them. The difference is that in 1979 Clara looked for political community but was unable to find it. In 1997 she felt called upon to justify her lack of political involvement.

Despite her reticence, Clara discovered that she could witness the political face of breast cancer from within the privacy of her own living room. That summer, while reclining on her couch and recovering from chemotherapy, Clara watched as cancer activists marched in the 1997 Lesbian-Gay-Bisexual-Transgender Pride Parade in San Francisco. One-breasted, two-breasted, and bare-breasted women marched at the front of the procession, carrying the parade banner. That year, as the banner carried by the activists indicated, the parade was officially dedicated "to our sisters with cancer." This time around, instead of searching the streets in vain for signs of other women with breast cancer, Clara watched comfortably from her couch as images of breast cancer activists taking over the streets of San Francisco were beamed into her living room.

The contrast between the first and second regimes of breast cancer was dramatic. In the earlier regime of practices, Clara attempted to take breast cancer to the streets by making visible its inscription on her body. But she did so alone, and her impact was necessarily limited. Instead of sisterhood and solidarity, she crashed into the rigid structure of isolation, stigma, and invisibility—the architecture of the closet. The second time she was diagnosed with breast cancer, Clara maintained her distance from the diverse cultures of action that populated the Bay Area field of contention. They changed her experience of illness nonetheless, because they transformed the terrain of breast cancer and reshaped the public contours of disease.

Although Clara was and is a truly exceptional individual, what she encountered and endured when she was diagnosed with breast cancer in the late 1970s was neither exceptional nor extreme. In that regime (which was in the process of transition), her experience of breast cancer was relentlessly individualized. She looked for a sisterhood of survivors but never found one. She engaged in acts of civil disobedience but remained isolated. Surgeons were the undisputed sovereigns of the kingdom, and the only role scripted for women with breast cancer was that of the compliant patient. Almost inevitably, the power inequalities structured into the physician–patient relationship were deepened by the gender inequalities between male surgeons and female patients. Even an atypical patient like Clara, who was involved in consciousness-raising, women's liberation, and lesbian feminism (and whose partner was a physician) found the power dynamics and disparities overwhelming. The women's movement and lesbian feminism provided her with the intellectual, social, and emotional resources to maintain

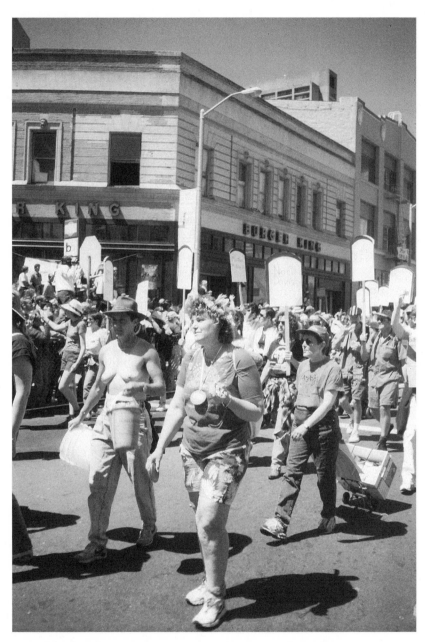

Activists marching in the Women and Cancer contingent at the 1998 San Francisco Lesbian-Gay-Bisexual-Transgender Pride Parade. Photograph by Maren Klawiter.

a critical distance from some of the technologies of normalization that she faced, but there were practical limits to her resistance. Those limits were set by the disease regime.

By 1997, however, a new regime of breast cancer had emerged in the San Francisco Bay Area. Clara was treated in a feminist- and lesbian-friendly cancer center. She decided between medical alternatives, attended patient-education workshops, participated in her treatment as a member of a "health care team" that consisted of a range of health care professionals, and relied upon an assortment of support personnel. Books by lesbian feminist patients and physicians magically appeared in her hands as gifts from family and friends. Support groups, medical information, and practical resources for women with breast cancer were freely available.

Not only had the clinical contours of the disease changed, but the public face of breast cancer had undergone a remarkable transformation. Women with breast cancer had become a visible presence in the public domain and were now heralded as heroes instead of pitied and shunned as victims. Breast cancer had been politicized along multiple dimensions and reframed, among other things, as a feminist issue and an environmental disease. To top it all off, the Lesbian-Gay-Bisexual-Transgender Pride Parade, which was dedicated to women with cancer, marched right into her living room.

# Breast Cancer
# in the Twenty-first Century

Breast cancer fits into a twenty-first century phenomenon. . . . The critical
shared issue of our time is moving from an age of extinctions to an age
of renewal and sustainability. One of the principal hopes for this is the
environmental health movement. . . . the role of the breast cancer movement
as a vanguard of the environmental health movement is not just of parochial
interest to breast cancer patients; it is core to the future of life on earth.

—MICHAEL LERNER, "Breast Cancer and the Environment"

Breast cancer, as Michael Lerner declared at the International Summit on
Breast Cancer and the Environment in 2002, is a twenty-first-century phenomenon. By this the founder of Commonweal (the highly respected cancer and environmental health center in Bolinas, California) meant not that
breast cancer is a disease new to the twenty-first century but, rather, that
breast cancer engages twenty-first-century issues of environmental health
that are crucial to the future of life on earth. In Lerner's planetary vision,
the women's movement holds the greatest potential for building a global
environmental health movement, and within the women's movement it is
the reproductive rights and breast cancer movements that hold the greatest
promise. The breast cancer movement, in Lerner's view, has been more successful in "moving a specific health agenda in the United States" than any
other group in recent decades. Further, as Lerner noted elsewhere, a "significant minority" of breast cancer activists "are already deeply committed
to environmental health concerns."[1] Thus, as Lerner declared at the summit, the breast cancer movement "is not just of parochial interest."[2]

I agree with Lerner's assessment. I also believe, however, that the strength of the breast cancer movement lies in the tremendous diversity of its goals and the tremendous dynamism that is fed by its internal differences. Even as key sectors of the breast cancer movement deepen their commitment to a healthy environment, other cultures of action continue to press for early detection, access to treatment, and patient empowerment. What I find so remarkable about the breast cancer movement—and I believe this is what makes the breast cancer movement so powerful—is the wide range of institutional spaces in which it successfully advocates for change. It is, on the one hand, the narrowest of single-issue movements, organized as it is around one specific disease. It is, on the other, the broadest of movements—bridging across institutional domains, disease regimes, fields of contention, and cultures of action. In this chapter I highlight several key developments in the contemporary regime of breast cancer and the breast cancer movement, paying particular attention to California and the Bay Area field of contention.

## The Bay Area Field of Contention

The most important development in California's culture of early detection occurred in 2001, when the governor, Gray Davis, signed legislation establishing the California Breast and Cervical Cancer Treatment Program, which committed the State of California, after years of resistance, to pay for the medical treatment of low-income, uninsured, and underinsured women diagnosed with breast cancer within its borders. The program was an outgrowth, in part, of the federal Breast and Cervical Cancer Prevention and Treatment Act (BCCPTA), which was conceived and promoted by the National Breast Cancer Coalition and signed into law by President Clinton in 2000.[3] It was also, however, shaped by the character of the breast/cancer movement in California. Just as the California Breast Cancer Early Detection Program exceeded the scope and ambition of the federally funded screening program, California activists successfully lobbied for treatment legislation that expanded the scope of this federal initiative.

Federal restrictions embedded in the BCCPTA limited program eligibility to U.S. citizens and legal residents. Instead of accepting these terms, however, women's health activists and sympathetic politicians pushed for an additional treatment program, wholly funded by the State of California, for women whose immigration status disqualified them from the federal treatment program. The legislation that was signed into law in California authorized the state's Department of Health Services to provide medical treatment to all eligible women, regardless of their citizenship or immigration status.[4] This was an important victory, and it was spearheaded by the collaborative efforts of the cultures of screening and of feminist treatment activism.

Along with the culture of early detection, the culture of feminist treatment activism continued its development during the twenty-first century by creating new images and representations of women with breast cancer, pushing corporate sponsors and social-issues marketing campaigns to shift their funding practices and priorities, expanding direct services and access to information within underserved communities, conducting community-based participatory research projects to document the needs of women living with cancer, and expanding the social spaces, group activities, and networks of solidarity that fed and sustained the women's cancer community.

In January 2000, for example, the Breast Cancer Fund launched its "Obsessed with Breasts Educational Campaign." In bus shelters, on buildings, and in other public places around the Bay Area, the BCF placed posters satirizing the "breast obsession" of the fashion, fitness, and beauty industries. The posters featured several different images. One poster spliced the nude torso of a woman with a double mastectomy (Andrea Martin, the executive director of the BCF onto the body of a model on the cover of a magazine that looked like *Mademoiselle, Glamour,* or *Cosmopolitan.* Instead of the usual magazine title and article teasers about diet, sex, and beauty, however, the magazine was titled *Mastectomy* and included front-cover teasers like "1 in 8: Your Chances of Getting Breast Cancer," "Breast Cancer Epidemic: What's behind It?" "Breast Cancer Quiz: Are You at Risk?" and "Your Breasts: Not Just for Looks." A second poster in the campaign was designed to mimic the photographic style and staging of Calvin Klein advertisements. A third poster was designed as a send-up of catalogs and advertisements for Victoria's Secret. Both of these posters featured images of one-breasted women. The goal of the campaign, as the BCF indicated in its press release, "was to capture the viewer's attention and change the way we think and act about breast cancer."[5] This was a very different kind of breast cancer awareness than the awareness promoted by early detection campaigns. The "Obsessed with Breasts" campaign, which was part of the BCF's larger program of "Art-Reach," caused such a public outcry that the

BCF was forced to remove the offending images from public spaces within a matter of days—which only served, ironically, to enhance the campaign's visibility.[6]

A second campaign, "Think before You Pink," was launched by Breast Cancer Action in 2002 through a full-page advertisement in the *New York Times.* The ad, which featured an image of a Eureka vacuum cleaner, drew attention to corporate "pinkwashers" that BCA charged were "cleaning up" by exploiting the good will of consumers and using the issue of breast cancer to sell products, often without contributing much, if anything, of value to the breast cancer movement. The campaign received a great deal of positive publicity around the country and continues to be one of BCA's most popular public-education campaigns. BCA helped coin the term "pinkwashing" to characterize these corporate promotional campaigns.

In its 2006 "Parade of Pink," for example, BCA developed a partial list of close to forty corporate marketing campaigns that were cashing in on the popularity of breast cancer as a feel-good cause. These products included Cartier's Roadster Watch ($3,800), Breast Cancer Awareness Tweezers ($20), Pink Ribbon Tic Tacs ($0.79), an Estée Lauder lipstick named Elizabeth Pink ($22), Essie Pink Ribbon nail polish ($7), 3M Pink Ribbon Post-it Notes ($1.99–$4.95), an assortment of Ralph Lauren Pink Pony Products ($10–$498), Playtex Passion for Living pink gloves ($2.99), Pink M&Ms ($2.99), Qwest and Sanyo pink cell phones (from $79.99), and Everlast pink boxing gloves (from $30).[7]

"Navigating the sea of pink ribbon promotions," BCA explained, "requires consumers to ask a few critical questions." How much money actually goes toward breast cancer–related causes? Is the corporate donation a percentage of the purchase price, or is it based on the number of items sold or the net profits or some other formula? Are there minimum and maximum limits? To whom and to what is the money being donated? Does any of it directly aid or improve the lives of women living with breast cancer or women without access to basic services, treatment, and screening? Does the philanthropic promotion contribute more to the corporation's bottom line than it does to the intended beneficiaries? In a 2005 article in *PR,* for example, 3M bragged that its seventy-foot-tall pink ribbon of Post-it Notes, which was erected in New York City's Times Square in 2004, reached more than three million people and exceeded by more than 80 percent the anticipated increase in sales. Although 3M reportedly spent

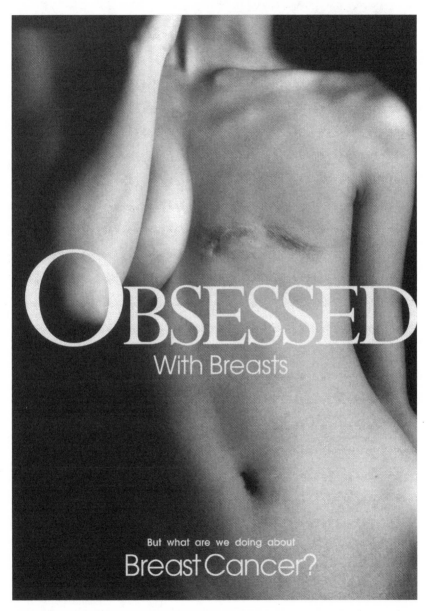

Obsessed with breasts. Image courtesy of the Breast Cancer Fund's "Obsessed with Breasts" ad campaign, http://www.breastcancerfund.org/obsessedwithbreasts.

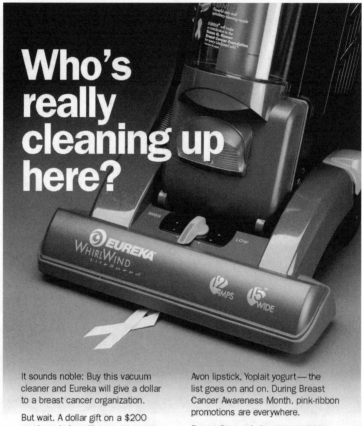

# Who's really cleaning up here?

It sounds noble: Buy this vacuum cleaner and Eureka will give a dollar to a breast cancer organization.

But wait. A dollar gift on a $200 purchase is less than one percent— and Eureka caps its annual contribution from the sales at $250,000.

Is the company spending more on its "Clean for the Cure" ads than it's donating to the cause?

It's not just Eureka. American Express donates a penny per transaction when you "Charge for the Cure." BMW kicks in a buck per mile when you test-drive its cars, which produce chemical compounds linked to breast cancer.

Avon lipstick, Yoplait yogurt—the list goes on and on. During Breast Cancer Awareness Month, pink-ribbon promotions are everywhere.

Breast Cancer Action urges you to "think before you pink." Will your purchase make a difference? Or is the company exploiting breast cancer to boost profits?

Preventing, curing, and guaranteeing quality treatment for breast cancer will require real change—and not the kind you carry in your pocket.

**BREAST CANCER ACTION**

55 New Montgomery St., Suite 323, San Francisco, CA 94105 • www.ThinkBeforeYouPink.org

"Who's really cleaning up here?" Courtesy of Breast Cancer Action, http://www.bcaction.org; part of BCA's "Think before You Pink" campaign, http://www.thinkbeforeyoupink.org.

$500,000 on the marketing campaign and contributed $300,000 to breast cancer–related causes, the company did not disclose how much it profited from its pink-ribbon promotion.[8]

The Bay Area culture of environmental cancer activism also matured and expanded during this period, achieving a number of significant successes. In 1999, for example, a consortium of cancer and environmental organizations formed the Bay Area Working Group on the Precautionary Principle. The group—whose organizational members included Bayview–Hunters Point Community Advocates, Breast Cancer Action, Center for Environmental Health, Clean Water Action, Commonweal, Greenaction, Healthy Building Network, Healthy Children Organizing Project, Physicians for Social Responsibility, Redefining Progress, Science and Environmental Health Network, the Breast Cancer Fund, Urban Habitat, and Women's Cancer Resource Center—worked to raise awareness and promote the adoption of the precautionary principle, focusing on city and county governments. In 2003 San Francisco became the first city in the nation to formally adopt the precautionary principle. The city of Berkeley followed suit shortly thereafter. Both cities, in adopting the precautionary principle, committed themselves to seeking safer alternatives to the use of toxic, carcinogenic, and environmentally destructive products and practices.

In 2000 the BCF redefined its organizational mission as "identifying—and advocating the elimination of—the environmental and other preventable causes of the disease." The BCF's decision to redefine its mission around the environmental causes of breast cancer signaled its abandonment of an earlier strategy that centered on its role as a funder of innovative research and direct services for women with breast cancer. The BCF's intensified commitment to the environmental dimensions of breast cancer fed and reflected the popularity of the precautionary principle and other environmental initiatives within the women's cancer community.

In 2002, for example, the BCF and BCA collaborated on an influential new report entitled *State of the Evidence: What Is the Connection between Chemicals and Breast Cancer?* (in its fourth edition in 2006). The report documented and discussed the growing body of evidence linking exposure to radiation and synthetic chemicals to an increased risk of breast cancer. The report also outlined a series of recommendations for new directions in research, including the reorientation of public policy around the precautionary principle, arguing that "the public's health cannot and should not have to wait for absolute proof that certain chemicals cause breast cancer before moving to reduce the risk of such harm occurring."[9] Unlike the broader definition of "environment" used by researchers and public health professionals—a definition that usually encompassed and often emphasized individual lifestyle behaviors such as nutrition, alcohol consumption, obesity, smoking, and exercise—this report explicitly focused on the "involuntary exposures" to which people are subjected, such as chemically contaminated water, soil, air, and consumer products.

As part of this approach, the BCF and BCA also launched a "precautionary purchasing" campaign called the Healthy Cosmetics Campaign (now called the Campaign for Safe Cosmetics). The campaign targeted the manufacturing processes of cosmetics companies, many of whom had burnished their corporate images through their public displays of support for breast cancer research and for early detection drives. It was designed to educate consumers about the hazardous ingredients in many cosmetics and the industry's refusal to disclose or remove these ingredients. By tarnishing the public image of these corporations, the campaign pressured cosmetics companies to sign "a voluntary compact to prove that their concern for their customers is more than just skin deep."[10] The campaign was also waged on the terrain of the state, and in 2005 Governor Arnold Schwarzenegger signed legislation requiring cosmetics companies selling products in California to disclose and remove hazardous ingredients from their products.

The year 2002 also witnessed the successful staging of the International Summit on Breast Cancer and the Environment, which convened in Santa Cruz, California. The summit, which was funded by the Centers for Disease Control and Prevention, was the brainchild of Andrea Martin, the executive director of the BCF, and Patricia Buffler, then the dean of the School of Public Health at the University of California, Berkeley.[11] The structure, content, and format of the summit were determined by a steering committee that included a mix of activists, scientists, and public health professionals. Although it was billed as an international summit, the vast majority of organizational representatives and individual participants were based in the Bay Area, ground zero of the environmental breast cancer movement.

The summit, according to the painstakingly produced conference report, "was infused with underlying themes such as population monitoring [biomonitoring], the precautionary principle, health disparities, community-based participatory research, the definition of community, and historical tensions between advocates and the community, and the community and scientists."[12] These themes were reflected in the recommendations that emerged from the summit, including the recommendations that lay communities play a central role in all phases of public health research, that the precautionary principle be integrated into policy making, and that a national biomonitoring program be established to measure levels of bioaccumulative chemicals in human bodies and to monitor environmental culprits such as industrial and vehicle emissions, pesticides, and drinking-water contaminants. I will return to a discussion of the summit below, but let me turn first to a related development sponsored by the National Institute of Environmental Health Sciences.

In October 2003 the National Institute of Environmental Health Sciences (NIEHS) and the National Cancer Institute launched a seven-year, $35 million initiative to establish four multidisciplinary research centers to investigate the relationship between environmental factors and breast cancer. Members of the Bay Area breast cancer community—including representatives from medical, scientific, and advocacy organizations—collaborated on a proposal that resulted in the establishment of one of the four Breast Cancer and the Environment Research Centers (BCERC) in the Bay Area. Marin Breast Cancer Watch, which played a key role in developing the proposal, was appointed to lead the Community Outreach and Translational Core (COTC) of the initiative.[13] This community component, which all environmental research centers were required to include, was "tasked with ensuring that the views and concerns of the breast cancer advocate community are heard and that the researchers' findings are disseminated to the public."[14]

The development and design of the NIEHS/NCI initiative signified, at the very least, the growing legitimacy of environmental research on breast cancer within federal agencies and the growing status of environmental health sciences within the domain of breast cancer research. It also signified and further legitimized the increasingly central role of breast cancer advocacy organizations and "the public" in the design, implementation, diffusion, and interpretation of breast cancer research. Although the NIEHS interpreted "environment" quite broadly to mean the "social, chemical, and physical environment," the focus of the research it sponsored through this initiative was heavily weighted toward gene–environment interactions, focusing in particular on breast maturation and vulnerabilities during puberty. Likewise, the stated goals of the initiative were cast in strikingly narrow terms.[15] "The overall outcomes of the BCERC," according to the project's Web site, "are to develop public health messages designed to educate young girls and women who are at high risk of breast cancer about the role(s) of specific environmental stressors in breast cancer and how to reduce exposures to those stressors."[16] The central goal of BCERC research, in other words, was articulated in terms of managing the behavior of "high-risk" girls and women, not in terms of identifying and reducing carcinogens in the physical environment or changing the behavior of corporations and governments. For this reason, the response to BCERC by participants in the cultures of feminist and environmental activism has been mixed.[17]

The International Summit on Breast Cancer and the Environment, on the other hand (to pick up the thread of my earlier discussion), fed the momentum already gathering behind the precautionary principle and a policy initiative sponsored by Commonweal and the BCF to establish a statewide biomonitoring program in California. Biomonitoring, or "body burden," studies are scientific methods for detecting and measuring the presence of chemical compounds or their metabolites in the body. When Governor Schwarzenegger, in 2005, vetoed the legislation to establish a state-funded and state-administered biomonitoring program, his veto was widely interpreted as evidence that he was in the pocket of the chemical industry, which had strenuously lobbied again such legislation. In 2006, however, after the legislation was once again passed by the California Assembly and Senate, Governor Schwarzenegger acceded to mounting public pressure and signed into law the California Environmental Contaminant Biomonitoring Program (SB 1379). The vast expansion of biomonitoring signals, at least potentially, the emergence of a new public health and regulatory regime.[18] Just as the environmentalization of breast cancer has gained momentum in the twenty-first century, so too has the biomedicalization of breast cancer.

THE BIOMEDICALIZATION OF BREAST CANCER
IN THE TWENTY-FIRST CENTURY

During the late 1990s and the first years of the twenty-first century, the regime of breast cancer continued to expand through and within the institutional domains of public health and medicine. It did so primarily by colonizing new domains of risk and constituting new categories of risky subjects. The regime of breast cancer expanded along both axes of biomedicalization—the biopolitics of populations and the anatomo-politics of bodies. Over time, however, the analytic distinction between these two axes has become less salient as the boundary between the biopolitics of public health and clinical medicine has grown increasingly fuzzy, blurry, and blended. At the same time, the practices of the regime have increasingly taken shape through a partly chosen and partly forced negotiation with the various COAs that make up the U.S. breast cancer movement.

## The Biopolitics of Breast Health Promotion

Although the discourse of *breast health* first appeared in the early 1990s, for the first few years breast health was just another name for breast cancer screening—no different in kind from the campaigns for "breast cancer awareness" and "early detection." During the second half of the 1990s, however, the discourse of breast health promotion became more prominent, and the semiotics of breast health campaigns began to change. Instead of breast cancer screening practices oriented toward early detection, the meaning of breast health promotion became more expansive and proactive. Although the precise meaning of breast health was by no means fixed, it increasingly indexed a growing list of health-promoting behaviors that women were told could reduce their risk of breast cancer: following a diet low in fat and high in fruits and vegetables, engaging in regular exercise, maintaining a body mass index (a measure of body fat) that was neither too low nor too high, and limiting the consumption of alcohol. When the final results from the hormone-replacement therapy (HRT) trials of the Women's Health Initiative were announced in 2002, HRT emphatically joined the list of risky behaviors.[19] In sum, although the discourse of early detection referred to a discrete set of screening practices—breast self-exam, clinical exams, and mammographic screening—the discourse of breast health advocated an entire lifestyle designed around the twin goals of nurturing and preserving healthy breasts.

Interestingly enough, during roughly this same period, the American Cancer Society, the Centers for Disease Control and Prevention, and the National Cancer Institute quietly backed away from their long-term policies of promoting monthly breast self-exam by all women over the age of eighteen. When the early results from the first large-scale clinical trials of BSE (which were conducted in China and Russia) began to appear in the second half of the 1990s, the compelling logic of BSE was thrown into doubt. During the late 1990s many cancer agencies and organizations quietly shifted the content and tone of their message. Instead of promoting BSE as one of three key steps in early detection, women were encouraged, in much milder tones, to become familiar with their breasts and consult a physician if they noticed any unusual lumps or discharge or physical change. They were, however, no longer enjoined to go on monthly hunting expeditions using the precise breast examination techniques taught in magazines, brochures, instructional videos, group classes, and one-on-one sessions. By the time the final results from these trials were published years later—demonstrating that BSE had no effect on breast cancer mortality or stage of diagnosis, although it did increase the number of benign lumps detected and the number of benign breast biopsies performed—the tide had already turned against the promotion of a rigid adherence to BSE.[20]

At the same time, conflicts and disagreements over mammography screening guidelines continued unabated. Recall that in 1993 the NCI had changed its recommended age for initiating annual mammographic screening from forty to fifty. In 1997 the National Institutes of Health held a consensus development conference to examine the state of the evidence for mammography screening of women in their forties. After reviewing the evidence, the NIH concluded that the data were inconclusive, and that women between the ages of forty and forty-nine should decide for themselves whether or not to begin mammographic screening before the age of fifty. Although many feminist breast/cancer organizations applauded the willingness of federal agencies to acknowledge the uncertainty and ambiguity of the evidence, the NIH's recommendation, or lack thereof, inspired a great deal of outrage from the screening establishment. A month later, the National Cancer Advisory Board (NCAB)—the advisory body to the National Cancer Program—convened a working group to make guideline recommendations to the NCI. Before NCAB could arrive at a recommendation, Congress entered the debate. In February 1997 the U.S. Senate passed a resolution urging NCAB to endorse universal screening for women between the ages of forty and forty-nine. NCAB did so, and shortly thereafter the NCI issued new screening guidelines, recommending that mammographic screening begin at age forty.

The war of the guidelines continued into the twenty-first century. In December 2001 mammographic screening once again erupted into a headline-grabbing controversy when the *Lancet* published a meta-analysis of clinical trials. Its well-respected authors concluded that there was no convincing evidence that mammographic screening reduced the risk of dying from breast cancer for any age group of women. The *New York Times* referred to the controversy as "a passionate debate among doctors in Europe and the United States," but this was clearly an understatement.[21] Just as it had on numerous occasions in the past, the debate over mammographic screening quickly leapfrogged beyond the covers of medical journals.

Over the course of the next few months the *New York Times* published more than a dozen articles, editorials, and letters debating the conclusions and implications of the latest study. Public agencies, expert advisory panels, professional associations, cancer charities, and research foundations issued press releases and formal statements in support of mammographic screening. An ACS spokesperson commenting on the *Lancet* study, for example, promised that the organization would review the study but stated that there did not appear to be anything in the study that would lead the ACS "to question the evidence and wisdom of screening mammography for women 40 and older."[22] An alliance of public agencies and private organizations (including the ACS, the American Society of Clinical Oncology, and the American Academy of Family Physicians) even placed a full-page advertisement in the *New York Times* reassuring the public of the life-saving benefits of mammographic screening.

Organizations active in the breast/cancer movement also issued press releases and posted position papers on their Web sites. Not surprisingly, organizations that were actively involved in the promotion of breast cancer screening criticized the study and renewed their support for mammography. Organizations that were critical of mammographic screening used the study, and the media attention it garnered, to press their point. Fran Visco, the president of the NBCC, for example, told a *New York Times* reporter that the NBCC welcomed the mammography dispute. "We know that mammography screening has serious limitations," Visco stated, "yet it has been sold as the be-all and end-all for breast cancer. . . . When someone says, 'We have to question that assumption,' we're thrilled. We've been questioning it from the beginning."[23] Nonetheless, a 2004 study on Americans' attitudes toward screening revealed that the public's enthusiasm for cancer screening (of various kinds, for various cancers) was "not dampened," and neither was its tendency to pass judgment on people who did not get screened. This was particularly true in the case of mammographic screening, where 41 percent of the respondents believed that an eighty-year-old woman who chose not to be screened was "irresponsible."[24] A study published in 2004 showed that the benefits and risks of mammographic screening were routinely and systematically misrepresented (i.e., exaggerated) on the Web sites of cancer organizations.[25]

More recently, a 2005 study commissioned by the NCI and published in the *New England Journal of Medicine* sought to estimate the relative importance of screening mammograms and drug therapies (primarily cytotoxic chemotherapies and tamoxifen) in producing the 24 percent decline in breast cancer mortality that, according to recent statistics, had occurred in the United States between 1990 and 2000. Seven different research teams, including researchers with a history of skepticism regarding the benefits of mammographic screening, developed seven different statistical models to answer the question. Although their results varied widely—from a 65/35 split in favor of the contribution of mammography screening to a 72/28 split in favor of the contribution of drug therapies—all seven teams concluded that mammographic screening had played a significant role in the declining death rate from breast cancer. The study was not, however, designed to answer the question of whether or not mammographic screening benefited women in their forties.[26] This question remains, after several decades of promotion unanswered.

In an editorial announcing, rather optimistically, that "long-simmering doubts" about the benefits of mammography screening "should be dispelled" by the study discussed above, the *New York Times* nonetheless refrained from encouraging women to get screened. As the *New York Times* editorial averred, "Women still need to make their own judgments as to whether the usefulness of screening outweighs the risks, which include false positives and possibly needless treatment to remove tiny tumors that might never have caused a problem if left alone."[27]

This message of uncertainty and ambiguity, however, continues to be rejected by the overwhelming majority of health providers and public health professionals. This rejection is illustrated by a flyer I received at a doctor's appointment in 2006.

The recommendations in the flyer come from Kaiser Permanente of

Georgia. First, despite the absence of evidence of its effectiveness, Kaiser instructs women to perform monthly breast self-exams. Second, despite the conflicting evidence, Kaiser instructs women to "get routine mammograms beginning at age 40 or earlier, if you fall into a high risk category." Third, even though I received the flyer four years after the release of the results from the HRT trials of the Women's Health Initiative, Kaiser's flyer fails to inform women that HRT is a risk factor for breast cancer. Likewise, no mention is made of the dangers of medical radiation, a potent risk factor for breast cancer. Nor is any mention made of common environmental carcinogens. Finally, the Kaiser flyer embraces the individual lifestyle emphasis of breast health promotion: "Maintain a healthy diet. . . . If you drink alcohol, limit the amount. . . . Be active. Try to get 30 minutes of exercise at least 5 days a week." It finishes with: "Know the warning signs. If you notice any symptoms, contact your doctor immediately." Sometimes the more things change, the more they stay the same.

In 2006 researchers from the M. D. Anderson Cancer Center reported a 15 percent drop in the most common form of invasive breast cancer diagnosed during 2003, arguing that the dramatic decrease in estrogen-positive tumors was a result of the sudden and dramatic decline in the use of hormone therapy by women in the United States during the previous year. It was well known that women had abandoned the use of HRT in droves following the July 2002 announcement that women taking Prempro (the drug tested in the HRT trial sponsored by the Women's Health Initiative) had a significantly increased risk of breast cancer. It will be interesting to see the extent to which the admonition to "avoid and reduce the use of HRT" messages will be incorporated into future campaigns promoting breast health.

*Blurring the Lines*

Two additional developments fed the expansion of the regime of biomedicalization, blurring the boundaries between the biopolitics of breast health promotion and the anatomo-politics of breast cancer. First, genetic screening for breast cancer became an option for women with strong family histories of the disease. Second, the first breast cancer chemopreventive drug was approved by the Food and Drug Administration to reduce the risk of breast cancer among healthy, "high-risk" women. Like the shift from early detection to breast health promotion, these new technologies further expanded the reach of the disease regime. Each of these is briefly discussed below.

First, following researchers' discovery of BRCA1 and BRCA2—the "breast cancer genes"—earlier in the decade, Myriad Genetic Laboratories developed and patented a commercially viable genetic screening test. In 1998 Myriad introduced this new risk-assessment technology into the U.S. market, primarily through promotional activities aimed at doctors. In 2002 Myriad launched a controversial new direct-to-consumer advertising campaign that promoted genetic testing for breast cancer to healthy women for a cost of between $745 and $2,760 for each woman tested.[28] Genetic testing and its promotion through direct-to-consumer marketing raised a number of legal, ethical, political, clinical, and scientific questions concerning the privacy of health care records, insurance coverage, insurance discrimination, access to risk-assessment counseling, access to prophylactic treatment, ethical obligations to inform close relatives, and so on. The key point for the purposes of this discussion, however, is a simple one: Genetic screening further expanded the regime of breast cancer and created a new category of risky subjects.[29]

The impact of genetic screening, however, is never limited to the individuals who undergo testing. A BRCA alteration in one family member, for example, increases the risk profile of close male and female relatives— both those who are living and those who have not yet been conceived. Thus, knowledge of an alteration in one or more of the breast cancer genes heightens the experience of risk and anxiety among the carrier and the carrier's extended family.[30] Although the vast majority (90 to 95 percent) of breast cancer diagnoses do *not* involve inherited genetic mutations, the presence of a genetic mutation raises the risk of being diagnosed with invasive breast cancer to somewhere between 36 and 85 percent, depending on the studies consulted.[31] The presence of a BRCA alteration also signals a much higher risk of developing breast cancer at a young (premenopausal) age, and it subjects the carrier to the risk of genetic discrimination by potential employers and insurance carriers.[32] The only effective treatment option available to women with BRCA1 or BRCA2 alterations, when they were first discovered, was a double prophylactic mastectomy, an oophorectomy, or both—the same options that women with strong family histories of breast cancer had been offered for more than a century.[33] This changed in 1998.

In 1998, following the early termination of the Breast Cancer Prevention Trial (BCPT), the FDA approved the breast cancer treatment drug tamoxifen for a supplemental indication: to reduce the risk of breast cancer among cancer-free but "high risk" women.[34] For the purposes of the BCPT, which tested tamoxifen against a placebo, "high risk" was defined as having a 1.7 percent (or higher) risk of being diagnosed with breast cancer in the next five years. This number, it turned out, was the average risk of a sixty-year-old woman. The results indicated that the group of women who received tamoxifen was 49 percent less likely to develop invasive breast cancer than the control group, who received a placebo (early results and announcements indicated that the reduction was a slightly more modest 45 percent). Women taking tamoxifen were also, however, approximately twice as likely to develop endometrial cancer (cancer of the lining of the uterus), three times as likely to develop pulmonary embolisms (blood clots in the lungs), 50 percent more likely to suffer a stroke, and equally likely to die (but less likely to die from breast cancer).

The FDA's decision to approve tamoxifen for this supplemental use was controversial. Feminist cancer organizations, consumer organizations, and women's health organizations testified against the approval of tamoxifen for healthy women at the September 1998 meeting of the FDA's Oncology Drugs Advisory Committee (ODAC) and publicly criticized the FDA's decision to license the drug for use in this new patient population. Activists representing eight different women's health and breast cancer organizations urged ODAC to advise the FDA not to approve tamoxifen for use on healthy women. Only one activist recommended approval, and she acknowledged that the organization she represented was funded by the pharmaceutical industry. The other seven, who represented organizations that did not accept funding from the pharmaceutical industry, argued that the study should not have been prematurely terminated, that the results provided convincing evidence not of prevention but, rather, of short-term risk reduction, that the interim results of similar trials in Italy and the United Kingdom showed no evidence of risk reduction, and that tamoxifen's risk–benefit ratio was not sufficiently strong to warrant its use on healthy women.

AstraZeneca launched an advertising campaign following the FDA's decision to license tamoxifen for this new use. Advertisements placed in medical journals promoted this new use of tamoxifen to physicians, and direct-to-consumer advertisements in popular magazines promoted this new technology to healthy women—in part by promoting a new risk-assessment tool that women could access online. This simple, do-it-yourself risk-assessment technology—which was available on the NCI's Web site and which could be ordered for free—enabled women, with just a few clicks of the mouse, to assess their breast cancer risk and determine whether or not they qualified as "high risk" and might benefit from breast cancer chemo-prevention. The theme of AstraZeneca's advertising campaign was "There *is* something you can do."

Here too, however, AstraZeneca's efforts met with resistance and served as a lightning rod for negative publicity, heightened surveillance, consumer complaints to the Division of Drug Marketing, Advertising, and Communications (DDMAC) of the FDA, and counterattacks—all of which were launched by the women's breast/cancer movement and its organizational allies in the women's health and consumer rights movements.

One advertisement from *Parade* magazine, for example, shows a young woman from her neck down to her black lace bra. The text reads, "If you care about breast cancer, care more about being a 1.7 than a 36B." Then, directly beneath the picture: "Know your breast cancer risk assessment number. Know that NOLVADEX® (tamoxifen citrate) could reduce your chances of getting breast cancer if you are at high risk."

This ad and others like it were particularly offensive to breast cancer and women's health activists because it drew upon a superficial, stereotyped image of women's desires to be seen as sexually attractive (referring to women's presumed concern with their cup size and, perhaps, with shopping for lacy black bras?) and followed this up with the patronizing message that women should be less concerned with the number that signified their bra size and more concerned with finding out—through the "new risk assessment test"—the number that signified their risk of breast cancer. The National Women's Health Network took the lead on this issue and responded to the advertisement by recirculating it—but in a different form. Across the top of its flyer, the Network wrote in bold caps: "WHAT'S WRONG WITH THIS AD?" On the reverse side the question is posed again, followed by a list of answers, including the analysis that AstraZeneca "is trying to scare healthy women into taking a drug that is known to cause life-threatening health problems, including endometrial cancer and blood clots. Their ads won't tell you that healthy women who took Nolvadex died of pulmonary embolism during the clinical trial." The Network's response was widely circulated within the breast cancer movement.

Around this same time, BCA and its executive director, Barbara Brenner, took the lead in bringing together a group of organizations that were developing critical analyses of direct-to-consumer advertising and that shared an interest in promoting a view of public health that stressed cancer prevention through the elimination of toxic substances from the environment rather than through what they saw as a narrowly focused agenda on "risk reduction through pharmaceutical interventions"—remedies, they argued, that "are individual precautions not available to everyone." This collection of organizations became a new coalition, Prevention First. Prevention First applied for and received a two-year, $300,000 grant from the San

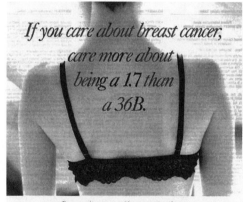

Nolvadex advertisement in *Parade* magazine, April 4, 1999.

Francisco–based Richard and Rhoda Goldman Fund, a foundation with a history of funding projects connected to breast cancer and the environment.

In October 2001 Prevention First produced a flyer, which each member organization circulated via their communication networks (inserting in newsletters, posting on their Web sites, and so on). The flyer constituted the public launching of their project against the pharmaceutical industry, and specifically against direct-to-consumer advertising of tamoxifen to healthy women. The flyer begins with a question—"Will Breast Cancer Prevention ever come in a pill?"—and supplies an answer:

> Billions of dollars are spent annually on cancer research—but the vast majority of that research is on drug development, not on prevention. Pills touted to "prevent" cancer can at best only lower the risk of developing the disease—and they often increase the risk of other health problems. True cancer prevention requires understanding and eliminating environmental causes of the disease.

The flyer goes on to name names:

> Americans are bombarded with ads for pills to "prevent" diseases like breast cancer. . . . Eli Lilly has promoted Evista® (raloxifene) for breast cancer benefits though the drug has been approved only for osteoporosis. And Astra-Zeneca, which manufactures the breast cancer drug Nolvadex® (tamoxifen), has marketed the drug to healthy women, even though it's more likely to hurt than help most of them.

The flyer asserts that drug ad campaigns such as those conducted by Eli Lilly and AstraZeneca hurt everyone by generating "misinformation" and driving up the cost of drugs, and then concludes by identifying the authors of the flyer as health organizations that maintain their independence from drug companies by refusing to accept funding from them. A 2½-inch-wide column running down the left side of the flyer, labeled "THE FACTS," makes three bulleted claims: that drug companies spend twice as much on marketing and administration as they do on research and development, that the FDA forced AstraZeneca to withdraw several ads, and that "by focusing on pills for breast cancer 'prevention,' the drug ads divert attention from the *causes* of disease."

Despite the media hype generated by the BCPT and AstraZeneca's advertising campaign, the adoption of tamoxifen by healthy high-risk women and their doctors proved remarkably anemic. Few primary care physicians demonstrated an interest in prescribing tamoxifen to healthy women, and it appears that relatively few women decided to incorporate chemoprevention into their breast health regimens.

Despite the anemic adoption of tamoxifen by healthy women, however, additional trials testing tamoxifen, raloxifene (brand name Evista), and anastrozole (brand name Arimidex) on healthy high-risk women were launched in the United States, Canada, Western Europe, and Australia. Results from the International Breast Cancer Intervention Study–I (IBIS-I), announced in 2002, showed a one-third reduction in the development of invasive breast cancer among women on tamoxifen compared to the control group. These women also, however, experienced a fourfold increase in endometrial cancer and fatal heart attacks and a threefold increase in thromboembolic events. Longer-term results released in December 2006, on the other hand, showed that the protective benefit of tamoxifen persisted after ten years, whereas the side effects and major risks ceased as soon as treatment was ended. Overall mortality, however, was slightly higher among the group of women on tamoxifen than among the women on placebo, and the effectiveness of tamoxifen was drastically reduced among women who used HRT. Results from IBIS-II, which is testing tamoxifen against anastrozole, are expected in 2010.[35] Meanwhile, results from the NIH-funded Study of Tamoxifen and Raloxifene (STAR), which was launched after the completion of the BCPT, showed that raloxifene was as effective as tamoxifen in reducing the short-term incidence of invasive breast cancer but slightly less effective in reducing the short-term incidence of ductal carcinoma in situ. Raloxifene was less likely, however, to cause life-threatening thromboembolic events, though the risk of other cancers, fractures, heart disease, and stroke was similar for both drugs.[36]

The development and promotion of these new technologies of risk assessment and risk reduction had an effect similar to that of genetic screening: It expanded the regime of breast cancer further back in time, to a place of pure risk, when breast cancer represented one of many possible futures. Like genetic screening, the use of tamoxifen for this purpose constituted a new risk domain and a new category of risky subjects. Ongoing clinical trials and the almost-certain approval of new forms of cancer chemo-prevention will undoubtedly feed this trend.

*The Anatomo-Politics of Individual Bodies*

Moving inside the clinic, there have also been a number of changes in the medical management of breast cancer in individual bodies. The growing use of sentinel node biopsies instead of axillary node dissections to help "stage" invasive breast cancer has improved the lives of thousands of women. Instead of making an incision and removing between one dozen and three dozen lymph nodes from the underarm area, only one lymph node, the "sentinel node" (or nodes) is removed and examined. The sentinel node biopsy reduces the pain and discomfort associated with an axillary (armpit) node dissection, which is a standard part of breast cancer surgery in the United States. The sentinel node biopsy also reduces the risk of long-term complications such as lymphedema, which is a painful condition of swell-ing in the arm that can be partially disabling. Estimates of the frequency of lymphedema complications vary from 5 to 20 percent of women who undergo axillary lymph node dissection.

A new class of breast cancer treatment drugs have been approved by the FDA. Unlike traditional cytotoxic chemotherapies, these drugs are designed to target and interrupt specific biological processes necessary to the growth of cancer cells. These drugs include trastuzumab (Herceptin), a new class of hormone therapies known as aromatase inhibitors (Arimidex, Aromasin, and Femara), and a new class of selective estrogen receptor modulators (SERMS). Herceptin, which is administered by infusion on an outpatient basis, was initially approved by the FDA in 1998 to treat women with meta-static breast cancer whose tumors "overexpressed" a protein called HER2. More recent studies have shown that Herceptin can also be effective in treating women with earlier-stage breast cancer whose tumors overexpress HER2. Arimidex (anastrozole), the most popular aromatase inhibitor (AI), is self-administered in pill form and is currently prescribed primarily to post-menopausal women with hormone-positive tumors who cannot tolerate tamoxifen or who have suffered a recurrence, or a new primary breast can-cer, while taking tamoxifen. Like other AIs, Arimidex helps block the growth of estrogen receptor positive tumors in postmenopausal women by lower-ing the amount of estrogen circulating in the body. These drugs have not, however, replaced surgery, radiation, or traditional chemotherapy. Rather, they are used *in addition* to these older therapeutics. They have expanded the available treatment options, but they have simultaneously expanded the range of choices, side effects, and complications.

In the estimate of many women, however, the development that has had the greatest impact on the experience of breast cancer patients is a technological innovation whose origins lie completely outside medical research and clinical practice: the rise of Internet-based support and information. During the second half of the 1990s, the proliferation of cancer Web sites, Internet mailing lists, chat boards, blogs, medical databases, and online support groups democratized access to resources, support, and information in ways previously unimaginable. The Internet dramatically transformed the way women experienced and navigated the regime of breast cancer. Let me illustrate this point with three examples.[37]

*Example 1.* When I became a volunteer at WCRC in 1994, the most popular service WCRC offered was research assistance. Women in the Bay Area visited WCRC's small library, where they searched for information in a handful of old-fashioned filing cabinets and a few bookcases. Other women phoned the WCRC hotline from around the country to ask for information. The information and referral hotline volunteer made a record of the caller's research request and passed that request along to the librarian, Margo Mercedes Rivera (now Margo Rivera-Weiss), and her small army of library volunteers. They, in turn, searched through the available books and paper files, made copies of the relevant information, put the hard copies in large envelopes, and mailed them to women across the country. There was no online access to medical databases through WCRC. There were no Web sites to consult. There were no abstracts of recent studies available at the click of a mouse. WCRC's information and referral hotline was an incredibly popular and valuable service, and it was free, but compared to the resources now available online, 24-7, at the click of a mouse in the privacy of one's own home, it was positively archaic.

*Example 2.* Shortly after I began my research in 1994, I joined one of the first breast cancer Internet mailing lists. The list, which did not restrict its membership, included women with invasive and in situ breast cancer, family members and friends of women with breast cancer, health care professionals, and various others. I lurked on this list for a period of months, receiving e-mail digests of new postings on a daily basis and posting an occasional comment or question. There was such a high volume of e-mail, however, that I withdrew from the list after a few weeks, unable to keep up.

One of the hottest topics of discussion on the list during that period was a controversy that involved one of the more active and generous contributors to the list, a man by the name of Loren Buhle, who was an assistant professor of medical physics at the University of Pennsylvania School of Medicine. The controversy, which erupted in November 1994, concerned the fate of OncoLink, an electronic cancer information service that the computer-savvy Buhle had created in March of that year. Buhle's three-year-old daughter had been diagnosed with leukemia several years earlier, and he wanted to use his computer skills and his access to cancer research and information to assist other families and individuals facing cancer. In addition to peer-reviewed research reports, the site included patient experiences and advice, support services and resources, information on alternative medicine, information on research in progress and research under review, postings from government agencies, newspaper articles, lists of clinical trials, art by children with cancer, and so on.

OncoLink grew rapidly, to around ten thousand hits per day from as many as ninety-two countries, before Buhle was ordered by the University of Pennsylvania to relinquish control of the Web site (which was run on a University of Pennsylvania server) and disciplined for posting "medically-irresponsible" materials that had not been vetted and approved by a medical advisory committee (Buhle was a Ph.D. in medical physiology, not an M.D.). The controversy sparked by Buhle's dismissal was fanned by the fledgling online community of cancer patients, family, friends, advocates, and other health care professionals, including the breast cancer Internet mailing list that I joined and to which Buhle regularly contributed. By April 1995 the controversy had made it onto the front page of the *Scientist*. "For better or for worse," wrote Franklin Hoke, "physicians' control over the information reaching patients and the public may be ebbing." "There won't be a monopoly on knowledge anymore," observed a researcher interviewed by Hoke. "It's an interesting phenomenon, the democratization of expertise."[38]

Members of the Internet list that I belonged to responded with expressions of support (for Buhle), outrage (at the University of Pennsylvania), and clear-sighted analyses of the politics of science, knowledge, and expertise. The issue, as the list members and the magazine the *Scientist* accurately noted, extended well beyond the turf wars between M.D.'s and Ph.D.'s in medical research. The controversy raised questions about the rights and responsibility of experts to control the public's access to information and, indeed, raised the question of who qualified as an expert. What about the experiential expertise of patients? What about their right to information?

I use this example to illustrate the point that as late as the mid-1990s, it was still possible for university administrators, medical researchers, and physicians to function—or to believe they could function—as gatekeepers to medical knowledge, research, and information. Clearly, their gatekeeping abilities were breaking down, but this breakdown was still being resisted by some of the most powerful and prestigious medical schools and research universities in the country. The fact that a science journalist could write, in 1995, that "physicians' control over the information reaching patients . . . *may* be ebbing" (my emphasis) indicates the phenomenal speed at which the tables turned during the second half of the 1990s. As Web sites proliferated during the second half of the 1990s and the ability to limit access to information began to evaporate, the restrictions imposed on this Internet mailing list and others were subsumed by the tidal wave of medical data and information available online to anyone who wanted it. The democratization of access to information did not, however, simplify the role of breast cancer patients or lead to a greater sense of security. In fact, quite the opposite was true, as I illustrate with one final example.

*Example 3.* At the end of 2004, one of my closest friends was diagnosed with stage 2 breast cancer. Mary, who lives in San Francisco with her long-term lover and partner Ruby, is a white, well-educated, medically savvy lesbian who was forty-three years old when she was diagnosed with breast cancer. Her diagnosis came at the end of a "normal" chain of events that included a routine screening mammogram, a "recall" round of additional mammographic images, a surgical biopsy performed by a reassuring and optimistic surgeon, and the surprising announcement that, unfortunately, the pathology report did not support the surgeon's optimism.

Next came the second opinions, and the consultations with multiple specialists, and of course the medical research. For computer-literate people with access to the Internet and a basic fluency in the languages of science and medicine, there are no natural limits to the amount of information that can be accessed and the depth and breadth of research that can be conducted. One's lover/spouse/partner, family, friends, friends of friends, and coworkers often jump right in. There are also no limits whatsoever to the conflicts, contradictions, confusions, and uncertainties yielded by unlimited access to medical databases, Web sites, and other women's experiences. Furthermore, because it is impossible to know for certain whether treatment, once completed, has been completely successful or whether any success is simply temporary (certainty is easier to achieve in the case of obvious treatment failures), every diagnosis of breast cancer launches the recipient into permanent limbo—where, if she is an information-seeking person, she will continue to research her condition and pay attention to the results of new studies for the rest of her life. There is no natural end—no temporal limit—to the confusion and the uncertainty.

Medical confusion and uncertainty were certainly not invented by the Internet, but the democratization of access to information and the ease of access for educated, middle-class women eliminated all professional, physical, social, spatial, temporal, and financial barriers to the pursuit of scientific knowledge and medical expertise. What is relatively recent is that now, at the tip of the fingers, there lies a gateway to knowledge that is constantly being regenerated and supplemented. This means that all decisions are subject to continual reassessment because the risk role never ends—not prior to, not during, and not even after treatment is completed. As the treatment options and combinations expand, the complexity of the questions and answers grows geometrically, often accompanied by declining clarity and hence by a rising uncertainty, insecurity, and a sense of permanent risk. "I'm really glad I was diagnosed 13 years ago," Barbara Brenner quipped sardonically in a recent *New York Times* article on new options in chemotherapy, "when there were fewer choices."[39]

The questions never end, nor does the pursuit of the ever-elusive answers. Do the effects of radiation ever disappear? Was chemotherapy necessary? Should I have done one without the other? One before the other? Was reducing the risk of recurrence a fair trade-off for increasing the risk of other health problems? Did chemotherapy permanently damage my mind as well as my body? Will the neuropathy ever disappear? Will I ever regain my energy? Should I take tamoxifen? Should I get an oophorectomy? Should I do both or none or one without the other? Would it help if I took tamoxifen for one year instead of five? Would that improve my odds of not having a recurrence enough to justify the added risk of taking a drug known to be a uterine carcinogen? Furthermore, new information can retroactively change the calculus of risk, confirming or calling into question previous decisions.

Joining the "remission society," in other words, does not bring the risk role or even the patient role to an end. It simply repositions the patient along the breast cancer continuum, where she is now saddled with the permanent responsibility of making choices in the face of incomplete, contradictory, and changing information, practicing "breast health," doing everything she can to lower her risk of recurrence, and feeling guilty and irresponsible if she does not. The democratization of knowledge, information, and expertise thus, paradoxically, has deepened the penetration and expanded the reach of these moralizing and individualizing discourses of risk and responsibility. After attending one meeting of a support group, Mary wrote,

> The most striking thing to me was how many of the women expressed some kind of self-recrimination, or sentiment that made it clear that they feel responsible for their cancer: because they drank wine and ate chocolate, because they were stressed, because they didn't get a bone scan, because they didn't go to yoga, because they didn't get their ovaries out, because they didn't get a mastectomy, because they weren't eating right, because they weren't taking their tamoxifen, because they didn't have the right attitude, and on and on.[40]

Thus, the process of democratization is both a burden and a blessing. The price it exacts is peace of mind and the right to view breast cancer as nothing more than a random stroke of bad luck.

Nevertheless, two years after her diagnosis, Mary's journey through breast cancer treatment was widely viewed—by Mary, her partner, her doctors, and her friends—as a success story, and given the alternatives, it probably was. Mary loves her new oncologist, who, she enthuses, views acupuncture, herbs, nutrition, and psychotherapy as integral parts of her treatment. Unfortunately, she continues to suffer from neuropathy, a side effect of Taxol, which causes neuropathic pain in her hands, which makes it difficult to write and perform daily tasks. She also suffers from post herpetic neuralgia (PHN), which was caused by an episode of shingles, which was occasioned by a weakened immune system, which was the result of chemotherapy, and which may never go away. She receives monthly injections of Lupron, a hormonal treatment, and she can look forward to a lifetime of weekly physical therapy appointments to treat her lymphedema—which was caused

by her breast cancer surgery, which included an axillary lymph node dissection, which was performed to accurately "stage" her cancer so that she
received the best possible treatment.

At the same time, as Mary wrote a little over a year ago, "I can't believe
how much respect breast cancer gets. Doctors call me back RIGHT AWAY
every time I call—even the gynecologist who has always been impossible
to see. In the past, I waited six months for a pelvic ultrasound but yesterday the doctor got me in on the same day. Drugs? Therapy groups? Visiting nurse? Dietician? Yoga classes? Anything I want. It's amazing." Her
doctor even talked to her about the benefits of marijuana for managing
nausea. "I told her," quipped Mary, "that I didn't think I would have too
much trouble with that particular aspect of the treatment regimen."[41]

In addition to the range of resources and services provided through the
health care system that Mary, who was covered by her partner's health
insurance policy, was able to access, she benefited from transformations in
the political culture and social relations of disease that were particularly pronounced in the Bay Area lesbian and gay community, where breast cancer
had joined AIDS as a top-priority health issue. In addition to her regular
support group, Mary attended a hybrid activist/support group called BAYS
(Bay Area Young Survivors). BAYS was organized by Deb Mosley and
facilitated by Merijane Block, who had been living with metastatic disease
for more than a dozen years and whose contributions to the women's cancer community bridged across many organizations.

Although neither Mary nor her partner Ruby lived near their families-
of-origin, they were part of an extensive friendship network that was quickly
mobilized, upon Mary's diagnosis, to help them through the long ordeal.
Their friends delivered home-cooked meals to their door on a rotating sched-
ule and provided massages, companionship on walks, rides to appointments,
emotional support, caring, laughter, and fun. Their support proved invalu-
able to Ruby, who had recently begun a new job with a long commute,
and to Mary, who, as noted above, developed serious side effects from the
various drugs she was prescribed: two different chemotherapy cocktails,
each prescribed over the course of several months, preceded by drug injections to increase her white blood cell count, followed by drugs to help
control her nausea so that she could eat.

Months after she finished the chemotherapy, Mary discovered on the
Internet that medical oncologists were beginning to question the wisdom

of prescribing toxic chemotherapy regimens to all eligible breast cancer patients. She also discovered that oophorectomies were frequently offered to women in Europe as an alternative to chemotherapy—a treatment option that Mary was never offered and that, in hindsight, she believes might have saved her a great deal of suffering, some of which, like the painful nerve damage to her arms and hands, might never disappear. Unlike the first few generations of women who endured chemotherapy, however, there were numerous forums available to Mary for turning her anger into action. Mary made contact with BCA and explained her interest in working on this issue, and when the *New York Times* journalist Gina Kolata wrote an article examining oncologists' changing views of chemotherapy, Mary was interviewed for the article and quoted extensively.[42] Mary's story thus reveals the extent to which, in the Bay Area regime of biomedicalization, breast cancer has increasingly become a springboard to new forms of social support, solidarity, and collective action.

*c o n c l u s i o n*

# The Body Politics of Social Movements

The language of biomedicine is never alone in the field of empowering
meanings, and its power does not flow from a consensus about symbols
and actions in the face of suffering.

—DONNA HARAWAY, "The Biopolitics of Postmodern Bodies"

At the tail end of the 1980s and the beginning of the 1990s, women with
breast cancer began marching out of medical clinics and family closets. They
were joined in this journey by hundreds of thousands of ordinary women
and men who became their supporters and allies in social change. Breast
cancer—as a politicized discourse and an anchor of new identities, networks, solidarities, and sensibilities—became the linchpin of a new social
movement. Over the course of the next decade a wide range of patient support and advocacy organizations, partnerships, and coalitions arose that
challenged and changed the regime of practices through which breast cancer had been publicly framed, institutionally managed, and subjectively
experienced. Although this was not the first time that breast cancer had
been politicized, the cultures of action that mushroomed during the 1990s
introduced onto the historical landscape a new set of social actors and agendas. The breast cancer movement quickly became—and remains—one of the
most popular and influential social movements of the last twenty-five years.

I began this book with a few simple questions: First, how and why, in
the late 1980s and early 1990s, did thousands of women with breast cancer suddenly emerge from the individualizing and "invisibilizing" architecture of the closet and reconstitute themselves as political actors? Second,
why did this movement resonate with so many women who had never faced
a diagnosis of breast cancer and most likely never would? Third, what did

this movement look like outside the rarefied field of national politicking and policy making? And finally, what might we learn about the dynamics of social movements by shifting our analytic vision from the Beltway to the Bay Area?

I argued that if we want to understand the origins and success of the breast cancer movement, instead of concentrating on state- and economy-centric theories and movement narratives of medical marginalization, we need to look carefully at the ways this disease and its involuntary subjects— a category whose occupants have changed over time—were constituted through the discourses and practices of medicine, public health, and their allied sciences. This requires, first, that we abandon state- and economy-centric theories of power by "cut[ting] off the head of the king."[1] It requires, second, that we develop new ways of theorizing the relationship between biopower—power without the king—and social movements. It requires, third, that we bring bodies more fully into the study of social movements.

Thus, in an effort to move beyond simple acts of regicide and behead-ings, I developed an alternative approach to studying this new terrain, an approach I termed "social movements without the sovereign." First, in place of the centralized, repressive state or the economy, I examined two histor-ically specific regimes of practices and the ways they shaped the social rela-tions of breast cancer; the visual, spatial, and temporal dimensions of the disease; and the bodies and embodied experiences of the involuntary sub-jects of these regimes. Second, in place of local-to-national trajectories and the Beltway activism of the National Breast Cancer Coalition (the sym-bolic head, or sovereign, of the breast cancer movement), I examined the lateral relationships and interactions among social actors in a region far removed from the political center, the Bay Area field of contention. Third, instead of examining monolithic movements and disembodied conceptu-alizations of movement culture, I disaggregated the Bay Area field of con-tention into three full-bodied COAs. Let me briefly summarize the lessons that emerged from each of these analytic moves.

BREAST CANCER IN TWO REGIMES

As I showed in part I, the first regime of breast cancer, the regime of medicalization, institutionalized the sick role, constituted women exhibit-ing the "danger signals" of breast cancer as temporarily sick and sympto-matic subjects, and subsequently reconstituted a subset of those patients as "mastectomees"—a term that referred to a type of surgery, not a collective identity. The first regime isolated women with breast cancer from each other, segregated them from the rest of society, "protected" them from knowledge of their diagnoses and prognoses, prevented them from participating in decision making about their treatment, treated them with a one-step, one-size-fits-all radical surgery, encouraged them to hide the evidence of their treatment and maintain a normal, heterofeminine appearance, and channeled them back into their precancer roles and responsibilities. Although discussions of early detection and "curative" surgery periodically appeared in health publications and women's magazines, the first regime of practices reinforced the architecture of the closet so effectively that flesh-and-blood women with breast cancer histories were invisible to the public, sometimes to members of their own families, and often to each other.

Thus, although the regime of medicalization reconstituted a subset of women as symptomatic subjects and charged them with the responsibility of seeking prompt medical attention ("Do Not Delay"), asymptomatic women were not expected to go in search of hidden signs of disease and were only loosely and superficially incorporated into the first regime of breast cancer. Thus, the regime's relatively limited reach, combined with the temporary nature of the sick role, medical-professional norms of nondisclosure, and the social invisibility, isolation, and segregation of mastectomees effectively inhibited the formation of disease-based identities, social networks, and solidarities among women with breast cancer. In fact, it is fair to say that the internal logic of the first regime effectively functioned to prevent mastectomees from knowing each other and to prevent public awareness of the existence of mastectomees in their midst.

During the 1970s and 1980s the regime of breast cancer began to change along a number of dimensions. Although mortality rates did not improve, treatment did not become more effective, and revolutionary new technologies were not invented, the changes that occurred facilitated the development of new forms of biosociality among women with breast cancer and between women with breast cancer and healthy, asymptomatic women at risk. These changes expanded the spatial and temporal boundaries of the regime of breast cancer in four different directions: outward into the asymptomatic populations, inward into territories of women's bodies not colonized by the previous regime, backward in time to the presymptomatic and precancerous stages of disease development, and forward in time via the calculation and management of risky futures. These changes were tied to the rise of a new regime, the regime of biomedicalization.

During the 1970s and 1980s the dramatic expansion of breast self-examination, clinical breast exams, and mammographic screening into populations of asymptomatic, healthy women expanded the boundaries of the disease regime and blurred the boundary between positions inside and outside of the regime. This, in turn, transformed the disease from an either-or condition to a breast cancer continuum.[2] Through screening, the regime of biomedicalization permanently incorporated asymptomatic women into the breast cancer apparatus and reconstituted them as risky subjects. In addition to the changed and charged relationship to one's body and breasts that participation in breast self-exam and mammographic screening entailed, the high recall rate and the high rate of false positive mammograms meant that a large number of cancer-free women shared the emotionally charged experience of returning to the imaging facility, having additional pictures taken, perhaps consulting with a surgeon, and perhaps undergoing a breast biopsy. In addition, the diagnosis of DCIS among asymptomatic women, as noted earlier, grew by more than 700 percent during the 1980s and 1990s. Recall that treatment for this condition is surgery, often followed by radiation and/or hormone therapy (beginning in 1998, with the approval of tamoxifen for the treatment of DCIS). The incorporation of asymptomatic women into the regime of breast cancer thus dramatically and radically changed their relationship to this disease. Encouraged to practice breast self-exam from an early age and to obtain routine mammograms beginning at age forty, a growing number of healthy, asymptomatic women with no signs of disease not only learned to *think* of breast cancer as a possible future, but *physically experienced* breast cancer surgery, radiation, and even hormone therapy as a result of their adherence to these future-oriented risk management practices.

Simultaneously, inside the clinic, treatment options for women with breast cancer multiplied, norms of nondisclosure were replaced by informed consent, and the space of patient decision making expanded. The Halsted radical mastectomy was gradually replaced by less radical surgeries, adjuvant chemotherapy and radiation therapy were added to standard treatment regimens, and the length of treatment was dramatically increased. Instead of undergoing a one-step procedure, women diagnosed with breast cancer returned over and over again for months—often for well over a

CONCLUSION                                    281

year—to be irradiated and to receive infusions of chemicals with harsh side effects. Thus, the temporal expansion of the regime was accompanied by an intensification and a spatial expansion of treatment deeper into the bodies and further into the lives of breast cancer patients. With the routinization of adjuvant therapy, the curative language of surgery was increasingly displaced by discourses of risk reduction. Finally, new rehabilitation practices emerged that, over time, helped transform the isolation and invisibility of breast cancer patients into new forms of biosociality—supportive relationships, social networks, group solidarity, and the construction of new collective identities.

The regime of biomedicalization thus expanded and deepened the circulation of power and reconstituted all women as risky subjects. The anatomopolitics of clinical medicine facilitated the development of disease-related identities, social networks, and solidarities among women with breast cancer. The biopolitics of screening created new subjectivities and sensibilities—namely, a widespread sense of risk and responsibility among healthy women who now occupied shifting positions on a breast cancer continuum. The issue of breast cancer resonated with these women because they were no longer outsiders looking in.

At the same time, my analysis privileged the subject position and experiences of white, middle-class, insured women who were diagnosed with non-metastatic breast cancer. This raises a number of important questions that I cannot answer but that I hope others will pursue. What, for example, did the regime of practices look like and how was it experienced by medically marginalized women (namely, women of color and women without insurance), by women diagnosed with advanced disease, and by women in different parts of the country? How did these different subject positions and experiences affect the emergence of new forms of biosociality? How were these forms of biosociality linked to processes of identity formation and collective action?

FIELDS OF CONTENTION

As we bring the body into the analysis of social movements and abandon top-down, disembodied, state-centric theories of power, we also need to abandon the images of social movements that grew out of those theories. Popular narratives of the breast cancer movement trace a teleology of development that begins in the local spaces of support groups and culminates in the formation of national organizations and their federal policy-making activities. Although this narrative is not untrue, it privileges one trajectory and freeze-frames one moment in a complex history. Instead of picturing social movements as pyramids with pinnacles or circles with centers, we would do better, I argue, to reenvision social movements as interacting and overlapping cultures of action operating within multiple fields of contention.

This leads to the conclusion that there is no single history of the breast/cancer movement but, rather, different *histories* of COAs and fields of contention that overlap and interact in different locations. The history of the breast/cancer movement in Washington, D.C., is not the history of the breast/cancer movement in the Bay Area, in the Boston-Cambridge area, or in New York City and Long Island—and these, in turn, are not the history of the breast/cancer movement in Dallas, Texas, or Sioux Falls, South Dakota. Likewise, the history of the breast/cancer movement in the Bay Area is not the history of the movement in the governor's office or the California State Legislature. In other words, we need to appreciate, as the saying goes, the importance of location, location, location!

Just as Beltway activism and the national arena of policy making should not be viewed as the highest expression or the most representative dimension of a given social movement, regional hot spots like the San Francisco Bay Area likewise should not be reduced to microcosms of the larger movement, smaller tributaries feeding into it, or even the "authentic grassroots." My point is not that we need to do a better job of finding representative arenas and organizations or that we need to do a better job of generalizing from part to whole or whole to part. My point is that we need to pay careful attention to context and specificity. If we do not do so, we will miss the opportunity to notice important differences and ask questions about their meaning, source, and significance.

The NBCC, for example, grew out of the nascent feminist cancer movement. Four out of seven of the founding members of the NBCC were feminist *cancer*, not *breast cancer*, organizations. Likewise, the first feminist cancer anthologies, which were published in the early 1990s, did not privilege the voices and perspectives of women with breast cancer above those of women with other types of cancer.[3] That the movement narrowed around breast cancer in the national arena is thus something to be examined and explained, not overlooked or assumed. Likewise, the fact that the Bay Area movement did *not* narrow to the same degree or with the same degree of rigidity is a fact worth explaining. The explanation of these differences, as my analysis suggests, can be found through an examination of the different actors and relationships that shaped and were shaped by the COAs and fields of contention in each location.

Reconceptualizing social movements as overlapping and interacting COAs operating in distinct fields of contention also makes it easier to discern the *interpenetration* of social movements by the state, private corporations, and philanthropic organizations. This interpenetration does not look the same, however, in different fields of contention, at different moments in time, or in different cultures of action. Sometimes public agencies and private firms function as collaborators and participants; sometimes they are the targets and antagonists. Likewise, philanthropic foundations and charitable organizations can be key movers and shakers in the development of social movements, playing different roles in different cultures of action. Traditional notions of co-optation, outsiders versus insiders, and "the state" versus "the social movement" are wholly incapable of unpacking this complexity. The boundaries of social movements—just like the boundaries of disease—are sometimes narrow and rigid, sometimes expansive and uncertain. There is a great deal about these differences and transformations that we have yet to explore. This book barely begins to scratch the surface.

When I began my fieldwork in 1994, the Bay Area was a "fragmented" field of contention (to return to Raka Ray's typology)—a field in which power is relatively widely dispersed and political culture is heterogeneous. This dispersal and heterogeneity prevented any one organization or network of organizations from dominating the field, enforcing one set of boundaries, or supporting one and only one COA. Over the course of my fieldwork, the fragments crystallized into three COAs. This alignment of fragments increased their effectiveness without compromising the diversity of the field. The enduring dynamism of the Bay Area field of contention, I suspect, is due in no small measure to the heterogeneity and hybridity of the field, as well as to the fluidity and fuzziness of its boundaries.

In contrast, the Washington D.C.–based breast cancer movement in which the NBCC acted was what Ray terms a "hegemonic" field—a field in which power is concentrated among a relatively small number of players who share a common understanding of the field's boundaries and rules of engagement. The NBCC grew ever more powerful over the years within the field of national policy making. The Susan G. Komen Foundation was the only women's cancer organization with the infrastructure, resources, and reputation to compete with the NBCC in the Washington, D.C., field of contention.

Since the late 1990s, there has been a great deal of fretting (in some quarters), relief (in others), and speculation (in the media) that the breast cancer movement is in decline, if not already dying. This, I believe, is a profound misreading of the tea leaves. At the level of national policy making it *may* be the case (though it is far from certain) that the NBCC has declined somewhat in power and lost some of its momentum (due in no small measure to its success). This is not true, however, of the Susan G. Komen Foundation, whose Race for the Cure events continue to draw millions and whose corporate contributors now compete for the privilege of becoming "official sponsors" of their events. The Komen Foundation is composed of more than one hundred local affiliates. In many parts of the country, the Komen Foundation *is* the breast cancer movement, and it is not declining.[4] Likewise, the COAs that operate within the Bay Area field of contention have by no means declined or lost momentum—in fact, quite the contrary.

The larger point is that the definition of movement boundaries is the outcome of political struggles and negotiations that take place in specific fields of contention. The outcomes of these struggles are not necessarily the same across fields, and there is no reason to believe that these boundaries, once established, are fixed. In the San Francisco Bay Area, as we know, this collapse around breast cancer did not happen in the same way or to the same degree as it did in the Washington, D.C., field of contention. Even as Beltway activism narrowed around breast cancer, the Bay Area field of contention sustained a productive tension among breast cancer–specific organizations, women's cancer organizations, and environmental health organizations. In the Bay Area, as we know, three COAs, not one, congealed.

## CULTURES OF ACTION

The Bay Area movement did not, of course, invent itself out of whole cloth. It flourished in part because it was able draw upon the political discourses, material resources, social networks, solidarities, and collective identities of preexisting social movements. The Bay Area movement thus directly benefited from the common phenomenon of "social movement spillover."[5] One of the most important sources of this spillover was the AIDS movement. First, the success of AIDS activists' appeals to federal legislators, funders, and regulatory agencies was used by breast cancer activists as evidence of the government's neglect of women's diseases like breast cancer. Because AIDS was implicitly coded as a men's disease, breast cancer activists were able to argue that their disease deserved an equal measure of public compassion and an equal level of political commitment to addressing it.[6] In addition to the framing opportunities that the AIDS movement offered to savvy breast cancer activists, breast cancer activists also benefited from the practical knowledge, networks, and experience of AIDS activists. In the Bay Area, for example, activists from ACT UP Golden Gate taught members of Breast Cancer Action how various agencies worked and helped them organize a protest against Genentech to gain access to the then experimental drug Herceptin.

In addition to the AIDS movement, the Bay Area breast/cancer movement was fed by the long tradition of civic engagement and volunteerism that the American Cancer Society and other major health voluntaries had relied upon and promoted throughout the twentieth century. The Bay Area breast/cancer movement was also fed by the women's health movement, the lesbian community, and the widespread diffusion of feminist identities, feminist organizations, and feminist convictions that "the personal is political" and that women's oppression often takes the form of the domination and control of women's bodies.[7] Finally, the Bay Area breast/cancer movement was fed by the environmental movement as a whole, and by the environmental justice and environmental health movements in particular.[8]

In addition, the breast/cancer movement flourished in the Bay Area because it was made up of different COAs that effectively channeled this spillover and competed, cooperated, and clashed in ways that fed the movement's dynamism and visibility. The first, the culture of early detection, expanded the biopolitics of screening into medically marginalized communities, privileged the identity of breast cancer survivor, and blurred the boundaries between the state, private industry, civic organizations, and social movements. The second, the culture of patient empowerment, privileged the voices of women living with cancer and provided them with information, support, practical services, and community. In addition, this COA pressured the state, public health and medical researchers, the health care industry, the pharmaceutical industry, the cosmetics industries, corporations that engaged in cause-related marketing, and other breast/cancer organizations to more effectively address the needs of women living with this disease. The third, the culture of cancer prevention, was the outcome of a synthesis between feminist breast/cancer activism and the environmental movement. This COA privileged the voices of cancer victims and members of contaminated communities, drew attention to the cancer industry, and organized various campaigns to reduce the level of carcinogens and other toxic substances in communities, consumer products, and industrial processes.

These COAs mobilized different emotions, privileged different identities, constructed different relationships to heteronormative femininity, and developed different responses to racial, ethnic, and class inequalities. They also maintained different relationships to science and medicine, authority and expertise, private industry, other social movements, the state, and even global capitalism. In my analysis of these three COAs, I emphasized their public faces and emotions, their points of contact and intersection, and the centrality of bodies—not only as sites for the inscription of power and sources of suffering but as the material anchors of new collective identities and communities and the visual signifiers of new political agendas.

The combination of conflict and cooperation between these three COAs is vividly expressed in the poem "Alive/To Testify," which was written by Bay Area activist Wanna G. Wright. Wright was an eighteen-year survivor of breast and cervical cancer when she composed this poem in 1997. She was also a health educator in a screening outreach project funded by the National Cancer Institute, a member of the board of directors of the Women's Cancer Resource Center, a peer reviewer for the Department of Defense's breast cancer research program, and the leader of an African American task force connected to a local breast cancer partnership. In short, Wright was an activist who wore many hats and moved with fluidity within the Bay Area field of contention.

Wright explained that "Alive/To Testify" was inspired by a retreat for low-income women with cancer that was organized by the Charlotte Maxwell Complementary Clinic. According to Wright, one of the guest speakers, a leader in the Bay Area movement, "talked about pink ribbons being mere fluff, a distraction from the real solutions to the breast cancer epidemic," and carried a banner that read, "'We can't afford to save one life at a time.'" "Although I agree with [her] in principle," Wright explained, "the lives of low-income women have to be saved one at a time and pink ribbons provide a soft reminder of how precious each of their lives are."[9]

## Alive/To Testify

I's got to reach out to keep 'em alive
din you can teach 'em to testify
'bout de air an de waters
dat's killin us daughtus'.

So pleas don't dis me caus my ribbon's pink
I wears it to make my sista's think
bout breakin' down barriers, bout choosin life
bout early detection—maybe even da knife.

We got problems you don't know
we shedin layers, we tryin to grow
to trust—to believe—to claim our power
to save lives lost hour after hour.

We hafta save lives one at a time
we's got to catch up—we's behind
so save us a place, we's on our way
gettin stronga ev'ry day by day.

We's making it known, makin it unda-stood
soon no toxins/Dioxins a-llowed in da Hood
but first we's got to stay alive—
din we will stand—(wid you) to testify.

This poem, and Wright's accompanying comments, offer a richly textured view of the different body politics and emotion cultures in the Bay Area field of contention and of the way those differences were played out in the ongoing tension over the symbolism and significance of pink ribbons.

These differences cannot be disentangled from the long history of racially stratified (bio)medicalization that runs through both regimes of breast cancer. This poem, Wright's contextualizing comments, and Wright's own history within the breast/cancer movement reveal the mutual shaping and interaction between COAs, as well as the flow of people, resources, discourses, and information within the Bay Area field of contention. Although the poem's narrator positions herself within the culture of screening activism, it is clear that she is also responding to and engaging with the cultures of feminist and environmental activism.

As a work of art, the poem traveled far and wide within the Bay Area field of contention. Thus, "Alive/To Testify" not only served as a window onto the local field of contention, it also acted within it. For example, it was publicly read and reprinted in multiple venues and publications. As a cultural object, and product, of the Bay Area field of contention, Wright's poem gave voice to and helped shape the local contours of breast cancer in the Bay Area.[10]

This leads me to a final point, which is that the production of culture was not separate from or subsidiary to the "real" work of the movement. Rather, the real work of the movement was, from the beginning, bound up in the construction and diffusion of new visual images, collective identities, emotional vocabularies, and forms of embodiment—new ways of being risky subjects and cancer patients within the regime of biomedicalization.[11] These new meanings were encoded in new policies and legislation, enacted through new kinds of lay–expert collaborations, and inscribed on the bodies of breast cancer survivors and women living with cancer. They were also encoded in films, photographs, drawings, paintings, performances, poetry, and other forms of writing and artistic expression. The spirit of the movement lived, as Clara Larson's story demonstrates, in the ability of a "Cancer Sucks" button to capture and nourish an otherwise suppressed sensibility.

Last but not least: In the final, concluding section, I want to extend outward from the case of breast cancer to the larger terrain of bodies, disease regimes, and social movements.

## BODIES, DISEASE REGIMES, AND SOCIAL MOVEMENTS

Bodies are both a product of and a mediating link between the practices of power, the construction of historical subjects, and the formation of collective identities, solidarities, and social movements. Social movements may not have heads, as I have argued, but they do have bodies, and in the case of health- and disease-based activism, they have bodies that are medicalized, bodies that are marginalized, bodies that are "riskified," bodies that are socialized, and bodies that are stigmatized, as well as bodies that fear, bodies that suffer, bodies that shock, bodies that inspire, bodies that hope, bodies that desire, bodies that emote, bodies that signify, bodies that resist, bodies that suffer, and bodies that expire.

Although bodies are a part of every social movement, movements that explicitly foreground the body have multiplied exponentially during the last several decades. Embodied social movements include the black power movement, the women's liberation movement, the lesbian and gay movement, the transgender movement, body modification movements, and the multiracial movement. Embodied social movements also include a wide variety of health-, disability-, and disease-based social movements, such as the antipsychiatry movement, the patients rights movement, the women's health movement, the disability rights movement, the reproductive rights/anti-abortion movement, the environmental health movement, the AIDS movement, and many others.[12]

These embodied health movements range from mass-participation mobilizations that draw tens of thousands of supporters to their public events (like the breast cancer movement) to self-help movements that consist of a handful of Web sites and Web-based organizations that provide information, support, and advice to people suffering from different illnesses and genetic risks. Although largely ignored by political process theorists, health- and disease-based social movements have become increasingly central to the efforts of medical sociologists and other scholars of science, medicine, and technology to understand the ongoing transformation of bodies, biomedicine, and health care, on the one hand, and our experiences of health, risk, disability, illness, and disease, on the other.[13]

It is by now abundantly clear that biomedicine has become one of the most powerful languages for managing and expressing forms of suffering and social distress of an almost-endless variety. Increasingly, however, instead of inscribing bodies as healthy or diseased and constituting temporarily sick and symptomatic subjects, the authoritative institutions of science, medicine, and public health inscribe bodies through the discourses and practices of risk reduction and its doppelgänger, health promotion. The United States and many other wealthy Western democracies have become nations of risky subjects who occupy shifting positions on numerous disease continuums that extend, on both ends, well beyond the territory of identifiable disease and into the prehistory and posthistory of diagnosis and treatment—that is, into the terrain of pure risk. The diagnostic parameters of many diseases are unfixed, unstable, and, as we are learning, increasingly subject to contestation by the voluntarily and involuntarily incorporated subjects of disease regimes—pharmaceutical companies, physicians and other health care professionals, insurance companies and managed care organizations, people at risk, people in treatment, and members of the remission society. They are also, however, contested by people who suffer from illnesses and disease conditions that are not fully recognized or legitimized by the medical establishment, employers, government agencies (which administer Social Security and disability benefits programs), or the insurance and health care industries—people who suffer from chronic fatigue syndrome, fibromyalgia, sick-building syndrome, chemical sensitivity, Gulf War syndrome, and many other illnesses believed to be of environmental origin.

The concept of disease regimes can help map the shifting relationship between the practices of public health and biomedicine and the proliferation of social movements led by "diseased," "disabled," "deviant," "sick," and "risky" subjects. I focus on the practices through which individual bodies and populations are medically managed and publicly administered not because they are the only practices that matter but because they are the practices that have passed under the radar, the practices whose significance has largely gone unrecognized.

At the same time that we draw on Foucault's insights about bodies, biopower, and regimes of practices, however, we need to maintain a critical perspective. Biopower is portrayed by Foucault in overly totalizing and individualizing terms. Yet, paradoxically, Foucault also claims that "where there is power there is resistance." He is wrong on all counts. Power is rarely totalizing; it is not necessarily individualizing; and it is pure folly to claim that it always elicits resistance. At times it does. At times it does not. The trick is figuring out which practices of power foreclose collective forms of resistance and which facilitate them. To do so, we need to study biopower within specific regimes of practices. The concept of disease regimes, not biopower writ large, is thus a more useful approach to mapping the relationships among bodies, biopower, and social movements.

Some disease regimes are relatively (though never absolutely) totalizing, others are less so. Some regimes are deeply anchored in multiple institutions. Others are less expansive. Although they are relatively structured and stable, disease regimes inevitably change over time because they are subject to a wide variety of overlapping and crosscutting pressures. Some of these pressures originate within the powerful industries, institutions, and professions in which disease regimes are anchored—the health care, insurance, and pharmaceutical industries, for example, as well as the institutions of science, public health, biomedicine, and the state. Others originate in sectors and professions that have been displaced or excluded—folk medicine, alternative treatment modalities, unorthodox science, and non-Western epistemologies of health, disease, and the body. Still others originate among the involuntary subjects of disease regimes—the individuals and small groups who contest specific practices, as well as the multiorganizational fields of contention and differentiated COAs that are the flesh and blood of social movements. The relationship between disease regimes and social movements thus is never fixed because, as we have seen, disease regimes can both inhibit and enable the development of social movements.

At the same time, we need to remember that disease regimes never penetrate equally everywhere, nor do they generate uniform experiences of disease. The stratified history of (bio)medicalization maps onto stratified histories of gender, race, class, and sexuality. These forms of differentiation and inequality result in significant variations in the ways subjects are incorporated into and constituted within different disease regimes. Finally, we need to remember that although bodies are shaped by the humanly created technologies of science, public health, and medicine, they are also shaped by the biological character of disease and its manifestations within individual bodies. The body is a site for the inscription of power, but it is also a site of organic suffering that preexists and can never be wholly constituted or controlled by this, or any other, regime of practices.

Finally, if we expand further outward, the concept of regimes of practices holds a great deal of promise, I believe, for studying a wide range of social movements that are *not* directly connected to health, disability, or disease. Because the concept of regimes of practices does not limit the relevant practices to specific institutions, it can help social movement scholars move beyond unproductive discussions about the role and relative contributions of different institutions. The concept of regimes of practices shifts the focus from specific institutions (namely the state) to the multi-institutional practices that manage and discipline the bodies of individual subjects and coordinate, control, and administer large populations, the body politic. It also shifts the focus from formal policies to the actual practices through which they are implemented and experienced by individual subjects and subject populations. Using this approach, we might, for example, examine the relationship between parent-led education-reform movements and the regimes of practices through which parents are constituted as subjects who are expected to participate in their children's education. Likewise, we could examine the relationship between a religious movement and the practices through which members of that religion are constituted as religious subjects, or we could compare religious-reform movements in two different places by examining differences in the regimes of practices from which they emerged and to which they respond. These are just two possibilities. There are many others.

## THE BODY POLITICS OF SOCIAL MOVEMENTS

This book began with a description of RavenLight marching in the San Francisco Lesbian-Gay-Bisexual-Transgender Pride Parade, and it is to that image we now return. I have often wondered why that image affected me so profoundly. Why did it permanently embed itself in my heart and my mind's eye? Was my response typical or idiosyncratic?

My response, I now know, was neither typical nor idiosyncratic. The groundswell of support for RavenLight at the 1993 parade and subsequent parades made it clear that I was not alone. Yet the reactions of many women I met over the years made it equally clear that the reaction of the man standing next to me was not unique. Although he expressed his resentment and disgust in a much more obnoxious manner than most, he was not alone in these sentiments. RavenLight inspired some women to disrobe and others to turn away in horror and disgust. Some believed that RavenLight's body politics were effective. Others believed they were counterproductive. Some felt liberated by her public performances. Others felt exposed and ashamed.

The same range of reactions was apparent, as well, in the outpouring of letters to the editor following the publication of the image of one-breasted Matuschka on the cover of the *New York Times Magazine* (previously discussed). Most of the letters, Matuschka later wrote, were "full of praise." One woman wrote that it was "like finding a fellow human on the backside of the moon." Another simply wrote, "Fantastic! A cover girl who looks like me!"[14]

There were also negative responses, however, and they fell into two categories. One group of women, as Matuschka described it, "spoke of feeling that their privacy had been violated. They said that the ability to see themselves as 'normal' was essential to their self-esteem, and they accused me and the *Times* of having run the photo only for shock value." Another group of women, Matuschka revealed, "worried that the photograph would prevent women from getting their breasts checked or from going for mammograms out of a fear that they would end up with a chest like mine."[15]

I recently discovered that the body politics of breast cancer activism, despite its controversial nature, has seeped into the marketing campaigns of pharmaceutical corporations. While waiting in line at a grocery store, thumbing through an issue of *Good Housekeeping*, I came across a three-page advertisement for Aloxi, an antinausea drug prescribed to cancer patients undergoing chemotherapy. An image of a bald woman in her fifties or sixties, looking squarely into the camera, dominated one full page of the advertisement. She looked simultaneously powerful, vulnerable, calm, and determined. Later that same night, I watched a television commercial whose pharmaceutical sponsors chose a bald woman to visually represent the company's commitment to cancer patients, on the one hand, and to promote cancer patients' consumption of their cancer-fighting drugs, on the other. The woman in the television commercial appeared to be relatively young (in her late twenties or early thirties), healthy, self-confident, and full of verve. This commercial was part of a larger "Bald is beautiful" direct-to-consumer campaign launched by the pharmaceutical company.

There are many ways to interpret these advertisements. One could view them as evidence of the pharmaceutical industry's co-optation or dilution of politically provocative images that were originally wielded by breast cancer activists to shock and educate the public about the true face, the true embodiment of breast cancer. This interpretation, however, would miss the larger point. An important part of the cultural work performed by health-, disability-, and disease-based social movements is, first, the creation of new public images and forms of embodiment, and second, the diffusion of these images and forms of embodiment. One of the most important accomplishments of the breast cancer movement, in my view, has been its remarkable success in changing the culture of breast cancer so that women diagnosed with this disease no longer believe that their only option is silence, shame, and concealment, and they no longer believe that public disclosure will inevitably lead to their stigmatization. The diffusion of these new images and corporeal styles into pharmaceutical advertisements is a sign of the breast cancer movement's success in reshaping the public sensibilities and the visual practices of the regime of breast cancer. If it is a sign of co-optation, the arrow points in the opposite direction. In this case, the movement has co-opted the visual vocabulary of pharmaceutical advertising. The invention of a new visual vocabulary, in turn, shapes the social relations and cultural meaning of the disease. In addition, visual vocabularies offer an important resource for the development of new risk- and disease-based identities, solidarities, and sensibilities.

This tension between the politics of respectability and the politics of provocation is a tension that runs through every movement of politically disempowered people whose forms of embodiment and behavior are socially stigmatized and disparaged. This tension runs through the civil rights and black power movements, the women's and women's health movements, the movements of sexual minorities, the mental health movement, the disability rights movement, the reproductive rights movement, the AIDS movement, the breast cancer movement, and many other smaller-scale mobilizations of illness sufferers and people at risk. We often seem to forget, however, that the flip side of the politics of provocation is often a politics of beauty and bodily reclamation. RavenLight and Matuschka, for example, did not simply provoke strong reactions, although they certainly did do that. They also strove to create new images of beauty and sexuality, new ways of living in one-breasted bodies. They were not the first to do so, but they were among the first to do so as part of a broad-based movement that, during the 1990s, reshaped the cultural contours of disease.

As one millennium came to a close and another began, Jon Carroll, a journalist at the *San Francisco Chronicle,* published a column entitled "The Image of the Century."[16] In this, his "millennial" column, Carroll described an experience that occurred "about a half a decade ago," when he was volunteering as a safety monitor for the Lesbian-Gay-Bisexual-Transgender Pride Parade. "A single woman marched down the middle of Market Street," wrote Carroll. "She was bare to the waist. She had a mastectomy scar. She did not (in my memory at least) carry any sign or provide any instructions on how to view her presence—she was testifying on her own terms. . . . I do not know her name, [but] I have thought of her often. . . . The more I remembered her . . . the more I decided that she had to be, for me, the image of the century."

Carroll's reaction to RavenLight was eerily similar to my own when he wrote, "I cannot pretend to understand the psychological impact of all this. . . . Words do not convey that much. . . . I can understand the issue in a dry political or social sense, [but] that's as far as my brain takes me. . . . And that is why . . . that single image keeps coming back. It transcends reason and speaks to the heart. That marching woman, head up, eyes bright, her lips an enigmatic line—she speaks candidly about the reality of pain and loss, and she says also: I am a woman. I am real. I am your mother or your daughter. Deal with me. Love me. I am among you now. I always have been."

# Multisited Ethnography and the Extended Case Method

Ethnography is the only social scientific method that relies upon the observation of people, power, and processes in their "natural setting"—that is to say, in the time, space, and contexts in which human beings live their lives. The technique of participant observation, in the words of Michael Burawoy, involves studying people "in their corporeal reality, in their concrete existence, in *their* space and time"—entering into the social worlds and relationships in which they are embedded and in which they act in order to develop grounded insights, understanding, and explanation.[1] Formal interviews can provide additional insight and information, but even the most free-flowing interview is at least partially prescribed and decontextualized. As sociologist Millie Thayer recently observed in an essay on the use of ethnographic methods for studying social movements: "Though ethnographers often complement their work with other methods, their particular contribution is an understanding of how power is embedded and contested in relationships, how subjectivities are constructed and resisted, and how collective meanings are imposed and reinvented."[2]

Traditional ethnography, such as was practiced by North American and European anthropologists studying preliterate, non-European societies, positioned the participant-observer as a neutral, objective, detached outsider. Many contemporary ethnographers, however, have abandoned these earlier modes of ethnographic inquiry. My research strategy—and I think it was more intuitive than deliberate—was one of multisited participant observation and emotional engagement. In retrospect, I do not think it ever occurred to me to strive for distance or to even attempt a stance of objectivity, and in many respects I probably erred more on the side of participation than observation. As a result of this style of participant observation, however, the experiential, relational, emotional, and physical dimensions of my research served as a central source of my own meaning-making practices and understanding. In my view, this is what is unique about ethnographic research, and it should not be shied away from or minimized.

There are, to my mind, three additional qualities that make multisited ethnography the ideal approach for studying social processes of all kinds and social movements in particular. First, ethnography does not depend upon the momentary "capture" of prespecified data but relies, instead, on the ongoing process of observation, interpretation, and engagement—what Burawoy terms the "extension of observations over time and space."[3] Instead of preconstituting the terms of discourse and limiting in advance the data that will be counted and collected, long-term ethnographic research provides an opportunity to reject, rethink, amend, and reshape one's analysis. Other methods allow this, but only ethnographic research (at least the style of ethnographic research that I was taught) demands it. It was the ongoing process of questioning and exploration over an extended period of time (in my case, more than four years) that allowed me to try different ideas and interpretations and discard the ones that did not fit. This would have been a very different book if I had written it after three months or six months or even two years of fieldwork.

Second, it was not ethnography alone, but roving, *multisited ethnography* that allowed me to develop the analysis set forth in this book.[4] If I had decided in advance what the breast cancer movement was and then systematically gone about interviewing representatives from key breast cancer organizations, I would never have discovered that the boundaries of the movement are unstable, uncertain, and contested. It was only by following the intertwining threads of cancer activism and the women's cancer community across and within different sites that I began to recognize the distinctiveness of the Bay Area field of contention and to conceptualize the Bay Area movement in terms of three overlapping cultures of action. Likewise, if I had stopped after observing one breast cancer support group, I would never have learned to ask new questions and listen differently. Thus, the study of dynamic and emergent social formations is best served, in my view, by multisited ethnographic modes of inquiry.

Third, the process of turning ethnographic research into field notes and

turning field notes into a public (and publishable) narrative forces the ethnographer who possesses even a modicum of self-awareness and humility
to directly confront the partial, situated, "non-innocent," and deeply constructed nature of the stories one crafts and the knowledge claims one
makes—and this, I believe, is a good thing, both ethically and intellectually.[5]
What I found most exciting, daunting, and humbling about ethnographic
storytelling was the multiplicity of stories that I could have constructed in
the service of very different arguments and agendas. I firmly believe that I
could have written a dozen different books from the research I conducted,
and each one of them would have been empirically and interpretively
sound and defensible. The ethnographic field, after all, does not speak for
itself, and it does not speak in one voice. It must be shaped into "true," insightful, and empirically sound accounts, and there is no inherent limit on
the number of accounts that ethnographic analyses of the field can yield.

Although the multivocality of ethnographic data is acknowledged in
some quarters, ethnographers tend to minimize the interpretive flexibility
and instability of their fieldwork when it comes to professional publications. This interpretive instability and flexibility, we fear, will undermine
our status and claims as social scientists. This strikes me as an unhelpful
and unnecessary professional fiction. We know from the burgeoning field
of science studies, for example, that even the experimental subjects, objects,
and processes on which laboratory scientists fix their gaze are inherently
unstable and that much of the practical knowledge of scientists consists of
learning techniques to stabilize their experiments and standardize their
interpretive lenses. If the objects and data of the laboratory sciences are
unstable, is there any reason to pretend otherwise with ethnographic fieldwork? Ethnographic data are inherently unstable. Instead of resisting this
reality by forcing sociological data into immutable forms, I propose that
we come to terms with the permanent messiness of the material we work
with. Ethnographers know this better than anyone, so why play along with
the professional fiction? My body of ethnographic data shape-shifts when
I look for different things, it morphs as my thinking changes, and it is further transformed when I craft different stories for different audiences. The
more stable the body of data, in my view, the greater its distance from the
unstable realities of the social world—and the greater the researcher's self-
delusion and distance from the sources of scientific creativity.

If we think of participant observation or ethnographic research as a technique for gathering data, we might think of scientific methodology as a theory of the relationship between techniques for gathering data and the production of knowledge. Different methodologies are based on different theories of knowledge production. The methodology that informed the data gathering and knowledge production of this book is known as the *extended case method.*

## THE EXTENDED CASE METHOD

The extended case method, as elaborated by Michael Burawoy, is based upon a reflexive model of science that attempts to steer a course midway between positivist science and postmodern nihilism.[6] Unlike positivist methods, reflexive science embraces and seeks to take advantage of the inevitably and undeniably partial, situated, biased, interactive, and social nature of data collection and knowledge production. Unlike postmodernist methods, reflexive science is not willing to relinquish its scientific status.

The extended case method, in Burawoy's vision, is the quintessential model of reflexive science. It is a recursive model that involves a constant movement back and forth along two axes. Movement along the first axis demands repeated excursions into the ethnographic field—her primary object of study and source of data. Movement along the second axis demands repeated excursions into the academic field—the field of scholarship and social theory. The extended case method thus consists of a dance with two steps that repeat ad infinitum until the music stops or the dancer tires. First, the extended case method compels the social scientist to choose a popular or compelling theory, any theory, to help focus her attention on something in the ethnographic field. Second, the extended case method compels the ethnographer to use her experiences in the field to complicate, challenge, extend, improve, reject, or rework the chosen theory. The ethnographer who chooses to reject her chosen theory, however, goes back to the drawing board and begins again with another theory. The point is that theory building and fieldwork are coconstitutive. Each shapes the other, and each is altered and transformed in the process of writing. Thus, unlike many research methods in which the theory (in theory) emerges from the data and the analysis of data does not begin until all the data have been gathered, the extended case method requires ethnographers to begin with a theory and continuously analyze their data as they go.

Thus, ethnographers working with the extended case method make no pretense of approaching the field as a blank slate, without preconceptions, without guiding questions, without concepts and theories that shape what they see and know and how they see and know it. They know they approach the field full of ideas, biases, preconceptions, preexisting commitments, and personal ambitions. Knowing this, they try to make explicit the concepts, theories, questions, assumptions, commitments, and ambitions that they carry with them into the field. "As social scientists we are conventionally taught to rid ourselves of our biases, suspend our judgments so that we can see the field for what it is," writes Burawoy. "We cannot see the field, however, without a lens, and we can only improve the lens by experimenting with it in the world."[7] Only by making the lenses—the theories—explicit can the ethnographer productively examine, challenge, rethink, and sometimes abandon them, only to start all over again with new theories to examine, challenge, rework, rebuild, and extend.

Finally, the extended case method requires that ethnographers locate the ethnographic field by "extending out from micro processes to macro forces, from the space-time rhythms of the site to the geographical and historical context of the field."[8] Traditional ethnography restricts its focus to micro and ahistorical sociology, as Burawoy argues, but the extended case method "bursts the conventional limits of participant observation" by insisting that the ethnographic field be grounded in a larger story about history and structural forces, but one that is spatially located and grounded geographically.[9]

Let me explain how this process played out during my four years of ethnographic research in the San Francisco Bay area. In 1994 I embarked upon an ethnographic study of breast cancer activism in the Bay Area. I began my fieldwork in two places: a breast cancer support group and the Women's Cancer Resource Center. Over the course of the next few years one support group grew into four, and one organization grew into a larger field of contention. I explore each of these trajectories in the sections that follow.

## WOMEN'S CANCER SUPPORT GROUPS: THE INVISIBLE POLE OF THE MOVEMENT

There were a number of reasons that motivated my desire to observe women's cancer support groups. First, I read in journalists' and activists' accounts that support groups had played an important role in the emergence of the breast cancer movement. Second, I knew that the Women's Cancer

Resource Center and Breast Cancer Action had originated in the social networks and friendships forged in support groups. Third, I knew that cancer support groups were proliferating in Bay Area hospitals and health care
facilities.

Based on these factors, it seemed reasonable to assume that support groups
were functioning as what social movement theorist Alberto Melucci had
termed the "invisible pole" of social movements. In Melucci's view the "invisible pole," or "latency structure," of social movements is a honeycomb
of protected enclaves where new identities and interpretive schemata are
formed and nurtured. It is these new identities and schemata, in turn, that
feed the "visible pole" of collective action.[10] Black churches, for example,
fed the civil rights movement, gay bars fed the gay liberation movement,
and consciousness-raising groups fed the women's liberation movement
and second-wave feminism.[11] Following this logic, it seemed likely that an
analogy could be drawn, for example, between the role that consciousness-
raising groups played in the women's liberation movement and the role
that support groups were playing in the breast cancer movement.

At the same time, however, there were good reasons for questioning the
assumption that cancer support groups were necessarily spaces of politicization, or even latency structures feeding the more visible forms of collective
action. First, in the sociological literature, case studies of medicalization
painted a uniformly bleak picture of the dominating, individualizing, and
depoliticizing effects of medicine. The women's health movement of the
1960s and 1970s was, after all, a movement against medical domination—
a movement, in many respects, against medicalization.

Second, support groups were a highly gendered type of self-help, and at
the time I began my fieldwork, many feminists viewed self-help with suspicion. Some feminists argued, for example, that the self-help movement and
"therapeutic feminism" were forces of depoliticization and individualization.
Self-help, according to this logic, had diluted and demobilized the social
change agenda of the women's movement and second-wave feminism.[12]

Third, the main source of growth in support groups, when I began my
fieldwork, was the health care industry, not the autonomous, largely feminist spaces of grassroots organizations. Following this logic, then, it seemed
equally plausible to me that the proliferation of support groups created by
the health care industry might be serving more of a medical than a social
or political function. Were support groups, then, an instance of medical

domination? Were medicalized support groups diluting and demobilizing the breast cancer movement?

These, then, were the ideas that I was grappling with when I began observing women's cancer support groups. I wanted to know whether support groups were spaces of therapeutic domination, medicalization, and depoliticization or whether, instead, they were spaces that fostered resistance to the individualizing, authoritative discourses and practices of biomedicine. Were they strengthening or disrupting the architecture of the closet? Did they encourage or inhibit the development of disease-based identities? Were they "rehabilitating" patients and returning them to their predisease statuses and identities (as the Parsonian sick role would have it), or were they feeding them into the organizations and activities of the breast cancer movement?

The first breast cancer support group I attended was a professionally led group held at a private, for-profit hospital. I knew next to nothing about the medical dimensions of breast cancer when I began attending this group. More revealing—and embarrassing—is the fact that it never *occurred* to me that my ignorance might be a problem. The reason it never occurred to me, however, was that I viewed the medical details of treatment discussed by support group participants essentially as "background noise" to the question motivating my research: What was the relationship between support groups and the breast cancer movement?

As I quickly discovered, however, I could understand very little of what the women in the support group were saying. I wrote down the barrage of medical terms and procedures that I found baffling, and my friend Dee, whom I accompanied to the group, translated the comments and terms for me afterward. This worked pretty well as a temporary solution, but it was clear that if I wanted to understand what was going on in breast cancer support groups, I would need to become more fluent in this foreign language.

Because of my inability to understand what the women in the support group were saying, I began reading the popular literature written for women with breast cancer, including Rose Kushner's *Why Me? What Every Woman Should Know about Breast Cancer* (1977) and *Dr. Susan Love's Breast Book* (1991), both of which I borrowed from the library of WCRC. I still, at this point, was not particularly interested in medical practices, technologies, or procedures, and I certainly was not interested in their history (why would a sociologist care about that?); I simply wanted to be able to follow the flow of conversation in the support group meetings so that I could construct a coherent narrative. To put a fine point on it, I did not attend support groups to learn about women's experiences of breast cancer per se. Rather, I attended support groups because I wanted to understand the relationship between support groups and the breast cancer movement. I studied the support group as a potential mobilizing structure, not as a window onto women's experiences of breast cancer. In fact I assumed, following political process theory, that women's lived experiences of breast cancer and medical technologies were not casually important.

In practice, this meant that I filtered out the substantive focus of group discussions and the stories women told about their experiences of breast cancer screening, diagnosis, and treatment—the ambiguities of diagnosis; the challenges of being diagnosed with a life-threatening disease; the difficulties of navigating treatment decisions and the relationships with physicians, other medical personnel, and insurance companies; the miserable, grueling, ongoing, overall wretchedness of treatment; the impact of breast cancer on their jobs, careers, families, and sex lives; the challenges of living with permanent risk and uncertainty.

After a few months I wrote a paper that drew on my research on support groups and my research on the visible pole of the breast cancer movement (which I discuss in the next section). I used social movements theory to construct a four-stage model of the breast cancer movement. It began, I argued, in support groups and culminated in the visible organizations of the breast cancer movement and their activities in the realm of formal politics and policy making. I never liked that paper. Nevertheless I presented it, with great ambivalence and more than the usual amount of trepidation, to a half-empty room at a professional conference. My ambivalence stemmed from the fact that, although I had constructed a factually true account, I knew I was doing an injustice to my fieldwork. I knew I was missing the point entirely. Soon thereafter I abandoned the theoretical framework on which it was based.

The movement from participant observation to field notes and from field notes to an ethnographic text is always, and necessarily, a process of reduction. But there are reductions that provide insight and illumination and reductions that hide and distort more than they reveal. My reductions belonged to the latter category. It was not so much that I was shoving a square peg into a round hole—which I most certainly was doing—it was that peering through that hole using the lens of social movements theory was so deeply dissatisfying.

Meanwhile, I began attending a second support group, and then a third and a fourth. Somewhere along the way my focus began to shift and I found myself paying more attention to the stories that women in the support groups told about their experiences of screening, diagnosis, treatment, doctors, and health insurance. These were the "mundane facts" and details that I had previously treated as background noise. I finally started listening more carefully, or rather, listening differently, to what the women were actually saying about their embodied experiences of breast cancer. What occurred was a gestalt shift in the way I listened and, as a consequence, in the registers I was able to hear. Although the physical location of the ethnographic field did not change, it was radically transformed. A door swung open, and I entered an entirely different terrain.

This shift was fed by two developments. First, it became clear to me that support groups in the Bay Area were indeed functioning as the invisible pole of the women's cancer movement, but they were also functioning as spaces of intensive and often patient-driven medicalization. I had assumed that the processes of medicalization and politicization were necessarily at odds with each other when in fact they were mutually reinforcing. It was the women who were most knowledgeable about the science and medicine of breast cancer and the most fluent in the discourse of oncology—the most medicalized, in a sense—who were also the most likely to challenge the authority of experts, raise political issues, attend public events, and volunteer with local organizations. Once I had answered the question that originally motivated my research, my attention began to shift.

Second, as I read more extensively in the clinical, epidemiological, and historical literature on breast cancer, I began to see that although breast cancer activists' claims regarding medical stasis and stagnation were not untrue at the level of mortality statistics and medical technologies—slash, burn, and poison still ruled the day, and the message of early detection was at least seventy-five years old—there had been a great deal of change at the level of patient experiences. Radiation and chemotherapy, for example, were not new discoveries or inventions, but their incorporation into the treatment regimens of large numbers of women with breast cancer was a relatively recent phenomenon. Similarly, although early detection was practically a turn-of-the-century discourse and diagnostic mammography was a 1950s invention, the use of mammography as a screening technology and its expansion into asymptomatic populations was a relatively recent development. These changes in the anatomo-politics and biopolitics of breast cancer (that is, the regime of practices through which breast cancer was medically managed and publicly administered) were deeply consequential—physically, psychologically, emotionally, and socially—for the experiences of women diagnosed with this disease *and* for the experiences of women at risk.

What made these stories so important, from a social movements perspective, was my sense—fed by historical research—that they indexed experiences significantly different from those of earlier generations. Biologically, perhaps, the disease had not changed. But at the level of women's embodied experiences, breast cancer had become a qualitatively different disease. Those differences mattered, and they mattered in ways that had important consequences for the development of new identities, social networks, solidarities, and sensibilities—key resources in the mobilization and success of social movements.

## The Visible Pole of the Breast/Cancer Movement

My research on the visible pole, the public face, of the breast cancer movement also began in the late summer and early fall of 1994, when I responded to an advertisement in the *East Bay Express* and entered a four-week volunteer training program at WCRC. The other volunteers in my training group ranged in age from their late twenties to their late fifties. Of the thirteen volunteers, there were nine white women, two African Americans, and one Latina. Three of the women in my volunteer group were lesbians, and three women had recently been treated for breast cancer. One was a sign-language interpreter.

The training consisted of a feminist crash course on the physical, psychosocial, and political dimensions of cancer, complete with a large packet of reading materials that most college students would have found daunting. The volunteer training program included a variety of guest speakers, introductions to WCRC services and programs, a day of "diversity training," lots of group discussions, role-playing exercises, sharing of fears and feelings, and a day trip to a small organic farm and a Buddhist retreat center. I loved some of these activities and disliked others, but even the activities that made me feel uncomfortable and uneasy—namely the role-playing and group-sharing exercises—took place in a social setting that was familiar to me. WCRC reminded me of other feminist organizations and women's communities that I had been involved with during the 1980s. I felt comfortable at WCRC. I liked it there.

The California Breast Cancer Act of 1993 had been signed into law eight months before I began my fieldwork, but the fourteen regional partnerships created by the Breast Cancer Early Detection Program were not yet up and running. Like the federally funded, CDC-administered screening program, the state-funded screening program barely made a blip on my radar screen during my first year of fieldwork. Unlike the federally funded Breast and Cervical Cancer Control Program, however, which remained an administrative abstraction to me, the state-funded BCEDP and the regional breast cancer partnership that I studied—the Bay Area Partnership (a pseudonym)—became an important part of my ethnographic research.

I had a very difficult time figuring out how to conceptualize the California BCEDP and its regional partnerships, and how to situate them within the local field of breast cancer activism. Within the feminist cancer and environmental organizations where I began my research, there was no enthusiasm for mammographic screening. In fact, organizations such as the American Cancer Society and the Susan G. Komen Breast Cancer Foundation were regularly attacked for their unflagging support of this screening technology, and National Breast Cancer Awareness Month soon became the focal point of a countercampaign organized by a local coalition of feminist cancer and environmental activists. Initially, my "view from a distance" of these publicly funded screening programs was consistent with—and derived from—local feminist and environmentalist perspectives: I viewed them as part of the "cancer establishment."

In my efforts to map the field of activism in the San Francisco Bay area, however, I kept running up against the limitations of the guiding assumptions that organized my own thinking and perceptions. In February 1996, for example, a full year and a half into my research, I wrote a progress report mapping the field as best I could. At this stage in my research I was particularly frustrated by the stubborn refusal (as I experienced it) of the BCEDP and the Bay Area Partnership, whose meetings I had been attending for quite some time, to fit neatly into my cognitive categories and conform to my expectations. "These categories," I wrote in my progress report, "are kind of shaky and . . . falsely separated." With regard to the BCEDP and its regional partnerships I simply rote, "I don't know how to think about them or how they're linked [to the breast cancer movement]."

Because the BCEDP Advisory Board was legislatively mandated to include representatives from key sectors of the breast cancer advocacy community, and because the regional partnerships were required by the California Department of Health Services to use a "community mobilization" approach to implement the program at the local level, the BCEDP and the regional partnerships were unusually open, both structurally and philosophically, to the input and influence of other groups and interests. Thus, my problem was not one of access, since membership in the Bay Area Partnership was open to the public and BCEDP reports, meetings, and events were a matter of public record. The problem was that I could not figure out how to think about what I was seeing. I wanted the screening program to settle down and "behave like a state" or "behave like the cancer establishment" so that I could treat it as a black box and focus my attention on what I viewed as the "real" breast cancer movement—the local groups, organizations, and coalitions involved in feminist and environmental activism. But this never happened, so I kept observing and participating in partnership activities, waiting for the pieces of the puzzle to slide into place.

Gradually, very gradually, it dawned on me that the Bay Area Partnership was *part* of the breast cancer movement rather than a force standing outside, over, or against it. The widely accepted notion that social movements have clear boundaries was simply not true in the case of the Bay Area breast cancer movement. But I remained confused, because it was clear to me that the early detection activism of the Bay Area Partnership was not "representative" of the breast cancer movement in general—in fact, some aspects of early detection activism (though not the BCEDP) were a *target* of other parts of the movement.

There were clearly many different things going on, and none of them matched the portrait of the national movement painted by the popular media or the picture of social movements I had learned from political process theory. In retrospect, although it was difficult to see this at first ("at first" meaning for about two years), part of the confusion stemmed from the fact that I was studying a field in formation, a field in which all the pieces were moving at once and the contours of the pieces themselves were changing. At bottom, however, it was my ongoing puzzlement over the Bay Area Partnership and my inability to make it fit the standard narrative of social movements that led me to question and eventually abandon the traditional framework for thinking about social movements. In turn, it was this abandonment that made it possible to discern new patterns in the chaos and a nascent logic in the dynamism. Cutting off the head of the king allowed me, finally, to explore this new terrain of social movements without the sovereign.

The production of this ethnography thus involved a constant movement back and forth along two axes, or fields. Movement along the first axis involved excursions into the local field of cancer communities and cancer activism—the complex field of human subjects, relationships, networks, organizations, normative practices, public events, and group activities, together with the cultural symbols, artifacts, texts, and discourses that circulated in different sites and locations of social movement activity. Movement along the second axis involved a parallel set of incursions into the field of sociology—the complex field of human subjects, relationships, networks, organizations, normative practices, public events, and group activities, together with the cultural symbols, artifacts, texts, and discourses that circulated in the different sites and locations of sociological knowledge production. Thus, just as I participated in the field of social movements and its processes of collective action, I also participated in the field of sociology and its processes of knowledge production.

My conceptualization of breast cancer as a regime of practices and my analysis of the relationship between disease regimes and social movements could not have developed without my observational research of women's cancer support groups. Likewise, my analysis of the San Francisco Bay area as a unique field of contention and my conceptualization of this field in terms of three overlapping cultures of action could not have occurred without long-term ethnographic research. Thus, although the analysis I developed in this book was shaped by multiple sources of data, it was made possible by multisited ethnographic research and the extended case method.

# NOTES

## INTRODUCTION

1. The phrase "kingdom of the ill" appears in Susan Sontag, *Illness as Metaphor* (New York: Vintage Books, 1979), 3.

2. Letters to the Editor, *New York Times Magazine,* September 5, 1993; Matuschka, "Why I Did It," *Glamour Magazine,* November 1993, 162–63.

3. Susan Ferraro, "'You Can't Look Away Anymore': The Anguished Politics of Breast Cancer," *New York Times Magazine,* August 15, 1993, 25–27, 58–60.

4. Michael T. Heaney, "Influential Groups in Health Policy Based on Interviews with Congressional Staffers," *Hill* 10 (October 1, 2003): 1.

5. Steven Epstein discusses the differences between AIDS-treatment activism in New York and San Francisco, for example, in his remarkable book *Impure Science: AIDS, Activism, and the Politics of Knowledge* (Berkeley and Los Angeles: University of California Press, 1996).

6. A more detailed description of my fieldwork and research methods is included in the appendix, "Multisited Ethnography and the Extended Case Method."

7. The activist-insider accounts of the breast cancer movement that informed my early research include Sharon Batt, *Patient No More: The Politics of Breast Cancer* (Charlottetown, Canada: gynergy books, 1994); Susan M. Love and Karen Lindsey, *Dr. Susan Love's Breast Book,* 2nd ed. (Reading, Mass.: Addison-Wesley, 1995); Roberta Altman, *Waking Up, Fighting Back: The Politics of Breast Cancer* (Boston: Little, Brown, 1996). The academic research on breast cancer activism that informed my early research included Theresa Montini, "Women's Activism for Breast Cancer Informed Consent Laws" (Ph.D. diss., University of California, San Francisco, 1991); Montini, "Gender and Emotion in the Advocacy of Breast Cancer Informed Consent Legislation," *Gender and Society* 10 (1996): 9–23; Kay Dickersin and Lauren Schnaper, "Reinventing Medical Research," in *Man-Made Medicine: Women's Health, Public Policy, and Reform,*

ed. Kary L. Moss, 57–76 (Durham, N.C.: Duke University Press, 1996); Mary K. Anglin, "Working from the Inside Out: Implications of Breast Cancer Activism for Biomedical Policies and Practices," *Social Science and Medicine* 44 (1997): 1403–15; Verta Taylor and Marieke Van Willigen, "Women's Self-Help and the Reconstruction of Gender: The Postpartum Support and Breast Cancer Movements," *Mobilization: An International Journal* 1 (1996): 123–43; Susan Yadlon, "Skinny Women and Good Mothers: The Rhetoric of Risk, Control, and Culpability in the Production of Knowledge about Breast Cancer," *Feminist Studies* 23 (1997): 645–77; Marilyn Yalom, *A History of the Breast* (New York: Alfred A. Knopf, 1997).

8. For a synthetic overview of political process models, see especially Doug McAdam, John D. McCarthy, and Mayer N. Zald, "Opportunities, Mobilizing Structures, and Framing Processes: Toward a Synthetic, Comparative Perspective on Social Movements," introduction to *Comparative Perspectives on Social Movements: Political Opportunities, Mobilizing Structures, and Cultural Framings*, ed. Doug McAdam, John D. McCarthy, and Mayer N. Zald, 1–20 (New York: Cambridge University Press, 1996).

9. See especially Nella Van Dyke, Sarah A. Soule, and Verta Taylor, "The Targets of Social Movements: Beyond a Focus on the State," *Research in Social Movements: Conflict and Change* 25 (2004): 27–51.

10. See especially James T. Patterson, *The Dread Disease: Cancer and Modern American Culture* (Cambridge, Mass.: Harvard University Press, 1987); Yalom, *A History of the Breast;* Ellen Leopold, *A Darker Ribbon: Breast Cancer, Women, and Their Doctors in the Twentieth Century* (Boston: Beacon Press, 1999); Barron H. Lerner, *The Breast Cancer Wars: Hope, Fear, and the Pursuit of a Cure in Twentieth-Century America* (New York: Oxford University Press, 2001); Walter S. Ross, *Crusade: The Official History of the American Cancer Society* (New York: Arbor House, 1987). For a fascinating historical account of cancer policy, see especially Mark E. Rushevsky, *Making Cancer Policy* (Albany: State University of New York Press, 1986); Robert N. Proctor, *Cancer Wars: How Politics Shapes What We Know and Don't Know about Cancer* (New York: BasicBooks, 1995).

11. The increase in breast cancer incidence that has occurred during the last thirty years, for example, has been confined to earlier-stage breast cancer. Approximately half of the cases of invasive breast cancer diagnosed in 1975 were localized. Today, that number is closer to 90 percent. Likewise, the incidence rate of smaller tumors (2.0 cm or less) has more than doubled since 1975, while the incidence of larger tumors has declined by 27 percent. American Cancer Society, "Breast Cancer Facts and Figures, 2005–2006," http://www.cancer.org/downloads/STT/CAFF2005BrF.pdf; trends in stage of diagnosis (graphs and discussion) are on 3–4. Cancer statistics are available online from the American Cancer Society; "Breast Cancer Facts and Figures" is published annually by the American Cancer Society and can be downloaded from their Web site.

12. I am using the term "medicalization" somewhat differently than it is commonly used. Typically, social scientists use the term "medicalization" to refer to the processes through which nonmedical issues and problems—often social problems and behavioral issues—come to be seen as medical problems, claimed by medical professionals, and

relocated within the domain of medicine. Medicalization theory and medicalization studies have thus tended to ignore (1) the practices through which conditions that are already commonly viewed as medical (breast cancer, for example) are shaped, managed, and contested by and within medicine, and (2) the way the practices through which medical conditions are continuously reproduced as medical conditions can change over time and, in changing, can produce new kinds of medical objects (breast cancer in the late 1800s versus breast cancer in the late 1900s) and new medical subjects (women diagnosed with breast cancer).

13. The term "biomedicalization," which I elaborate in chapter 1, is borrowed from Adele Clarke et al., "Biomedicalization: Theorizing Technoscientific Transformation of Health, Illness, and U.S. Biomedicine," *American Sociological Review* 68 (April 2003): 161–94.

14. Foucault's discussion of the twin poles of biopower, which he terms the "anatomo-politics of bodies" and the "biopolitics of populations" map onto what I refer to as the medical management of bodies and the public administration of populations. I return to this discussion in chapter 1. See Michel Foucault, *History of Sexuality*, translated from the French by Robert Hurley, vol. 1 (New York: Vintage Books, 1978).

15. I am using the term "risky subjects" (instead of "women at risk") to evoke a dual set of meanings. At the level of individual bodies, women at risk of being diagnosed with breast cancer are subjects of, and subject to, the anatomo-politics of risk management. At the level of populations, women at risk pose a threat to the orderly functioning of the body politic and thus are subject to the biopolitics of risk assessment, control, and regulation. The term "risky subjects" is intended to evoke this dual sense of being at risk and posing a risk.

16. The term "biosociality" is borrowed from Paul Rabinow, "Artificiality and Enlightenment: From Sociobiology to Biosociality," in *Incorporations*, ed. Jonathan Crary and Sanford Kwinter, 234–52 (New York: Urzone, 1992). I discuss the concept of biosociality in chapter 1.

17. The term "field of contention" is borrowed from the work of Nick Crossley. See especially Nick Crossley, "The Field of Psychiatric Contention in the UK, 1960–2000," *Social Science and Medicine* 62 (2006): 552–63. My analysis of fields is also indebted to the work of Raka Ray. See especially Raka Ray, *Fields of Protest: Women's Movements in India* (Minneapolis: University of Minnesota Press, 1999). Also see Nick Crossley, *Contesting Psychiatry: Social Movements in Mental Health* (New York: Routledge, 2006). I return to the discussion of fields of contention in chapter 1.

18. The concept "cultures of action," which I introduced in an earlier article, is developed in greater depth in chapter 1. See Maren Klawiter, "Racing for the Cure, Walking Women, and Toxic Touring: Mapping Cultures of Action within the Bay Area Terrain of Breast Cancer," *Social Problems* 46 (1999): 104–26.

19. Donna Haraway, "The Biopolitics of Postmodern Bodies: Constitutions of Self in Immune System Discourse," in *Simians, Cyborgs, and Women: The Reinvention of Nature* (London: Free Association Books, 1991), 203.

## 1. SOCIAL MOVEMENTS WITHOUT THE SOVEREIGN

1. Age-adjusted death rates going back to 1900 are available from the National Center for Health Statistics DataWarehouse, http://www.cdc.gov/nchs/datawh/statab/unpubd/mortabs/hist293.htm.

2. Unless otherwise noted, the source for all facts and figures in this chapter's discussion is "Breast Cancer Facts and Figures, 2005–2006."

3. All incidence and mortality rates cited in this book are age-adjusted unless otherwise noted. Between 1971 and 1993 the incidence of all cancer (excluding skin cancer) increased by 18 percent, and the mortality rate grew by 7 percent. National Cancer Advisory Board, *Cancer at a Crossroads: A Report to Congress and the Nation* (Bethesda, Md.: National Cancer Institute, 1994), 10.

4. For a historical analysis of the conflicting and competing theories of the relationship between cigarette smoking and lung cancer that were embraced by researchers in medical schools, on the one hand, and chronic-disease epidemiologists in schools of public health, on the other, see Colin Talley, Howard I. Kushner, and Claire E. Sterk, "Lung Cancer, Chronic Disease Epidemiology, and Medicine, 1948–1964," *Journal of the History of Medicine and Allied Sciences* 59 (2004): 329–74.

5. National Cancer Advisory Board, *Cancer at a Crossroads,* appendix D.

6. Ibid.

7. National Cancer Institute, *Cancer Facts* (Bethesda, Md.: National Cancer Institute, 2002), table IV-3.

8. For a recent overview of disparities in breast cancer, see Judy Ann Bigby and Michelle D. Holmes, "Disparities across the Breast Cancer Continuum," *Cancer Causes and Control* 16 (2005): 34–44. See also American Cancer Society, "Breast Cancer Facts and Figures, 2005–2006."

9. "Early Stage Breast Cancer Rates Are Rising," *Medical News Today,* April 12, 2005.

10. Barron H. Lerner, "Fighting the War on Breast Cancer: Debates over Early Detection, 1945 to the Present," *Annals of Internal Medicine* 129 (1998): 74–78.

11. Gregory D. Leonard and Sandra M. Swain, "Ductal Carcinoma in Situ: Complexities and Challenges," *Journal of the National Cancer Institute* 96 (June 2004): 906–20; Kefah Mokbel, "Contemporary Treatment of Ductal Carcinoma in Situ of the Breast," *Medical Science Monitor* 11 (March 2005): RA86–93.

12. American Cancer Society, "Breast Cancer Facts and Figures, 2005–2006," 3.

13. The first study to demonstrate a decrease in breast cancer incidence rates in the United States was published in 2007. The study showed that incidence rates declined by a dramatic 6.7 percent in 2003—the first significant decline in breast cancer incidence recorded by cancer registries participating in the National Cancer Institute's Surveillance, Epidemiology, and End Results (SEER) program. The study's authors concluded that the decrease in breast cancer incidence was probably caused by the sharp decline in the use of hormone-replacement therapy (HRT) in 2003 following the release of the Women's Health Initiative's study of HRT, which demonstrated that HRT was a risk factor for breast cancer among the study's participants. My larger point,

however, is that the recent decrease in breast cancer incidence rates was not tied to the increase in the diagnosis of preinvasive breast cancer. See Peter M. Ravdin et al., "The Decrease in Breast-Cancer Incidence in 2003 in the United States," *New England Journal of Medicine* 356, no. 16 (2007): 1670–74.

14. For an analysis of the public framing of breast cancer as an epidemic, see especially Paula M. Lantz and Karen M. Booth, "The Social Construction of the Breast Cancer Epidemic," *Social Science and Medicine* 46 (1998): 907–18.

15. The boundaries of the cancer establishment vary somewhat from text to text, but its basic history and general outline are not an issue of dispute within the literature. Building heavily on Samuel S. Epstein's controversial and influential *Politics of Cancer* (Garden City, N.Y.: Anchor Books, 1978), 253–75, Ralph W. Moss published *The Cancer Syndrome* in 1982. In it the former assistant director of public affairs at Memorial Sloan-Kettering Cancer Center, the flagship cancer research institution in the United States, defined the cancer establishment as the National Cancer Institute (NCI), the Food and Drug Administration (FDA), private and public research enterprises such as Memorial Sloan-Kettering, the pharmaceutical industry, and the American Cancer Society (ACS)—perhaps the oldest, largest, wealthiest, and most powerful voluntary health organization in the world. See Ralph W. Moss, *The Cancer Syndrome* (New York: Grove Press, 1982), 417; see also Moss, *The Cancer Industry,* 2nd ed. (New York: Paragon House, 1991). In a more recent article, Samuel Epstein defined the cancer establishment's members as the NCI, the ACS, a network of fifty-seven National Cancer Centers (including twenty-two Comprehensive Cancer Centers, of which Memorial Sloan-Kettering is the prototype), and the contractees and grantees of extramural research funding from the ACS and NCI—especially research universities and major pharmaceutical companies. Epstein, "Winning the War against Cancer? . . . Are They Even Fighting It?" *Ecologist* 28 (March–April 1998): 72. Writing from a less critical perspective, historian James Patterson, in *The Dread Disease,* details the collaborative and even symbiotic relationships of these same entities and industries but refers to them collectively as the "Alliance against Cancer" rather than the "cancer establishment." Whether conceived of as an establishment or an alliance, the story of the cancer establishment in the twentieth century is the story of what Lester Breslow refers to as "the triangular accommodation" of private industry, private medicine, and the biomedical research enterprise. Lester Breslow and Danile Wilner, *A History of Cancer Control in the United States with Emphasis on the Period 1946–1971,* prepared for the History of Cancer Control Project, Division of Cancer Control and Rehabilitation, National Cancer Institute, Department of Health, Education, and Welfare, publication no. 79-1516, 1979, 53.

16. For an analysis of the framing activities of the National Breast Cancer Coalition, see especially Emily S. Kolker, "Framing as a Cultural Resource in Health Social Movements: Funding Activism and the Breast Cancer Movement in the U.S., 1990–1993," *Sociology of Health and Illness* 26 (September 2004): 820–44.

17. The disease-specific NCI budgetary figures come from the National Cancer

Institute Financial Management Branch, "National Cancer Institute Research Dollars by Various Cancers, FY 1981–FY 1988," a fax of figures received March 14, 2001, prepared by staff member Karen Colbert in response to my inquiry.

18. This is not an entirely fair comparison, since the National Heart Institute, which was renamed the National Heart and Lung Institute in 1969 (now the National Heart, Lung, and Blood Institute, NHLBI), served as an additional source of funding for research on lung diseases. The NHLBI's research program on lung diseases, however, is very broad and includes research on dozens of lung, airway, and respiratory conditions.

19. These conferences included the following: Breast Cancer Screening (1977), The Treatment of Primary Breast Cancer and Management of Local Disease (1979), Steroid Receptors in Breast Cancer (also 1979), Adjuvant Chemotherapy for Breast Cancer (1980), Breast Cancer: A Measure of Progress in Public Understanding (1981), Adjuvant Chemotherapy for Breast Cancer (1985), and Treatment of Early-Stage Breast Cancer (1990).

20. In 1976 the Senate Subcommittee on Health held a hearing entitled *Breast Cancer, 1976* that was billed as "an examination on the treatment of breast cancer, what treatment is best, where physicians differ, and the risks and costs involved." U.S. Senate, Subcommittee on Health of the Committee on Labor and Public Health, *Breast Cancer, 1976: Examination on the Treatment of Breast Cancer, What Treatment Is Best, Where Physicians Differ, and the Risks and Costs Involved; Hearing before the Subcommittee on Health of the Committee on Labor and Public Health*, 94th Cong., 2nd sess., May 4, 1976. In 1984 a hearing titled *Progress in Controlling Breast Cancer* was held before the House of Representatives Subcommittee on Health and Long-Term Care, 98th Cong., 2nd sess. A year later, in 1985, a joint hearing was held titled *Breast Cancer Detection: The Need for a Federal Response*, 99th Cong., 1st sess.

21. The women's health movement of the 1960s and 1970s was, in large part, a reaction to the sexism and paternalism of the medical profession, which was reinforced and reflected in medical textbooks and medical training. In addition, medical research, as Sue Rosser has argued, was a "male-centered" endeavor whose male biases "led to the insufficient study and funding of diseases of women, the exclusion of women from experimental drug trials, and the failure to understand the health of the elderly." Sue Rosser, *Women's Health—Missing from U.S. Medicine* (Bloomington: Indiana University Press, 1994), ix. Women, for example, were systematically excluded from research on heart disease and from clinical trials of drugs designed to treat it. Likewise, women were largely ignored by AIDS researchers for the first ten years of the epidemic, and it was not until 1992 that the Centers for Disease Control (CDC) broadened the definition of AIDS to include the range of gynecologic conditions experienced by women with AIDS. Similarly, it was not until 1993 that the NIH, the world's largest funder of medical research, implemented policies requiring, first, that NIH funding recipients recruit and include women and racial and ethnic minorities in clinical trials, and second, that the data from clinical trials be analyzed for medically meaningful differences between men and women, on the one hand, and between members of different

racial and ethnic groups, on the other. Later that year (in 1993), as Steven Epstein points out, the FDA issued new guidelines that removed restrictions on the participation of "women of childbearing potential" in clinical trials of new drugs, restrictions that had been in place since 1977. Steven Epstein, "Bodily Differences and Collective Identities: The Politics of Gender and Race in Biomedical Research in the United States," *Body and Society* 10 (2004): 184. For an in-depth history of the FDA's treatment of female experimental subjects, see Jean A. Hamilton, "Women and Health Policy: On the Inclusion of Females in Clinical Trials," in *Gender and Health: An International Perspective*, ed. Carolyn F. Sargent and Caroline B. Brettell, 292–325 (Upper Saddle River, N.J.: Prentice Hall, 1996). For histories of women physicians in the United States and women's treatment by physicians, see especially Catherine Kohler Riessman, "Women and Medicalization: A New Perspective," *Social Policy* 14 (1983): 3–18; Regina Morantz-Sanchez, *Sympathy and Science: Women Physicians in American Medicine* (Chapel Hill: University of North Carolina Press, 2000); Rima D. Apple, ed., *Women, Health, and Medicine in America: A Historical Handbook* (New York: Garland, 1990); Carol S. Weisman, *Women's Health Care: Activism Traditions and Institutional Change* (Baltimore: The Johns Hopkins University Press, 1998); Barbara Ehrenreich and Deirdre English, *For Her Own Good: 150 Years of the Experts' Advice to Women,* reissue ed. (Garden City, N.Y.: Anchor Books, 1978); Elizabeth Fee, ed., *Women and Health: The Politics of Sex in Medicine* (Amityville, N.Y.: Baywood, 1983); Elizabeth Fee and Nancy Krieger, eds., *Women's Health, Politics, and Power: Essays on Sex/Gender, Medicine, and Public Health* (Amityville, N.Y.: Baywood, 1994). For histories of the women's health movement, see Sheryl Burt Ruzek, *The Women's Health Movement: Feminist Alternatives to Medical Control* (New York: Praeger, 1978); Weisman, *Women's Health Care;* Sandra Morgan, *Into Our Own Hands: The Women's Health Movement in the United States, 1969–1990* (New Brunswick, N.J.: Rutgers University Press, 2001).

22. See especially Leopold, *A Darker Ribbon;* Lerner, *The Breast Cancer Wars.*

23. An important exception to this rule is cervical cancer. The Pap smear, which was incorporated into medical practice as a screening technology in the post–World War II era, has had a dramatic effect on mortality rates from cervical cancer. See especially Monica Casper and Adele Clarke, "Making the Pap Smear into the 'Right Tool' for the Job: Cervical Cancer Screening in the USA, circa 1940–1995," *Social Studies of Science* 28 (1998): 255–90. For an evaluation of the National Cancer Program conducted during the early 1990s, see National Cancer Advisory Board, *Cancer at a Crossroads.*

24. Many of these social constructionist insights, it should be noted, were also present in NSMT. Scholars retained the social constructionist dimension of NSMT but did not pursue its structural claims. See, for example, Enrique Larana, Hank Johnston, and Joseph Gusfield, *New Social Movements: From Ideology to Identity* (Philadelphia: Temple University Press, 1994).

25. For a small sampling of work in this area, see especially Myra Marx Ferree and Patricia Yancey Martin, *Feminist Organizations: Harvest of the New Women's Movement* (Philadelphia: Temple University Press, 1995); Jeff Goodwin and James M. Jasper, eds.,

*Rethinking Social Movements: Structure, Meaning, Emotion* (New York, Rowman and Littlefield, 2004); Hank Johnston and Bert Klandermans, *Social Movements and Culture* (Minneapolis: University of Minnesota Press, 1995); Marcy Darnovsky, Barbara Epstein, and Richard Flacks, eds., *Cultural Politics and Social Movements* (Philadelphia: Temple University Press, 1995); Jeff Goodwin, James Jasper, and Francesca Polletta, eds., *Passionate Politics: Emotions and Social Movements* (Chicago: University of Chicago Press, 2001).

26. Imre Lakatos, *The Methodology of Scientific Research Programmes* (Cambridge: Cambridge University Press, 1977).

27. McAdam, McCarthy, and Zald, "Opportunities, Mobilizing Structures, and Framing Processes," 7.

28. Ibid., 6.

29. Charles Kurzman, "The Poststructuralist Consensus in Social Movement Theory," in *Rethinking Social Movements: Structure, Meaning, and Emotion*, ed. Jeff Goodwin and James M. Jasper, 111–20 (New York: Rowman and Littlefield, 2004).

30. McAdam, McCarthy, and Zald, "Opportunities, Mobilizing Structures, and Framing Processes," in *Comparative Perspectives on Social Movements*, 6. This essay and this book laid out the claims of the weak program.

31. For revisions of PPT around "contentious politics," see especially Doug McAdam, Sidney Tarrow, and Charles Tilly, *Dynamics of Contention* (Cambridge: Cambridge University Press, 2001).

32. Van Dyke, Soule, and Taylor, "The Targets of Social Movements."

33. Carol S. Weisman, "Breast Cancer Policymaking," in *Breast Cancer: Society Shapes an Epidemic*, ed. Anne S. Kasper and Susan J. Ferguson, 213–43 (New York: St. Martin's Press, 2000).

34. Maureen Hogan Casamayou, *The Politics of Breast Cancer* (Washington, D.C.: Georgetown University Press, 2001), 32.

35. Ulrike Boehmer, "Review of Maureen Hogan Casamayou, *The Politics of Breast Cancer*," *Journal of Health Politics, Policy, and Law* 27 (December 2002): 1034, 1035.

36. Taylor and Van Willigen, "Women's Self-Help and the Reconstruction of Gender."

37. Jennifer Myhre, "Medical Mavens: Gender, Science, and the Consensus Politics of Breast Cancer" (Ph.D. diss., University of California, Davis, 2001).

38. Ibid., iv.

39. Jeff Goodwin and James M. Jasper, "Caught in a Winding, Snarling Vine: The Structural Bias of Political Process Theory," in *Rethinking Social Movements: Structure, Meaning, Emotion*, ed. Jeff Goodwin and James M. Jasper, 3–30 (New York: Rowman and Littlefield, 2004), 4.

40. Van Dyke, Soule, and Taylor, "The Targets of Social Movements," 27.

41. See especially Steven Epstein, "Institutionalizing the New Politics of Difference in U.S. Biomedical Research: Thinking across the Science/State/Society Divides," in *The New Political Sociology of Science: Institutions, Networks, and Power*, ed. Scott Frickel and Kelly Moore, 327–50 (Madison: University of Wisconsin Press, 2006); Epstein,

*Inclusion: The Politics of Difference in Medical Research* (Chicago: University of Chicago Press, 2007).

42. Nancy Fraser, *Justice Interruptus: Critical Reflections on the "Postsocialist" Condition* (New York: Routledge, 1996).

43. See, for example, Joseph Gusfield, *Symbolic Crusade: Status Politics and the American Temperance Movement* (Urbana: University of Illinois Press, 1963); Linda Gordon, *Woman's Body, Woman's Right: Birth Control in America* (New York: Penguin, 1990); Michael Teller, *The Tuberculosis Movement: A Public Health Campaign in the Progressive Era* (New York: Greenwood Press, 1988).

44. For further discussion of the weaknesses of NSMT's empirical and historical claims, see Craig Calhoun, "New Social Movements of the Early Nineteenth Century," in *Repertoires and Cycles of Collective Action*, ed. Mark Traugott, 173–216 (Durham, N.C.: Duke University Press, 1995); Kenneth H. Tucker, "How New Are the New Social Movements?" *Theory, Culture, and Society* 8 (1991): 75–98. For a thorough critique of the central propositions of the new social movements paradigm, see Nelson Pichardo, "New Social Movements: A Critical Review," *Annual Review of Sociology* 23 (1997): 411–30.

45. See, for example, Jane Jenson, "Changing Discourse, Changing Agendas: Political Rights and Reproductive Policies in France," in *The Women's Movements of the United States and Western Europe: Consciousness, Political Opportunity, and Public Policy*, ed. Mary Fainsod Katzenstein and Carol McClurg Mueller, 64–88 (Philadelphia: Temple University Press, 1987); Scott Hunt, Robert Benford, and David Snow, "Identity Fields: Framing Processes and the Social Construction of Movement Identities," in *New Social Movements: From Ideology to Identity*, ed. Enrique Larana, Hank Johnston, and Joseph Gusfield, 185–208 (Philadelphia: Temple University Press, 1994); Verta Taylor and Nancy Whittier, "Collective Identity in Social Movement Communities: Lesbian Feminist Mobilization," in *Frontiers in Social Movement Theory*, ed. Aldon D. Morris and Carol McClurg Mueller, 104–29 (New Haven: Yale University Press, 1992); Susan Krieger, *The Mirror Dance: Identity in a Women's Community* (Philadelphia: Temple University Press, 1983). For a more recent review of this literature, see Francesca Polletta and James M. Jasper, "Collective Identity and Social Movements," *Annual Review of Sociology* 27 (2001): 283–305.

46. Structural approaches to identity that were introduced by NSMT, for example, have migrated into scholarship more closely aligned with the political process tradition, where they have been utilized to examine the relationship among states, identities, and social movements. See, for example, Mary Bernstein, "Celebration and Suppression: The Strategic Uses of Identity by the Lesbian and Gay Movement," *American Journal of Sociology* 103 (1997): 531–65; David S. Meyer, Nancy Whittier, and Belinda Robnett, eds., *Social Movements: Identity, Culture, and the State* (Oxford: Oxford University Press, 2002). Again, my point is not that states are unimportant, but that we need structural theories that do not reinforce inadequate conceptualizations of power and misguided claims about the state's primary or singular importance in the development of social movements (the strong program of PPT). Most second-generation scholars

who work within the political process tradition do not maintain that the state is singularly important, but this does not change the fact that the theory of power at the *foundation* of the political process paradigm is misguided and inadequate.

47. Alberto Melucci, "The New Social Movements: A Theoretical Approach," *Social Science Information* 19 (1980): 217.

48. Alberto Melucci, "The Symbolic Challenge of Contemporary Movements," *Social Research* 52 (1985): 789.

49. See especially Proctor, *Cancer Wars;* Rushevsky, *Making Cancer Policy;* Richard A. Rettig, *Cancer Crusade: The Story of the National Cancer Act of 1971* (Princeton: Princeton University Press, 1977); Epstein, *The Politics of Cancer;* Moss, *The Cancer Industry;* Arnold S. Relman, "The New Medical Industrial Complex," *New England Journal of Medicine* 303 (1980): 963–70.

50. To be fair, cancer patients have, in fact, actively participated in what David Hess describes as a "global social movement" for greater access to complementary and alternative medicines (CAM), calling for "greener" therapies based on dietary programs; supplements and herbs; nontoxic, immunity-enhancing drugs; and mind-body techniques. Hess traces the roots of the modern CAM movement for cancer treatment in the United States to a long line of "alternative cancer therapy traditions" that extends at least as far back as the 1890s, when "Coley's toxins" (invented by New York physician William Coley) gained a popular following. The modern CAM movement in the United States emerged in the 1970s to promote the legalization of laetrile, which was not licensed by the FDA. During the 1990s, as Hess shows, the CAM movement became more mainstream and achieved a number of important changes, including the establishment of the National Center for Complementary and Alternative Medicine (as an NIH agency) in 1998. David J. Hess, "Technology, Medicine, and Modernity: The Problem of Alternatives," in *Modernity and Technology,* ed. Thomas J. Misa, Philip Brey, and Andrew Feenberg, 279–302 (Cambridge: MIT Press, 2003), quotations on 283; also see Hess, "CAM Cancer Therapies in Twentieth-Century North America: The Emergence and Growth of a Social Movement," in *The Politics of Healing: A History of Alternative Therapies in Twentieth-Century North America,* ed. Robert D. Johnston, 231–43 (New York: Routledge, 2003). James Patterson, in *The Dread Disease,* also discusses the long history of "fringe" subcultures of cancer patients seeking and using unorthodox cancer therapies in the United States (that is, not licensed by the FDA, taught in medical schools, or practiced by mainstream physicians).

51. Sontag, *Illness as Metaphor,* 3.

52. Melucci, "The Symbolic Challenge of Contemporary Movements," 89.

53. Melucci, "The New Social Movements," 221.

54. Ibid., 219.

55. Ibid., 224 (emphasis added).

56. Ibid., 225 (emphasis added).

57. Michel Foucault, "Body/Power," trans. Colin Gordon, in *Power/Knowledge: Selected Interviews and Other Writings, 1972–1977,* ed. Colin Gordon, 55–62 (New York:

Pantheon Books, 1980), 62; Foucault, "Truth and Power," trans. Colin Gordon, in Gordon, *Power/Knowledge,* 109–33, at 122.

58. Centralized, repressive power does, however, remain the dominant form of power in many, perhaps most, societies in the world.

59. Foucault, *History of Sexuality,* 1:89–90.

60. Ibid., 1:90.

61. Michel Foucault, "Questions of Method: An Interview with Michel Foucault," trans. Alan Bass, in *After Philosophy—End or Transformation?* ed. Kenneth Baynes, James Bohman, and Thomas McCarty, 100–117 (Boston: MIT Press, 1987), 102–3.

62. Ibid.

63. Foucault, *History of Sexuality,* 1:89.

64. Foucault, "Body/Power," 59.

65. Michel Foucault, *Madness and Civilization,* trans. Richard Howard (London: Tavistock, 1965); Foucault, *The Birth of the Clinic: An Archaeology of Medical Perception,* trans. Alan Sheridan (New York: Vintage Books, 1973); Foucault, *History of Sexuality;* Foucault, *Discipline and Punish: The Birth of the Prison,* trans. Alan Sheridan (New York: Vintage Books, 1979); Foucault, "The Politics of Health in the Eighteenth Century," trans. Colin Gordon, in Gordon, *Power/Knowledge,* 166–82.

66. Michel Foucault, "Questions on Geography," trans. Colin Gordon, in Gordon, *Power/Knowledge,* 73–74.

67. Foucault, *History of Sexuality,* 140.

68. The anatomo-politics of populations is what Foucault elsewhere refers to as "disciplinary power." See for example Foucault, *Discipline and Punish.*

69. Foucault, *History of Sexuality,* 25.

70. As a general rule, Foucault's influence has been most significant in those disciplines and fields where feminist scholarship and questions were at the core of research programs and citation networks. In those fields where androcentric theories predominated and feminist scholarship was marginalized (for example, social movements theory), the Foucauldian turn never occurred. This does not mean that feminists have embraced Foucault with open arms. It means that feminist theory and gender studies are key sites in which the strengths, limitations, and implications of Foucault's contributions have been grappled with and critically examined. See, for example, Irene Diamond and Lee Quinby, eds., *Feminism and Foucault: Reflections on Resistance* (Boston: Northwestern University Press, 1988); Sandra Lee Bartky, "Foucault, Femininity, and the Modernization of Patriarchal Power," in *The Politics of Women's Bodies: Sexuality, Appearance, and Behavior,* ed. Rose Weitz, 25–45 (New York: Oxford University Press, 1998); Susan Bordo, "The Body and the Reproduction of Femininity: A Feminist Appropriation of Foucault," in *Gender/body/knowledge,* ed. Allison Jaggar and Susan Bordo, 13–28 (New Brunswick, N.J.: Rutgers University Press, 1989); Nancy Fraser, "Foucault's Body Language: A Posthumanist Political Rhetoric?" in *Unruly Practices: Power, Discourse, and Gender in Contemporary Social Theory,* ed. Nancy Fraser, 55–66 (Minneapolis: University of Minnesota Press, 1989); Fraser, "Foucault on Modern Power:

Empirical Insights and Normative Confusions," in Fraser, *Unruly Practices*, 17–34; Jana Sawicki, *Disciplining Foucault: Feminism, Power, and the Body* (New York: Routledge, 1991); Margaret A. McLaren, *Feminism, Foucault, and Embodied Subjectivity* (Albany: State University of New York Press, 2002); Linda J. Nicholson, ed., *Feminism/Postmodernism* (New York: Routledge, 1990); Ann Laura Stoler, *Race and the Education of Desire: Foucault's "History of Sexuality" and the Colonial Order of Things* (Durham, N.C.: Duke University Press, 1995).

71. See especially Boston Women's Health Course Collective, *Our Bodies, Our Selves* (Boston: New England Free Press, 1970); Claudia Dreifus, ed., *Seizing Our Bodies: The Politics of Women's Health* (New York: Vintage Books, 1977); Ruzek, *The Women's Health Movement;* Morgan, *Into Our Own Hands.*

72. Irving Kenneth Zola, "Medicine as an Institution of Social Control," *Sociological Review* 20 (1972), 487.

73. Peter Conrad, "Medicalization and Social Control," *Annual Review of Sociology* 18 (1992): 211.

74. For overviews of and key contributions to the scholarly literature on medicalization, see especially Barbara Ehrenreich and John Ehrenreich, "Medicine and Social Control," in *The Cultural Crisis of Modern Medicine,* ed. John Ehrenreich, 33–79 (New York: Monthly Review Press, 1978); Robert Crawford, "Healthism and the Medicalization of Everyday Life," *International Journal of Health Services* 10 (1980): 365–88; Nancy Scheper-Hughes and Margaret M. Lock, "The Mindful Body: A Prolegomenon to Future Work in Medical Anthropology," *Medical Anthropology Quarterly* 1 (1987): 6–41; Conrad, "Medicalization and Social Control"; Riessman, "Women and Medicalization"; Kathryn Pauly Morgan, "Contested Bodies, Contested Knowledges: Women, Health, and the Politics of Medicalization," in *The Politics of Women's Health: Exploring Agency and Autonomy,* ed. Feminist Health Care Ethics Research Network, 83–121 (Philadelphia: Temple University Press, 1998); Peter Conrad, "The Shifting Engines of Medicalization," *Journal of Health and Social Behavior* 46 (March 2005): 3–14; Clarke et al., "Biomedicalization"; Simon J. Williams and Michael Calnan, "The 'Limits' of Medicalization: Modern Medicine and the Lay Populace in 'Late Modernity,'" *Social Science and Medicine* 42 (1996): 1609–20; Elianne Riska, "Gendering the Medicalization and Biomedicalization Theses," in *Biomedicalization: Technoscience, Health, and Illness in the U.S.,* ed. Adele Clarke et al. (Durham, N.C.: Duke University Press, forthcoming).

75. For pioneering work on the medicalization of deviance, see especially Peter Conrad and Joseph Schneider, *Deviance and Medicalization: From Badness to Sickness* (Philadelphia: Temple University Press, 1980).

76. Three extremely influential feminist texts from this generation stand out. The first, muckraking journalist Barbara Seaman's *Doctor's Case against the Pill* (New York: Peter Wyden Books, 1969), launched a congressional investigation into the safety of the female contraceptive pill and led to dramatic lowering of dosage. The second is the Boston Women's Health Book Collective's *Our Bodies, Our Selves,* which was originally issued as a stapled workbook in 1970 and is still being updated and reissued

(most recently in 2005). The third, *For Her Own Good: 150 Years of Experts' Advice to Women* by Barbara Ehrenreich and Deirdre English, was originally published in 1978 and was recently updated and reissued with a new subtitle, *Two Centuries of Experts' Advice to Women* (Garden City, N.Y.: Anchor Books, 2005). In 1973, five years before publishing *For Her Own Good,* Ehrenreich and English collaborated on a pamphlet-length publication entitled *Witches, Midwives, and Nurses: A History of Women Healers* (New York: Feminist Press, 1973), which enjoyed wide distribution within the women's health movement. For a collection of historical studies that interrogates some of the historical claims of the first generation of feminist critiques of medicine, see especially Apple, *Women, Health, and Medicine in America.* None of the works cited above were framed by the authors as case studies of medicalization; rather, they were couched as feminist critiques of medicine. For key contributions to the women and medicalization perspective, see Riessman, "Women and Medicalization"; Susan E. Bell, "Sociological Perspectives on the Medicalization of Menopause," *Annals of the New York Academy of Sciences* 592 (1990): 173–78; Anne E. Figert, "The Three Faces of PMS: The Professional, Gendered, and Scientific Structuring of a Psychiatric Disorder," *Social Problems* 42 (1995): 56–73; Morgan, "Contested Bodies, Contested Knowledges"; Jacqueline Litt, *Medicalized Motherhood* (New Brunswick, N.J.: Rutgers University Press, 2002).

77. This shift toward theorizing gender and medicalization is part of a poststructuralist shift in medicalization studies, which I discuss later in this chapter. For studies of the medicalization of men's reproductive bodies, see Raymond C. Rosen, "Erectile Dysfunction: The Medicalization of Male Sexuality," *Clinical Psychology Review* 16 (1996): 497–519; Laura Mamo and Jennifer Fishman, "Potency in All the Right Places: Viagra as a Technology of the Gendered Body," *Body and Society* 7 (2001): 13–35; Elianne Riska, "Gendering the Medicalization Thesis," *Advances in Gender Research* 7 (2003): 61–89; Riska, "Gendering the Medicalization and Biomedicalization Theses." Also see Nelly Oudshoorn, *The Male Pill: A Biography of a Technology in the Making* (Durham, N.C.: Duke University Press, 2003).

78. For a more developed analysis of this point, see especially Riska, "Gendering the Medicalization and Biomedicalization Theses." For an excellent case study of women's active pursuit of medicalization, see Verta Taylor, *Rock-a-Bye Baby: Feminism, Self-Help, and Post-partum Depression* (New York: Routledge, 1996). Also see Mark Nichter, "The Mission within the Madness: Self-Initiated Medicalization as Expression of Agency," in *Pragmatic Women and Body Politics,* ed. Margaret Lock and Patricia A. Kaufert, 327–53 (Cambridge: Cambridge University Press, 1998). More recently, Joe Dumit has written with great insight about the struggles of people with "uncertain, emergent illnesses" to gain access to the resources and legitimacy that medicine can bestow as well as, at least potentially, access to effective treatment and relief from suffering. Joseph Dumit, "Illnesses You Have to Fight to Get: Facts as Forces in Uncertain, Emergent Illnesses," *Social Science and Medicine* 62 (February 2006): 577–90.

79. Peter Conrad and Deborah Potter, "From Hyperactive Children to ADHD Adults: Observations on the Expansion of Medical Categories," *Social Problems* 47 (2000): 560.

80. Riessman, "Women and Medicalization," 3–4.

81. For analyses of Foucault's influence, see especially David Armstrong, "Review Essay: The Subject and the Social in Medicine; An Appreciation of Michel Foucault," *Sociology of Health and Illness* 7 (1985): 108–17; Jennifer Harding, "Bodies at Risk: Sex, Surveillance, and Hormone Replacement Therapy," in *Foucault: Health and Medicine,* ed. Alan Petersen and Robin Bunton, 134–50 (London: Routledge, 1997); Deborah Lupton, "Foucault and the Medicalisation Critique," in Petersen and Bunton, *Foucault: Health and Medicine,* 94–112; Margaret Lock, Allan Young, and Albert Cambrosio, eds., *Living and Working with the New Medical Technologies* (Cambridge: Cambridge University Press, 2000).

82. See, for example, Colin Jones and Roy Porter, *Reassessing Foucault: Power, Medicine, and the Body* (New York: Routledge, 1994); Nelly Oudshoorn, *Beyond the Natural Body: An Archaeology of Sex Hormones* (New York: Taylor and Francis, 1994); Bryan Turner, *Medical Power and Social Knowledge,* 2nd ed. (London: Sage, 1995); Lisa Cartwright, *Screening the Body: Tracing Medicine's Visual Culture* (Minneapolis: University of Minnesota Press, 1995); Monica J. Casper and Marc Berg, "Constructivist Perspectives on Medical Work: Medical Practices and Science and Technology Studies," *Science, Technology, and Human Values* 20 (1995): 395–407; Monica Casper, *The Making of the Unborn Patient: A Social Anatomy of Fetal Surgery* (New Brunswick, N.J.: Rutgers University Press, 1998); Alan Petersen and Robin Bunton, eds., *Foucault, Health, and Medicine* (New York: Routledge, 1997); Stefan Timmermans and Marc Berg, "The Practice of Medical Technology," *Sociology of Health and Illness* 25, silver anniversary issue (2003): 97–114.

83. Casper and Berg, "Constructivist Perspectives on Medical Work," 400, 402 (italics removed).

84. David Armstrong, "Public Health Spaces and the Fabrication of Identity," *Sociology* 27 (1993): 393–410; Armstrong, "The Rise of Surveillance Medicine," *Sociology of Health and Illness* 17 (1995): 393–404; Robert Castel, "From Dangerousness to Risk," in *The Foucault Effect: Studies in Governmentality,* ed. Graham Burchell, Colin Gordon, and Peter Miller, 281–98 (Chicago: University of Chicago Press, 1991); Deborah Lupton, "Risk as Moral Danger: The Social and Political Functions of Risk Discourse in Public Health," *International Journal of Health Services* 23 (1993): 425–35; Lupton, *The Imperative of Health: Public Health and the Regulated Body* (Thousand Oaks, Calif.: Sage, 1995); Lupton, *Risk* (New York: Routledge, 1999); Alan Petersen and Deborah Lupton, *The New Public Health: Health and Self in the Age of Risk* (Thousand Oaks, Calif.: Sage, 1996).

85. See especially Anthony Giddens, *Modernity and Self-Identity: Self and Society in the Late Modern Age* (Stanford: Stanford University Press, 1991); Ulrich Beck, *Risk Society: Towards a New Modernity* (Thousand Oaks, Calif.: Sage, 1992).

86. See, for example, Castel, "From Dangerousness to Risk"; David Armstrong, *Political Anatomy of the Body: Medical Knowledge in Britain in the Twentieth Century* (Cambridge: Cambridge University Press, 1983); Armstrong, "Review Essay: The Subject and the Social in Medicine"; Armstrong, "Foucault and the Sociology of Health

and Illness: A Prismatic Reading," in Petersen and Bunton, *Foucault, Health, and Medicine,* 15–30; Petersen and Bunton, *Foucault, Health, and Medicine;* Alan Petersen, "Risk, Governance, and the New Public Health," in Petersen and Bunton, *Foucault, Health, and Medicine,* 189–206; Petersen and Lupton, *The New Public Health;* Lupton, *The Imperative of Health;* Lupton, "Foucault and the Medicalisation Critique"; Robin Bunton and Roger Burrows, "Consumption and Health in the 'Epidemiological' Clinic of Late Modern Medicine," in *The Sociology of Health Promotion: Critical Analyses of Consumption, Lifestyle, and Risk,* ed. Roger Burrows, Sarah Nettleton, and Robin Bunton, 206–22 (London: Routledge, 1995); Robin Bunton and Alan Petersen, "Foucault's Medicine," introduction to Petersen and Bunton, *Foucault: Health and Medicine.* Also see Jane Ogden, "Psychosocial Theory and the Creation of the Risky Self," *Social Science and Medicine* 40 (1995): 409–15; Lupton, *Risk;* Giddens, *Modernity and Self-Identity;* Beck, *Risk Society.*

87. Armstrong, "The Rise of Surveillance Medicine," 393, 395.

88. Armstrong, "Public Health Spaces and the Fabrication of Identity." See also Petersen and Bunton, *Foucault, Health, and Medicine;* Petersen and Lupton, *The New Public Health;* Jones and Porter, *Reassessing Foucault.*

89. Rabinow, "Artificiality and Enlightenment," 244.

90. Simon Williams and Michael Calman, "The 'Limits' of Medicalization: Modern Medicine and the Lay Populace in 'Late Modernity,'" *Social Science and Medicine* 42 (1996): 1609–20, quotation at 1609.

91. The term "biomedicalization" was actually proposed by Adele Clarke and Virginia Olesen in "Revising, Diffracting, Acting," in *Revisioning Women, Health, and Healing: Feminist, Cultural, and Technoscience Perspectives,* ed. Adele E. Clarke and Virginia L. Olesen, 3–48 (New York: Routledge, 1999), but Clarke and her colleagues developed and elaborated it in much greater detail in their 2003 essay "Biomedicalization."

92. Clarke et al., "Biomedicalization," 161; see also Clarke and Olesen, "Revising, Diffracting, Acting." More recently, in "The Shifting Engines of Medicalization," Peter Conrad has updated earlier versions of medicalization theory, arguing that the "shifting engines of medicalization" in the United States include the rise of managed care, the growing influence of the pharmaceutical industry, and the role of the lay populace.

93. I use the term "(bio)medicalization" as shorthand for "medicalization and biomedicalization."

94. In 1980 Peter Conrad and Joseph Schneider argued that medicalization can occur on three levels—the conceptual, the institutional, and the interactional. This way of thinking about medicalization proved quite durable, and Conrad reaffirmed it in 1992 (Conrad and Schneider, *Deviance and Medicalization;* Conrad, "Medicalization and Social Control"). In 1998 Kathryn Paul Morgan proposed adding two additional levels to their schema, the "micro-institutional" level of lived experience and the level of "ordinary lifeworlds" (Morgan, "Contested Bodies, Contested Knowledges"). I like Morgan's idea of incorporating individuals' lived experience of medicalization into the schema, but the "ordinary lifeworlds" that she describes seem to me redundant, which is why I describe medicalization along four, not five, dimensions.

95. Conrad, "Medicalization and Social Control," 210.

96. Conrad, "From Hyperactive Children to ADHD Adults," 560. Conrad is drawing here on Michael Balint, who, in his classic work, *The Doctor, His Patient, and the Illness* (New York: International Universities Press, 1957), drew attention to help-seeking behavior, arguing that individuals seek medical diagnoses in the hope of transforming disorderly agglomerations of complaints and inchoate symptoms into meaningfully ordered systems that assign labels and define conditions, even if they cannot eliminate human suffering.

97. For a recent articulation of these issues, see especially Dumit, "Illnesses You Have to Fight to Get."

98. Elizabeth Ettorre, "Reshaping the Space between Bodies and Culture: Embodying the Biomedicalized Body," *Sociology of Health and Illness* 20 (1998): 549.

99. See especially Fraser, *Unruly Practices;* Chris Shilling, *The Body and Social Theory* (London: Sage, 1993); Bryan Turner, *The Body and Society,* 2nd ed. (London: Sage, 1996); Hubert L. Dreyfus and Paul Rabinow, *Beyond Structuralism and Hermeneutics* (Chicago: University of Chicago Press, 1983); Diamond and Quinby, *Feminism and Foucault;* Nicholson, *Feminism/Postmodernism.* See also note 70 on feminism and Foucault.

100. Steven Epstein's synthetic overview of these issues and the scholarship on patient groups and health movements is exceptionally thoughtful and comprehensive. Steven Epstein, "Patient Groups and Health Movements," in *New Handbook of Science and Technology Studies,* ed. Edward J. Hackett et al., 499–539 (Cambridge: MIT Press, 2007).

101. See David S. Meyer and Nancy Whittier, "Social Movement Spillover," *Social Problems* 41 (1994): 277–98; Kristin Luker, *Abortion and the Politics of Motherhood* (Berkeley and Los Angeles: University of California Press, 1985); Phil Brown and Edwin J. Mikkelsen, *No Safe Place: Toxic Waste, Leukemia, and Community Action* (Berkeley and Los Angeles: University of California Press, 1990); Epstein, *Impure Science;* Doris Zames Fleisher and Frieda Zames, *The Disability Rights Movement: From Charity to Confrontation* (Philadelphia: Temple University Press, 2000); Phil Brown, *Toxic Exposures and the Challenge of Environmental Health* (Ithaca, N.Y.: Cornell University Press, 2007).

102. See Taylor, *Rock-a-Bye Baby;* J. Stephan Kroll-Smith and H. Hugh Floyd, *Bodies in Protest: Environmental Illness and the Struggle over Medical Knowledge* (New York: New York University Press, 1997); Kristin K. Barker, *The Fibromyalgia Story: Medical Authority and Women's Worlds of Pain* (Philadelphia: Temple University Press, 2005); Phil Brown et al., "The Health Politics of Asthma: Environmental Justice and Collective Illness Experience in the United States," *Social Science and Medicine* (2003): 453–64; Michelle Murphy, *Sick Building Syndrome and the Problem of Uncertainty: Environmental Politics, Technoscience, and Women Workers* (Durham, N.C.: Duke University Press, 2006); Dumit, "Illnesses You Have to Fight To Get"; Brown, *Toxic Exposures and the Challenge of Environmental Health.*

103. See, for example, Phil Brown et al., "Embodied Health Movements: New

Approaches to Social Movements in Health," *Sociology of Health and Illness* 26 (2004): 50–80; Stephen Zavestoski et al., "Embodied Health Movements and Challenges to the Dominant Epidemiological Paradigm," *Research in Social Movements, Conflict, and Change* 25 (2004): 255–80; Rachel Morello-Frosch et al., "Embodied Health Movements: Responses to a 'Scientized' World," in *The New Political Sociology of Science,* ed. Scott Frickel and Kelly Moore, 244–71 (Madison: University of Wisconsin Press, 2006).

104. Mark Wolfson, for example, has used the term "interpenetration" to conceptualize the relationship between the antitobacco movement and the state, arguing that it is sometimes difficult to figure out where the movement ends and the state begins. Mark Wolfson, *The Fight against Big Tobacco: The Movement, the State, and the Public's Health* (New York: Aldine de Gruyter, 2001). Steve Epstein has extended the concept of interpenetration to include additional social sectors and social actors, namely, science and medicine. Epstein, "Institutionalizing the New Politics of Difference in U.S. Biomedical Research"; Epstein, *Inclusion.* Approaching from a different angle, Sabrina McCormick, Phil Brown, and Steve Zavestoski have used the term "boundary movements" to draw attention to the increasingly blurry boundaries between movement and nonmovement actors and between laypeople and professionals. Sabrina McCormick, Phil Brown, and Steve Zavestoski, "The Personal Is Scientific, the Scientific Is Political: The Environmental Breast Cancer Movement," *Sociological Forum* 18 (2003): 545–76. Many others have also written on this issue.

105. In the late 1980s and early 1990s Rosenberg advocated shifting from the language of social constructionism to what he viewed as the "less programmatically charged metaphor of framing." Charles E. Rosenberg, "Framing Disease: Illness, Society, and History," in *Framing Disease: Studies in Cultural History,* ed. Charles E. Rosenberg and Janet Golden, xiii–xxvi (New Brunswick, N.J.: Rutgers University Press, 1992), xiii. I prefer the Foucauldian language of regimes to the social constructionist language of frames for two main reasons. First, the term "regime" evokes the weight of institutionalized practices that cannot be easily sidestepped or avoided by simply "reframing" the disease. Second, framing directs attention to the *framers* (the state, scientific communities, medical societies, public health departments, physicians, the media, patients, and so on), and while it is obviously important to identify the main actors in the regime, I want to shift attention instead to the institutionalized *practices* through which diseases are shaped and experienced.

106. I am borrowing the term "biosociality" from Paul Rabinow because I find it to be a useful shorthand for the identities, social networks, solidarities, and sensibilities that are enabled (or foreclosed) by different disease regimes. As I indicated earlier, however, my use of this term is broader than Rabinow's. In my usage, biosociality is not necessarily tied to what Rabinow termed the "new genetics" but rather is tied to disease regimes. Disease regimes include but are by no means limited to genetic discourses and technologies. Rabinow, "Artificiality and Enlightenment."

107. I am discussing the two axes in reverse order here so that I maintain consistency with the organization of the book and the development of my argument.

108. Clarke et al., "Biomedicalization."

109. Talcott Parsons, "Social Structure and Dynamic Process: The Case of Modern Medical Practice," in *The Social System,* 428–79 (New York: Free Press, 1951), 471.

110. Ibid., 477.

111. Foucault, "Questions of Method."

112. Arthur W. Frank, *The Wounded Storyteller: Body, Illness, and Ethics* (Chicago: University of Chicago Press, 1995).

113. Rabinow, "Artificiality and Enlightenment."

114. Frank, *The Wounded Storyteller.*

115. Crossley, "The Field of Psychiatric Contention in the UK, 1960–2000." Also see Crossley, *Contesting Psychiatry.*

116. Ray's innovative work on political fields deserves much more attention than I am able to give it here. Ray, *Fields of Protest.* Also see Ray, "Women's Movements and Political Fields: A Comparison of Two Indian Cities," *Social Problems* 45 (1998): 21–36. For Bourdieu's understanding of fields, see Pierre Bourdieu and Loïc J. D. Wacquant, "The Logic of Fields," in *An Invitation to Reflexive Sociology,* 94–114 (Chicago: University of Chicago Press, 1992). Although Jack Goldstone does not cite Ray's work, he also uses the concept of fields to move beyond the narrowness of political opportunity structures. See Jack A. Goldstone, "More Social Movements or Fewer? Beyond Political Opportunity Structures to Relational Fields," *Theory and Society* 33 (2004): 333–65. For an innovative use of the concept of fields to theorize the role of identity in social movements (in this case, bypassing the state and PPT), see Hunt, Benford, and Snow, "Identity Fields."

117. I use the construction "breast/cancer movement" when I want to remind the reader that I am talking about a movement whose boundaries are contested. It is a breast cancer movement, but it is also a women's cancer movement and an environmental cancer movement. Likewise, I sometimes refer to "women with breast/cancer" and the "breast/cancer community" to indicate that I these groups are not solely made up of women with breast cancer.

118. Ray, *Fields of Protest,* 11.

119. The proceeds from the California Breast Cancer Fund were earmarked to be distributed as follows: 50 percent for what became the BCEDP; 5 percent for epidemiological research and data collection by the Cancer Surveillance Section of the California Department of Health Services; the remaining 45 percent to the University of California to organize and administer the BCRP. The BCRP was mandated to fund "innovative" research related to the cause, cure, treatment, prevention, and earlier detection of breast cancer, including research on "cultural barriers to accessing breast cancer screening services." This is discussed in greater detail in chapter 5. The BCEDP was recently renamed Every Woman Counts and administratively merged with a federally funded breast cancer and cervical cancer screening program.

120. The bill was defeated on the Assembly floor of the California State Legislature in August 1992, was reintroduced in February 1993, and was eventually passed with

the bare minimum of votes in June. An intense lobbying effort ensued, and the governor, Pete Wilson, a Republican, signed the Breast Cancer Act in October 1993.

121. This is discussed in greater detail in chapter 7.

## 2. THE REGIME OF MEDICALIZATION

1. Yalom, *A History of the Breast,* 206.

2. The Federal Food and Drugs Act of 1906, known as the Pure Food and Drugs Act, was the first of several federal initiatives designed to regulate the content, labeling, sale, and safety (but not yet the effectiveness) of pharmaceutical drugs during the first few decades of the twentieth century.

3. Daniel De Moulin, *A Short History of Breast Cancer* (Boston: Martinus Nijhoff, 1983), 2.

4. Ibid.

5. Ibid.

6. Ibid., 5.

7. Ibid., 42.

8. Ibid., 44.

9. Ibid., 48.

10. Ibid., 45–55.

11. Ibid., 55.

12. Frances Burney, "A Mastectomy," in *Medicine and Western Civilization,* ed. David J. Rothman, Steven Marcus, and Stephanie A. Kiceluk, 383–89 (New Brunswick, N.J.: Rutgers University Press, 1995). See also Fanny Burney, *Selected Letters and Journals,* ed. Joyce Hemlow (Oxford: Oxford University Press, 1986).

13. In a fascinating article on Eakins's paintings *The Agnew Clinic* (1889) and *The Gross Clinic* (1873), Michael Frumovitz uses Eakins's paintings to trace changes over time in American medicine. See M. M. Frumovitz, "Thomas Eakins' *Agnew Clinic.* A Study of Medicine through Art," *Obstetrics and Gynecology* 100 (December 2002): 1296–1300.

14. Quoted in Robert Aronowitz, "Do Not Delay: Breast Cancer and Time, 1900–1970," *The Milbank Quarterly* 79 (2001): 365.

15. Paul Starr, *The Social Transformation of American Medicine* (New York: Basic Books, 1982), 39. See also Rosemary Stevens, *American Medicine and the Public Interest: A History of Specialization* (Berkeley and Los Angeles: University of California Press, 1998 [1971]), 9–20.

16. Starr, *The Social Transformation of American Medicine,* 37, 39.

17. Weisman, *Women's Health Care,* 48. Drawing on Paul Starr's work, Weisman adds that "seventeen women's medical schools were established, and women began to be admitted to such elite medical schools as Johns Hopkins, which agreed in 1890 to admit women on the same basis as men as a condition of receiving a substantial financial endowment from a group of prominent women."

18. Regina Morantz-Sanchez, "Physicians," in Apple, *Women, Health, and Medicine in America,* 477–95.

19. Weisman, *Women's Health Care*, 48.

20. Naomi Rogers, "Women and Sectarian Medicine," in Apple, *Women, Health, and Medicine in America*, 281–310.

21. Ibid., 288.

22. Starr, *The Social Transformation of American Medicine*, 32–37.

23. Ibid., 30–31.

24. Susan E. Cayleff, "Self-Help and the Patent Medicine Business," in Apple, *Women, Health, and Medicine in America*, 311–66.

25. Ibid., 320.

26. The term "ecology of medical practice" is borrowed from Starr, *The Social Transformation of American Medicine*, 77.

27. Nicholas Jewson, "Medical Knowledge and the Patronage System in 18th Century England," *Sociology* 8 (September 1974): 369–85. Discussed in Starr, *The Social Transformation of American Medicine*, 38–39.

28. Starr, *The Social Transformation of American Medicine*, 80.

29. Patterson, *The Dread Disease*, 20.

30. Ibid., 41.

31. Ibid.

32. Regular physicians did, however, greatly outnumber the irregulars. According to Paul Starr: "While unorthodox practitioners multiplied, they were still greatly outnumbered by members of the regular profession. Between 1835 and 1860 . . . sectarians represented roughly 10 percent of the total number of physicians. By 1871 they represented 13 percent. . . . In 1879 the sectarians operated 15 out of 75 medical schools. In 1880 the regulars conducted seventy-six medical schools, the homeopaths fourteen, the Eclectics eight. . . . These figures suggest a fairly stable distribution of strength among the rival groups, with the irregulars at roughly 20 percent or slightly lower." Starr, *The Social Transformation of American Medicine*, 99.

33. Foucault, *The Birth of the Clinic*, 120.

34. Ibid., xiii.

35. Starr, *The Social Transformation of American Medicine*, 72. See also Charles Rosenberg, *The Care of Strangers: The Rise of America's Hospital System* (Baltimore: The Johns Hopkins University Press, 1987); Rosemary Stevens, *American Medicine and the Public Interest: A History of Specialization* (Berkeley and Los Angeles: University of California Press, 1971).

36. Jens Lachmund examines this transformation in England, but a similar shift took place in the United States. Jens Lachmund, "Between Scrutiny and Treatment: Physical Diagnosis and the Restructuring of 19th Century Medical Practice," *Sociology of Health and Illness* 20 (1998): 779–801. Also see Foucault, *The Birth of the Clinic*.

37. Ibid., 795.

38. Ibid., 794. See also Stanley J. Reiser, "Technology and the Use of the Senses in Twentieth-Century Medicine," in *Medicine and the Five Senses*, ed. W. F. Bynum and Roy Porter, 262–73 (Cambridge: Cambridge University Press, 1993); Roy Porter,

"The Rise of Physical Examination," in Bynum and Porter, *Medicine and the Five Senses,* 179–97.

39. Lachmund, "Between Scrutiny and Treatment," 795.

40. Starr, *The Social Transformation of American Medicine,* 146.

41. Ibid., 116.

42. Ibid., 81.

43. Ibid., 116.

44. Ibid., 124. See also Weisman, *Women's Health Care,* 48.

45. Ibid., 124, 161.

46. Annie Riley Hale, *"These Cults": An Analysis of the Foibles of Dr. Morris Fishbein's "Medical Follies" and an Indictment of Medical Practice in General, etc.* (New York, National Health Foundation, 1926), available online through the Soil and Health Library, http://www.soilandhealth.org/03sov/0303critic/030315cults/cults-toc.htm.

47. Ibid.

48. Parsons, "Social Structure and Dynamic Process."

49. David Cantor, "Cancer," in *Companion Encyclopedia of the History of Medicine,* ed. B. F. Bynum and Roy Porter (New York: Routledge, 1993), 543.

50. Barron H. Lerner, "Inventing a Curable Disease: Historical Perspectives on Breast Cancer," in *Breast Cancer: Society Shapes an Epidemic,* ed. Anne S. Kasper and Susan J. Ferguson, 25–50 (New York: St. Martin's Press, 2000), 30.

51. Joan Austoker, "The 'Treatment of Choice': Breast Cancer Surgery, 1860–1985," *Society for the History of Medicine Bulletin* 38 (1985): 100–107; Lerner, "Inventing a Curable Disease." Also see Barron H. Lerner, "Great Expectations: Historical Perspectives on Genetic Breast Cancer Testing," *American Journal of Public Health* 89 (1999): 939.

52. Lerner, "Inventing a Curable Disease." Technically, breast cancer was actually "reinvented" as a curable disease, since it had already been invented as a curable disease by quacks and sellers of patent medicines.

53. Austoker, "The 'Treatment of Choice,'" 101.

54. Halsted first described this operation in W. S. Halsted, "Results of Operations for the Cure of Cancer of the Breast Performed at Johns Hopkins Hospital from June 1889–January 1894," *Annals of Surgery* 20 (1894): 497. For an excellent sociocultural history of breast cancer surgery, see Lerner, "Inventing a Curable Disease," 30. For less sociological histories of breast cancer surgery (history told as a straightforward story of medical progress), see Edward F. Scanlon, "The Evolution of Breast Cancer Treatment," *Journal of the American Medical Association* 266 (1991): 1280, 1282; David P. Winchester, Lucrecia Trabanino, and Marvin J. Lopez, "The Evolution of Surgery for Breast Cancer," *Surgical Oncology Clinics of North America* 14 (2005): 479–98; Alvin M. Cotlar, Joseph J. Dubose, and D. Michael Rose, "History of Surgery for Breast Cancer: Radical to the Sublime," *Current Surgery* 60 (May–June 2003): 329–37.

55. Gert Brieger, "Sense and Sensibility in Late Nineteenth-Century Surgery in America," in Bynum and Porter, *Medicine and the Five Senses,* 242.

56. Austoker, "The 'Treatment of Choice,'" 102.

57. Ibid. Pursuing this point further, Austoker argues, "A review of Halsted's original reports indicates little, if any, change in survival rates after the introduction of the radical procedure. That the Halstedian hypothesis resulted in a paradigm for breast cancer treatment enduring for over three-quarters of a century seems truly remarkable. A short tenure was all that could have been expected from the available evidence. Simply, the radical approach promoted by Halsted failed to cure the disease because the underlying hypothesis was wrong" (102).

58. Theresa Montini and Sheryl Ruzek, "Overturning Orthodoxy: The Emergence of Breast Cancer Treatment Policy," *Research in the Sociology of Health Care* 8 (1989): 3–32.

59. The average number of radical mastectomies performed each year at Johns Hopkins Hospital during the 1920s, for example, was only twenty-four—the exact same number, according to Ellen Leopold, as were performed on an annual basis between 1900 and 1910. Leopold, *A Darker Ribbon*, 76.

60. Surgical anesthesia was quickly adopted following the demonstration of ether at Massachusetts General Hospital in 1846. Anesthesia made slower, more complicated operations possible. But infection continued to exact a heavy price for the performance of surgery, according to Starr, and as a consequence, surgery "stood far behind medicine in the therapeutic arsenal." The principles of antisepsis were first demonstrated by Joseph Lister in 1867 but were not generally adopted until the 1880s. Antisepsis called for the use of disinfectants during surgery to kill microorganisms. Soon after antiseptic surgery was adopted, it was superseded by more effective aseptic techniques that relied on sterile procedures to exclude microorganisms from the field of operation. The principles of antisepsis were adopted during the 1880s, and their adoption greatly reduced the postoperative mortality rate due to infections. Starr, *The Social Transformation of American Medicine*, 156, 135.

61. All information regarding the AMA's cancer committee of 1905 and the formation of the ASCC comes from Ross, *Crusade*, appendix A. Dr. Frederick Hoffman's ten recommendations, delivered in an address to the American Gynecological Society, May 7, 1913, are reprinted as appendix B in Ross, *Crusade*.

62. Ross, *Crusade*, 19.

63. For discussions of physicians' reticence, see especially Leslie J. Reagan, "Engendering the Dread Disease: Women, Men, and Cancer," *American Journal of Public Health* 87 (1997): 1779–87; Kirsten E. Gardner, "'By Women, for Women, with Women': A History of Female Cancer Awareness Efforts in the United States, 1913–1970s" (Ph.D. diss., University of Cincinnati, 1999); Breslow and Wilner, *A History of Cancer Control in the United States with Emphasis on the Period 1946–1971;* Patterson, *The Dread Disease;* Ross, *Crusade;* Aronowitz, "Do Not Delay"; Leopold, *A Darker Ribbon;* Lerner, *The Breast Cancer Wars.*

64. Breslow and Wilner, *A History of Cancer Control in the United States with Emphasis on the Period 1946–1971*, 11.

65. Ross, *Crusade*, 21.

66. Aronowitz, "Do Not Delay," 358.

67. Breslow and Wilner, *A History of Cancer Control in the United States with Emphasis on the Period 1946–1971,* 780–81.

68. Ibid., 782.

69. Ross, *Crusade,* 23.

70. William F. Wild, "Danger Signals of Cancer," *Hygeia* (December 1926): 701.

71. Ibid., 700.

72. J. B. Carnett, "Cancer of the Breast," *Hygeia* (March 1930): 262.

73. Gardner, "'By Women, for Women, with Women,'" 88–89.

74. Ross, *Crusade,* 29.

75. Ibid.

76. Ibid.

77. Ibid., 30.

78. Ibid., 31.

79. Quoted in ibid., 31.

80. Patterson, *The Dread Disease,* 122.

81. Ibid.

82. Breslow and Wilner, *A History of Cancer Control in the United States with Emphasis on the Period 1946–1971,* 122.

83. Ibid., 124.

84. See Ross, *Crusade,* 31.

85. Ross, *Crusade,* 32. Although I have quoted extensively from Walter Ross, a more in-depth analysis and nuanced discussion of the WFA is found in Kirsten Gardner's dissertation, "'By Women, for Women, with Women'"; see especially 127–48. Gardner's estimates of the WFA's membership are much lower than Ross's. She argues that the WFA's membership ultimately exceeded 300,000. Gardner, "'By Women, for Women, with Women,'" 100.

86. Gardner, "'By Women, for Women, with Women,'" 100.

87. Patterson, *Dread Disease,* 72. For in-depth discussions of the transition from the ASCC to the ACS, see James T. Bennett and Thomas J. DiLorenzo, *Unhealthy Charities: Hazardous to Your Health and Wealth* (New York: BasicBooks, 1994); Patterson, *The Dread Disease;* Ross, *Crusade.*

88. Breslow and Wilner, *A History of Cancer Control in the United States with Emphasis on the Period 1946–1971,* 786.

89. Ibid.

90. Patterson, *The Dread Disease,* 174. For a discussion of this campaign in the context of cervical cancer, see Casper and Clarke, "Making the Pap Smear into the 'Right Tool' for the Job."

91. Ross, *Crusade.* According to Kirsten Gardner, *Good Housekeeping* claimed that five million women saw the breast self-examination (BSE) film during the first four years after its release. For a more detailed discussion of the promotion of BSE to healthy women, see especially Gardner, "'By Women, for Women, with Women,'" 160–71.

92. This photograph is reproduced in Gardner, "'By Women, for Women, with Women,'" 149.

93. Dorothy Abbott, *Nothing's Changed: Diary of a Mastectomy* (New York: Frederick Fell Publishers, 1981), 146.

94. See especially Lerner, "Inventing a Curable Disease."

95. Throughout the twentieth century there was a great deal of experimentation and innovation in the use of radiation therapy of various kinds on women diagnosed with breast cancer (external irradiation, implanted radium needles, preoperative radiation therapy, postoperative radiation therapy, radiation therapy for inoperable cases of breast cancer, high-dose radiation, low-dose radiation, and so on). See especially Gilbert H. Fletcher, "History of Irradiation in the Primary Management of Apparently Regionally Confined Breast Cancer," *International Journal of Radiation Oncology, Biology, Physics* 11 (1985): 2133–42; Eleanor D. Montague, "Radiation Therapy and Breast Cancer," *American Journal of Clinical Oncology* 8 (December 1985): 455–62.

96. Kirsten Gardner traced the history of the production of breast prostheses in the United States to 1874, when the first patent for a breast form was issued. By 1937 patents referred to the extensive removal of flesh associated with the Halsted radical mastectomy, and by the end of the century 178 patents for "artificial breasts" had been filed. Tracing the history of the early breast-prosthetic industry through patent applications, surgical trade journals, and trade literature on the bra and corset industry, Gardner discovered that prior to the 1950s most patent applications were filed by individuals or teams of two to three people, many of whom were women. Beginning in the early 1950s, however, there was a marked shift toward corporate applications and the transformation of small entrepreneurial ventures into a corporate industry. Gardner, "'By Women, for Women, with Women,'" 215.

97. Maxine Davis, "After Breast Surgery," *Good Housekeeping*, September 1954, 130.

98. Ibid., 28, 130 (all quotations).

99. Patterson, *The Dread Disease*, 69.

100. Charles C. Lund, "The Doctor, the Patient, and the Truth," *Annals of Internal Medicine* 24 (1946): 957–58.

101. Donald Oken, "What to Tell Cancer Patients: A Study of Medical Attitudes," *Journal of the American Medical Association* 175 (April 1, 1961): 1120–28.

102. Ibid., 1123.

103. Ibid.

104. Ibid.

105. Ibid.

106. Reagan, "Engendering the Dread Disease," 1784.

3. BIOMEDICALIZATION AND THE BIOPOLITICS OF SCREENING

1. As previously noted, the concept of biomedicalization is elaborated in Clarke et al., "Biomedicalization."

2. Throughout this chapter I use the locution "healthy women" to refer to women

who are asymptomatic, appear to be cancer-free, and have never been diagnosed or treated for breast cancer. This has the unfortunate consequence of implying that women who *are* symptomatic, who show evidence of cancer, or who have been diagnosed or treated for breast cancer are *un*healthy, and vice versa, that women who appear to be cancer-free and have never been diagnosed with cancer are necessarily healthy. Neither of these implications is true, obviously, and neither is intended. "Healthy," in the context of my usage, is an adjective used for a woman who has no known history of breast cancer.

3. For additional explorations of the social, cultural, and political dimensions of the discourses and practices of breast cancer risk and screening, see Deborah Lupton, "Femininity, Responsibility, and the Technological Imperative: Discourses on Breast Cancer in the Australian Press," *International Journal of Health Services* 24 (1994): 73–89; Cartwright, *Screening the Body;* Patricia A. Kaufert, "Women and the Debate over Mammography: An Economic, Political, and Moral History," in *Gender and Health: An International Perspective,* ed. Carolyn F. Sargent and Caroline B. Brettell, 167–87 (Upper Saddle River, N.J.: Prentice Hall, 1996); Yadlon, "Skinny Women and Good Mothers"; Patricia A. Kaufert, "Screening the Body: The Pap Smear and the Mammogram," in *Living and Working with the New Medical Technologies,* ed. Margaret Lock, Alan Young, and Alberto Cambrosio, 165–83 (Cambridge: Cambridge University Press, 2000); Ann Robertson, "Embodying Risk, Embodying Political Rationality: Women's Accounts of Risks for Breast Cancer," *Health, Risk, and Society* 2 (2000): 219–35; Jennifer Fishman, "Assessing Breast Cancer: Risk, Science, and Environmental Activism in an 'At Risk' Community," in *Ideologies of Breast Cancer: Feminist Perspectives,* ed. Laura Potts, 181–204 (New York: St. Martin's Press, 2000); Shobita Parthasarathy, "Regulating Risk: Defining Genetic Privacy in the United States and Britain," *Science, Technology, and Human Values* 29 (Summer 2004): 332–58. For breast cancer risk and chemoprevention, see Linda F. Hogle, "Chemoprevention for Healthy Women: Harbinger of Things to Come?" *Health* 5 (2001): 299–320; Maren Klawiter, "Risk, Prevention, and the Breast Cancer Continuum: The NCI, the FDA, Health Activism, and the Pharmaceutical Industry," *History and Technology* 18 (2002): 309–53; Margaret J. Wooddell, "Codes, Identities, and Pathologies in the Construction of Tamoxifen as a Chemoprophylactic for Breast Cancer Risk Reduction in Healthy Women at High Risk" (Ph.D. diss., Rensselaer Polytechnic Institute, 2004); Jennifer Fosket, "Constructing 'High-Risk Women': The Development and Standardization of a Breast Cancer Risk Assessment Tool," *Science, Technology, and Human Values* 29 (Summer 2004): 291–313; Maren Klawiter, "Regulatory Shifts, Pharmaceutical Scripts, and the New Consumption Junction: Configuring High Risk Women in an Era of Chemoprevention," in Frickel and Moore, *The New Political Sociology of Science,* 432–60.

4. There is a growing literature on the "individualization of risk" and the construction of new roles and subjectivities organized around—and derived from—the "riskification" of society and the medicalization of risk. Key contributions to this literature, briefly discussed in chapter 1, include Giddens, *Modernity and Self-Identity;* Beck, *Risk*

*Society;* Castel, "From Dangerousness to Risk"; Armstrong, "Public Health Spaces and the Fabrication of Identity"; Armstrong, "The Rise of Surveillance Medicine"; Burrows, Nettleton, and Bunton, *The Sociology of Health Promotion;* Petersen and Lupton, *The New Public Health.*

5. Cartwright, *Screening the Body,* 146.

6. See especially Bigby and Holmes, "Disparities across the Breast Cancer Continuum"; Nancy Krieger, "Defining and Investigating Social Disparities in Cancer: Critical Issues," *Cancer Causes and Control* 16 (2005): 35–44; J. Marchick and D. E. Henson, "Correlations between Access to Mammography and Breast Cancer at Stage of Diagnosis," *Cancer* 103 (April 15, 2005): 1571–80; Barry A. Miller, Benjamin F. Hankey, and Terry L. Thomas, "Impact of Sociodemographic Factors, Hormone Receptor Status, and Tumor Grade on Ethnic Differences in Tumor Stage and Size for Breast Cancer in US Women," *American Journal of Epidemiology* 155 (2002): 534–45; Donald R. Lannin et al., "Influence of Socioeconomic and Cultural Factors on Racial Differences in Late-Stage Presentation of Breast Cancer," *Journal of the American Medical Association* 279 (June 10, 1998): 1801–7; Rena J. Pasick, Carol N. D'Onofrio, and Regina Otero-Sabogal, "Similarities and Differences across Cultures: Questions to Inform a Third Generation of Health Promotion Research," *Health Education Quarterly* 23 (December 1996): S142–61.

7. See Aronowitz, "Do Not Delay."

8. Reagan, "Engendering the Dread Disease."

9. Stanley Joel Reiser, "The Emergence of the Concept of Screening for Disease," *Health and Society* 56 (1978): 403.

10. Ibid., 403–7.

11. The X-ray was discovered by Wilhelm Röntgen in 1895, but during the first half of the twentieth century, X-rays were more often used as a therapeutic treatment for breast cancer than as a technology for diagnosing and viewing breast lesions. For histories of imaging technologies, see Bettyann Holtzmann Kevles, *Naked to the Bone: Medical Imaging in the Twentieth Century* (New Brunswick, N.J.: Rutgers University Press, 1997), 250–53; Cartwright, *Screening the Body,* 159–70.

12. Kevles, *Naked to the Bone,* 253.

13. Cartwright, *Screening the Body,* 160.

14. Lerner, "Fighting the War on Breast Cancer."

15. Kevles, *Naked to the Bone,* 253.

16. Ibid.

17. Cartwright, *Screening the Body,* 168.

18. Philip Strax, Louis Venet, and Sam Shapiro, "Value of Mammography in Reduction of Mortality from Breast Cancer in Mass Screening," *American Journal of Roentgenology* 117 (1973): 668–89. See also R. N. Battista and S. A. Grover, "Early Detection of Cancer: An Overview," *Annual Review of Public Health* 9 (1988): 21–45.

19. Cartwright, *Screening the Body,* 169.

20. A. I. Holleb, letter to U.S. Congressman Harry Waxman, California, May 31,

1977 (on file at American Cancer Society, New York), as quoted in Ross, *Crusade*, 101–2. The bracketed term "asymptomatic" was inserted by Ross.

21. Ross, *Crusade*, 102–3.

22. Larry H. Baker, "Breast Cancer Detection Demonstration Project: Five-Year Summary Report," *CA: A Cancer Journal for Clinicians* 32 (1982): 194.

23. Ibid., 195.

24. Ibid.

25. Ibid., 196, table 191.

26. Ibid., 208; percentages calculated from data in table 209.

27. Ibid., 200, table 205.

28. Ibid., 201, table 206.

29. Quoted in Patterson, *The Dread Disease*, 258.

30. Happy Rockefeller was the wife of Nelson Rockefeller, heir to the Rockefeller fortune and the governor of New York.

31. Batt, *Patient No More*, 38.

32. In October 1975 Bailar approached ACS representatives and NCI officials overseeing the BCDDP with his analysis of the radiation risks that screening mammography posed to younger asymptomatic women. He went public the following July when he concluded that the ACS and NCI were not taking his analysis seriously. After Bailar went public with his findings, he was relieved of his duties as deputy associate director of NCI's cancer control program and was named editor of the *Journal of the National Cancer Institute*, at that time a relatively undistinguished journal. See John C. Bailar III, "Mammography: A Contrary View," *Annals of Internal Medicine* 84 (1976): 77–84; Bailar, "Screening for Early Breast Cancer: Pros and Cons," *Cancer* 39 (1977): 2783–95. Also see Ross, *Crusade*, 104; Susan Rennie, "Mammography: X-Rated Film," *Chrysalis* (1977): 21–33.

33. See Bailar, "Mammography," 77–84.

34. Ross, *Crusade*, 106.

35. Ibid., 107.

36. Rennie, "Mammography," 27.

37. Ibid., 24.

38. For discussions of these controversies and the politics of mammography, see "The Politics of Mammography Screening: Hard Sell, No Benefit—A History," *Health Facts: Center for Medical Consumers* 17 (June 1992): 5; R. Ruth Linden, "Writing the Breast: Contests over Screening Mammography, 1973–1995" (paper presented at the Program in History and Philosophy of Science Colloquium Series, Stanford University, Stanford, Calif., April 27, 1995); "National Breast Cancer Awareness Month—The Script Is Changing," *Health Facts: Center for Medical Consumers* 21 (October 1996): 1; Steven H. Woolf and Robert S. Lawrence, "Preserving Scientific Debate and Patient Choice: Lessons from the Consensus Panel on Mammography Screening," *Journal of the American Medical Association* 278 (December 17, 1997): 2105–8; Maryann Napoli, "What Do Women Want to Know?" (paper presented at the National Institutes of Health

Consensus Conference on Breast Screening for Women, Ages 40–49, Washington, D.C., January 21, 1997); Rennie, "Mammography."

39. Ross, *Crusade*, 107.

40. Barbara J. Culliton, "Mammography Controversy: NIH's Entree into Evaluating Technology," *Science* 198 (October 14, 1977): 171–73.

41. National Institutes of Health, "Breast Cancer Screening. NIH Consensus Statement Online," 1 (September 14–16, 1977), http://consensus.nih.gov/1977/1977Breast Cancer001html.htm.

42. All quotations are from National Institutes of Health, "Breast Cancer Screening."

43. In 1988, for example, the NCI changed its guidelines to conform to those of the ACS, recommending that women begin mammographic screening at age forty. In 1993 the NCI changed its guidelines again, resetting the bar for mammographic screening at fifty years of age. These changes did not, however, affect the use of mammographic screening among younger populations, who were consistently the highest users of this technology, relative to their risk.

44. Christina Marino and Karen K. Gerlach, "An Analysis of Breast Cancer Coverage in Selected Women's Magazines, 1987–1995," *American Journal of Health Promotion* 13 (1999): 163.

45. Reported by Rose Kushner in *Alternatives: New Developments in the War on Breast Cancer* (New York: Warner Books, 1986), 205. This survey was part of a report on breast cancer published by the NIH, *Breast Cancer: A Measure of Progress in Public Understanding*, Department of Health and Human Services, NIH publication no. 81-2306, 1981.

46. American Cancer Society, "Survey of Physicians' Attitudes and Practices in Early Cancer Detection," *CA: A Cancer Journal for Clinicians* 35 (July–August, 1985): 197.

47. American Cancer Society, "Guidelines for the Cancer-Related Checkup: Recommendations and Rationale," *CA: A Cancer Journal for Clinicians* 30 (1980): 193–240.

48. Ibid.

49. Ibid., 194, emphasis in original.

50. American Cancer Society, "Chronological History of ACS Recommendations on Early Detection of Cancer in Asymptomatic People" (n.d.), http://www.cancer.org/docroot/PED/content/PED_2_3X_Chronological_History_of_Cancer.asp?sitearea=PED (accessed January 15, 2004).

51. American Cancer Society, "Survey of Physicians' Attitudes and Practices in Early Cancer Detection."

52. Ibid., 198.

53. Diane J. Fink, "Community Programs: Breast Cancer Detection Awareness," *CA: A Cancer Journal for Clinicians* 64 (December 1989): 2674.

54. Ibid.

55. See, for example, H. Seidman, S. K. Gelb, and E. Silverberg, "Survival Experience in the Breast Cancer Detection Demonstration Project," *Cancer* 37 (1987): 256–89.

56. ACS BCDA program manual, quoted in Kate Dempsey et al., "Screening

Mammography: What the Cancer Establishment Never Told You" (unpublished report prepared for the Women's Community Cancer Project, Cambridge, Mass., 1992), 32.

57. Fink, "Community Programs," 2675.

58. Kaufert, "Women and the Debate over Mammography," 172.

59. Dempsey et al., "Screening Mammography," 32.

60. AstraZeneca International, Community and Company Projects: National Breast Cancer Awareness Month, U.S. (n.d.), http://www.astrazeneca.com/communityproject/110.aspx.

61. In 1993, ICI spun off, or "demerged," its bioscience business into an independent company, Zeneca PLC, which consisted of Zeneca Pharmaceuticals, Zeneca Agrochemicals, and Zeneca Specialties. Tamoxifen became the property of Zeneca Pharmaceuticals, and Zeneca Pharmaceuticals became the official sponsor of NBCAM. For a more detailed discussion of Zeneca's evolution and devolution, see Maren Klawiter, "Chemicals, Cancer, and Prevention: The Synergy of Synthetic Social Movements," in *Synthetic Planet: Chemical Politics and the Hazards of Modern Life*, ed. Monica Casper, 155–76. (New York: Routledge, 2003).

62. See National Breast Cancer Awareness Month (n.d.), http://www.nbcam.com/newsroom_nbcam_facts.cfm.

63. National Association of Breast Cancer Organizations, *Breast Cancer Resource List, 1996/97 Edition* (New York: National Association of Breast Cancer Organizations, 1996).

64. Zeneca Patient Education Service, *Zeneca Pharmaceuticals: Bringing Ideas to Life,* (Wilmington, Del.: Zeneca Pharmaceuticals, n.d.).

65. Dempsey et al., "Screening Mammography," 43–44; Batt, *Patient No More,* 243–46.

66. Dempsey et al., "Screening Mammography," 1.

67. Martin L. Brown, Larry G. Kessler, and Fred G. Rueter, "Is the Supply of Mammography Machines Outstripping Need and Demand?" *Annals of Internal Medicine* 113 (October 1990): 547–52.

68. Ibid.

69. Mandated insurance benefit laws, according to the definition of Kathryn Glovier Moore, are "laws that require third-party payers, such as health insurers (individual or group plans), disability insurers, Medicare supplemental insurance, or prepaid health plans (HMOs), to cover certain benefits or at least to offer the benefit to their policyholders as a condition of doing business in the state." Kathryn Glovier Moore, "States Enact Mammography Coverage Laws," *Women's Health Issues* 1 (Winter 1991): 102.

70. Centers for Disease Control and Prevention, "State Laws Relating to Breast Cancer: Legislative Summary January 1949 to May 2000" (2000), http://www.cdc.gov/cancer/breast/pdf/BCLaws.PDF.

71. Kathleen Horsch and Kerrie Wilson, "Legislative Issues Related to Breast Cancer," *Cancer* 72 (1993): 1483–85.

72. Lerner, *The Breast Cancer Wars,* 208. See also Barron H. Lerner, "Seeing What

Is Not There: Mammography and Images of Breast Cancer" (paper presented at "Intimate Portraits: Body Imaging Technologies in Medicine and Culture," University of California, San Francisco, April 4, 1998).

73. Lerner, *The Breast Cancer Wars*, 207, 208.

74. A recent study comparing mammography screening in the United States and the United Kingdom found that among women between the ages of fifty and fifty-four who underwent a first-screening mammogram, recall rates (for additional assessment) were almost twice as high in the United States as in the United Kingdom—14.5 percent and 12.5 percent in the two U.S. programs examined and only 7.6 percent in the UK program. This difference in recall rates was not the result of different detection rates, which were similar in both countries—5.8 per 1,000 mammograms in the United States compared to 6.3 in the United Kingdom. There were also twice as many negative biopsies performed in the United States, compared to the United Kingdom, and women in the United States were more likely to receive a surgical biopsy in the operating room, as opposed to a nonsurgical needle biopsy in the doctor's office. Rebecca Smith-Bindman et al., "Comparison of Screening Mammography in the United States and the United Kingdom," *Journal of the American Medical Association* 290 (2003): 2129–37.

75. Leonard and Swain, "Ductal Carcinoma in Situ."

76. For a thoughtful discussion of these issues, see Sue Rochman, "Figuring Out What a DCIS Diagnosis Really Means," *Mamm: Women, Cancer, and Community*, October 2000, 37–39. Also see Lerner, "Fighting the War on Breast Cancer." For a recent study that addresses these issues, see Leonard and Swain, "Ductal Carcinoma in Situ."

77. All numbers are taken from Virginia L. Ernster et al., "Incidence of and Treatment for Ductal Carcinoma in Situ of the Breast," *Journal of the American Medical Association* 275 (March 27, 1996): 913.

78. Lantz and Booth, "The Social Construction of the Breast Cancer Epidemic."

79. For recent additions to this literature, see especially Jill Quadagno, "Why the United States Has No National Health Insurance: Stakeholder Mobilization against the Welfare State, 1945–1996," *Journal of Health and Social Behavior* 45, extra issue (2004): 24–44. See also David Mechanic et al., eds., *Policy Challenges in Modern Health Care* (New Brunswick, N.J.: Rutgers University Press, 2005); David R. Williams and P. B. Jackson, "Social Sources of Racial Disparities in Health," *Health Affairs* 24 (2005): 325–34. Also see Ehrenreich and Ehrenreich, "Medicine and Social Control."

80. Clarke et al., "Biomedicalization."

81. See Cyllene R. Morris and William E. Wright, *Breast Cancer in California* (Sacramento: Cancer Surveillance Section, California Department of Health Services, 1996). The Cancer Surveillance Section of the California Department of Health Services and the Northern California Cancer Center publish an assortment of online reports that trace breast cancer trends in California, including patterns of mammography utilization. See Cancer Detection Section, http://www.dhs.ca.gov/cancerdetection, and Northern California Cancer Center, http://www.nccc.org.

## 4. BIOMEDICALIZATION AND THE ANATOMO-POLITICS
## OF TREATMENT

1. Dennis H. Novack et al., "Changes in Physicians' Attitudes toward Telling the Cancer Patient," *Journal of the American Medical Association* 241 (March 2, 1979): 897–900.

2. Oken, "What to Tell Cancer Patients"; Mary-Jo Del Vecchio Good et al., "American Oncology and the Discourse on Hope," *Culture, Medicine, and Psychiatry* 14 (1990): 1120–28.

3. Rose Kushner, *Breast Cancer: A Personal History and an Investigative Report* (New York: Harcourt Brace Jovanovich, 1975), 9. George Crile Jr., *What Women Should Know about the Breast Cancer Controversy* (New York: Pocket Books, 1973); Crile, "Breast Cancer: A Patient's Bill of Rights," *Ms.*, September 1973, 66.

4. Kushner, *Breast Cancer,* 17.

5. Ibid., 18.

6. When the second edition of her book was published in 1977, the title was changed to *Why Me? What Every Woman Should Know about Breast Cancer* because, according to Kushner, despite the book's tremendous popularity, many women were embarrassed to be seen reading a book called *Breast Cancer* in public. Her book *Alternatives,* which was first published in 1984, followed Kushner's second diagnosis in 1981 and included a great deal of information on new developments, especially chemotherapy.

7. Kushner, *Breast Cancer,* 23.

8. National Institutes of Health, "The Treatment of Primary Breast Cancer: Management of Local Disease. NIH Consensus Statement Online," 2 (June 5, 1979), http://consensus.nih.gov/1979/1979PrimaryBreastCancer015html.htm. For an excellent discussion of this consensus conference, see Montini and Ruzek, "Overturning Orthodoxy."

9. In May 1980 Kushner became a member of the National Cancer Advisory Board. She was a remarkable women who was, in almost every respect, at least a decade ahead of her time.

10. National Institutes of Health, "The Treatment of Primary Breast Cancer and Management of Local Disease."

11. Kushner, *Alternatives,* 211.

12. This was part of the broader patients' rights movement of the 1970s.

13. For analyses of the wave of breast cancer informed consent legislation that swept across the country during the 1980s, see, especially, Montini, "Women's Activism for Breast Cancer Informed Consent Laws"; Montini, "Gender and Emotion in the Advocacy of Breast Cancer Informed Consent Legislation"; Theresa Montini, "Resist and Redirect: Physicians Respond to Breast Cancer Informed Consent Legislation," *Women and Health* 26 (1997): 85–105.

14. Mary Fainsod Katzenstein, "Discursive Politics and Feminist Activism in the Catholic Church," in Ferree and Martin, *Feminist Organizations,* 33–52.

15. Montini, "Gender and Emotion in the Advocacy of Breast Cancer Informed Consent Legislation."

16. Ibid., 20.

17. In "Resist and Redirect," Montini argues that informed consent legislation was approved without a great deal of opposition and was stronger in the first few states where it was introduced, but that quickly thereafter the AMA and the ACS organized a strong opposition and successfully weakened subsequent proposed informed consent legislation and, in many cases, defeated it altogether.

18. Montini and Ruzek, "Overturning Orthodoxy."

19. Ibid., 19.

20. Ibid.

21. For a fascinating history of clinical trials as the gold standard of medical science and clinical judgment, see Harry M. Marks, *The Progress of Experiment: Science and Therapeutic Reform in the United States, 1900–1990* (Cambridge: Cambridge University Press, 1997). For an analysis of current controversies over clinical trials, experiential knowledge, and "evidence-based medicine," see Stefan Timmermans and Marc Berg, *The Gold Standard: The Challenge of Evidence-Based Medicine and Standardization in Health Care* (Philadelphia: Temple University Press, 2003).

22. Montini and Ruzek, "Overturning Orthodoxy," 19.

23. Lerner, "Inventing a Curable Disease," 25.

24. Ibid., 38, 39.

25. Ibid., 42, quoting from Albert Q. Maisel, "Controversy over Breast Cancer," *Reader's Digest*, December 1971, 151–56, quotation on 152.

26. Ruzek, *The Women's Health Movement*, 114.

27. Ibid.

28. Montini and Ruzek, "Overturning Orthodoxy," 12.

29. Ibid.

30. Crile, *What Women Should Know about the Breast Cancer Controversy*; Crile, "Breast Cancer"; George Crile Jr., "The Surgeon's Dilemma: The Built-In Conflict of Interest in Medical Fees," *Harper's*, May 1975, 30–38.

31. Boston Women's Health Book Collective, *Our Bodies, Ourselves: A Book by and for Women*, 2nd ed., completely rev. and expanded (New York: Simon and Schuster, 1976). For an analysis of the impact of *Our Bodies, Ourselves* on health movements, feminist theory, sociology, and mainstream medicine in the United States, see Linda Gordon and Barrie Thorne, "Women's Bodies and Feminist Subversion," *Contemporary Sociology* 25 (1998): 322–25.

32. National Institutes of Health, "The Treatment of Primary Breast Cancer and Management of Local Disease."

33. Ibid.

34. Montini and Ruzek, "Overturning Orthodoxy," 15.

35. Kushner, *Alternatives*, 295–309. Also see Philip P. Trabulsy, James P. Anthony, and Stephen J. Mathes, "Changing Trends in Postmastectomy Breast Reconstruction: A 13-Year Experience," *Plastic and Reconstructive Surgery* 93 (June 1994): 1418–27.

36. Bernard Fisher et al., "Surgical Adjuvant Chemotherapy in Cancer of the Breast:

NOTES TO CHAPTER 4

Results of a Decade of Cooperative Investigation," *Annals of Surgery* 168 (1968): 337–56. The Cancer Chemotherapy National Service Center of the NIH was established in 1955, two years before this trial began. For an analysis of the origins and development of the culture of clinical experimentation in oncology, see Ilana Löwy, *Between Bench and Bedside: Science, Healing, and Interleukin-2 in a Cancer Ward* (Cambridge, Mass.: Harvard University Press, 1996), 36–85.

37. Fisher et al., "Surgical Adjuvant Chemotherapy in Cancer of the Breast," 337. As Harry Marks's history of clinical trials reveals, it was not easy to convince functionally independent research hospitals and institutions to adopt standardized protocols so that large clinical trials enrolling thousands of patients could be conducted in multiple sites, nor did it occur automatically. See Marks, *The Progress of Experiment.*

38. G. Bonadonna, E. Brusamolino, and P. Valagussa, "Combination Chemotherapy as an Adjuvant Treatment in Operable Breast Cancer," *New England Journal of Medicine* 294 (1976): 405–10.

39. Rose Kushner, "Is Aggressive Adjuvant Chemotherapy the Halsted Radical of the '80s?" *CA: A Cancer Journal for Clinicians* 34 (1984): 346.

40. Kushner, *Alternatives,* 33.

41. Ralph W. Moss, *Questioning Chemotherapy* (Brooklyn, N.Y.: Equinox Press, 1995), 83.

42. National Institutes of Health, "Adjuvant Chemotherapy for Breast Cancer. NIH Consensus Statement Online," 3 (July 14–16, 1980), http://consensus.nih.gov/1980/ 1980AdjuvantTherapyBreastCancer024html.htm.

43. National Institutes of Health, "Adjuvant Chemotherapy for Breast Cancer. NIH Consensus Statement Online," 5 (September 9–11, 1985), http://consensus.nih.gov/1985/ 1985AdjuvantChemoBreastCancer052html.htm. An NIH consensus conference on "steroid receptors in breast cancer" that was held in 1979 recommended that steroid receptor assays be performed on the tumor tissue of all women diagnosed with breast cancer to help determine the best course of treatment (estrogen receptor positive tumors and estrogen receptor negative tumors respond differently to various chemotherapies). National Institutes of Health, "Steroid Receptors in Breast Cancer. NIH Consensus Statement Online," 2 (June 27–29, 1979), http://consensus.nih.gov/1979/1979Breast CancerReceptors016html.htm.

44. For histories of the use of chemotherapy for breast cancer and discussions of the impact of the NCI's 1988 clinical advisory on the use of adjuvant therapy, see Angela Mariotto et al., "Trends in Use of Adjuvant Multi-Agent Chemotherapy and Tamoxifen for Breast Cancer in the United States: 1975–1999," *Journal of the National Cancer Institute* 94 (November 6, 2002): 1626–34; B. E. Hillner and T. J. Smith, "Efficacy and Cost Effectiveness of Adjuvant Chemotherapy in Women with Node-Negative Breast Cancer: A Decision-Analysis Model," *New England Journal of Medicine* 324 (1991): 160–68; T. P. Johnson et al., "Effect of a National Cancer Institute Clinical Alert on Breast Cancer Practice Patterns," *Journal of Clinical Oncology* 12 (1994): 1783–88.

45. Löwy, *Between Bench and Bedside,* 44.

46. B. J. Kennedy, "Origin and Evolution of Medical Oncology," *Lancet* 354, special issue (1999): SIV41.

47. Figures based on a chart of board-certification numbers from ibid.

48. Löwy, *Between Bench and Bedside,* 63.

49. Sometimes radiation was sandwiched between multimonth regimens of chemotherapy. Sometimes chemotherapy was administered first.

50. Kushner, "Is Aggressive Adjuvant Chemotherapy the Halsted Radical of the '80s?" 345.

51. Interview by author, November 22, 1995.

52. Breast cancer support group meeting, February 1996.

53. National Institutes of Health, "Adjuvant Chemotherapy for Breast Cancer. NIH Consensus Statement Online," 5 (September 9–11, 1985). In 1998 tamoxifen became the first cancer chemotherapeutic drug approved by the FDA for the treatment of healthy high-risk women. Shortly thereafter, tamoxifen was approved by the FDA for the treatment of women with DCIS. I return to this point in the book's conclusion. Also see Klawiter, "Risk, Prevention, and the Breast Cancer Continuum."

54. Kushner, *Alternatives,* xii.

55. Frank, *The Wounded Storyteller,* 8.

56. Breslow and Wilner, *A History of Cancer Control in the United States with Emphasis on the Period 1946–1971,* 459. Also see Terese Lasser and William Kendall Clarke, *Reach to Recovery* (New York: Simon and Schuster, 1972).

57. For analyses of Reach to Recovery, see Kushner, *Breast Cancer,* 210–11, 220, 223–24, 256, 306–7, 349; Breslow and Wilner, *A History of Cancer Control in the United States with Emphasis on the Period 1946–1971,* 431–64; Audre Lorde, *The Cancer Journals* (San Francisco: Aunt Lute Books, 1980); Ross, *Crusade,* 161–71; Batt, *Patient No More,* 218–32.

58. The term "breasted existence" is borrowed from Iris Marion Young, "Breasted Experience: The Look and the Feeling," *Throwing Like a Girl and Other Essays in Feminist Philosophy* (Bloomington: Indiana University Press, 1990).

59. Ross, *Crusade,* 167–68.

60. For a discussion of guidelines for Reach to Recovery volunteers and the expulsion of volunteers who did not conform to the specifications, see Batt, *Patient No More,* 218–37.

61. Quoted in Breslow and Wilner, *A History of Cancer Control in the United States with Emphasis on the Period 1946–1971,* 460.

62. Again, Rose Kushner's pioneering efforts and writings are instructive. Kushner wrote about the obstacles she encountered when she began trying to gather information on the experiences of women who had been treated for breast cancer. Kushner wanted to contact women who were not immediately post-op, and she turned to the ACS and the Reach to Recovery program for help. They were unable to assist her, however, because Reach to Recovery did not maintain contact with women who had been served by their program. Kushner, *Breast Cancer,* 211. For a personal account of

the racial and heterosexual dimensions of Reach to Recovery during the late 1970s, see Lorde, *The Cancer Journals.*

63. Kushner, *Breast Cancer,* 211.

64. Quoted in Breslow and Wilner, *A History of Cancer Control in the United States with Emphasis on the Period 1946–1971,* 462.

65. Surveys conducted by the California Division of the ACS in 1976 and 1981, for example, reveal a steady growth in cancer support groups throughout the state during this period. The 1976 survey shows a total of 28 cancer support groups active throughout the state, but no mention was made regarding how many, if any, of these were designed for breast cancer patients in particular, nor was it possible to ascertain the degree to which the support groups had been institutionalized. By 1981 the number of cancer groups had grown to 161. Despite the nearly sixfold increase in the number of active groups, only 12 groups for the entire state of California, approximately 5 percent of the total number of cancer support groups, were categorized as "mastectomy groups." This indicates a very low level of institutionalization of support groups for women with breast cancer. Pat Fobair et al., "Considerations for Successful Groups," in *Western States Conference on Cancer Rehabilitation: Conference Proceedings, March 1982, San Francisco, California,* ed. Robert Segura, 105–23 (Palo Alto, Calif.: Bull, 1982); paper provided courtesy of Joan Bloom.

66. The founding of the *Journal of Psychosocial Oncology* in 1982 marks the emergence of psychosocial oncology as a distinct field of research and clinical practice. I am grateful to Joan Bloom, one of the pioneers of this field, for this observation (personal communication, April 27, 1999).

67. All names of breast cancer patients who are not otherwise public figures have been changed.

68. Interviewed by author, January 23, 1998.

69. Interviewed by author, September 9, 1996.

70. Interviewed by author, August 2, 1996.

71. Jacqueline R. R. Carter and Pamela Priest Naeve, eds., *Who and Where: A Guide to Cancer Resources* (Union City: Northern California Cancer Center, 1989).

72. Pamela Priest Naeve (personal communication, April 27, 1999).

73. For the earlier study, see D. Spiegel, J. R. Bloom, and I. Yalom, "Group Support for Patients with Metastatic Cancer: A Randomized Prospective Outcome Study," *Archives of General Psychiatry* 38 (May 1981): 527–33. For the follow-up study, see D. Spiegel, J. R. Bloom, and H. C. Kraemer, "Effects of Psychosocial Treatment on Survival of Patients with Metastatic Breast Cancer," *Lancet* 2 (1989): 888–91.

74. *Bay Area Breast Cancer Resource Guide,* sponsored by the Better Health Foundation and cosponsored by Y-ME Bay Area Breast Cancer Network (San Francisco: Better Health Foundation, 1992).

75. The doubling of the size of the resource guide occurred without any changes in the font or format. The 1998 revised edition of the *Guide* was 115 pages long. The first Spanish-language version of the guide was published in 1997: *Area de la Bahia*

346 NOTES TO CHAPTER 5

*Guía de Recursos para la Lucha Contra el Cáncer de los Senos* (San Francisco: Better Health Foundation, 1997).

76. This information was provided by Sherry Spargo, a member of the management team of the California Division of the ACS. Interviewed by author, March 5, 1999.

77. Musa Mayer, "Rethinking 'Cure,'" *Mamm: Women, Cancer, and Community,* March 2001, 42.

78. Frank, *The Wounded Storyteller,* 9.

## 5. EARLY DETECTION AND SCREENING ACTIVISM

1. Lisa Belkin, "How Breast Cancer Became This Year's Hottest Charity," *New York Times Magazine,* December 22, 1996, 40–57, quotation on 45.

2. For a thorough and thoughtful examination of corporate cause-related marketing and the breast cancer movement, see Samantha King, *Pink Ribbons, Inc.: Breast Cancer Culture and the Politics of Philanthropy* (Minneapolis: University of Minnesota Press, 2006).

3. Wolfson, *The Fight against Big Tobacco.* For further development of the concept of interpenetration, see Epstein, "Institutionalizing the New Politics of Difference in U.S. Biomedical Research."

4. Susan Braun, "The History of Breast Cancer Advocacy," *Breast Journal* 9 (2003): S103. For an analysis of the culture of volunteerism in a local chapter of the Komen Foundation, which included a rejection of an "activist" identity, see Amy Blackstone, "'It's Just about Being Fair': Activism and the Politics of Volunteering in the Breast Cancer Movement," *Gender and Society* 18 (2004): 350–68.

5. Suein L. Hwang, "Linking Products to Breast Cancer Fight Helps Firms Bond with Their Customers," *Wall Street Journal,* September 21, 1993.

6. Debra Goldman, "The Consumer Republic: Illness as Metaphor," *AdWeek,* November 3, 1997.

7. Samantha King, "An All-Consuming Cause: Breast Cancer, Corporate Philanthropy, and the Market for Generosity," *Social Text* 19 (2001): 115–43. Also see King, *Pink Ribbons, Inc.*

8. Sandy M. Fernandez, "Mamm's Guide to Breast Cancer Corporate Bucks," *Mamm: Women, Cancer, and Community,* December–January 1999, 34.

9. Belkin, "How Breast Cancer Became This Year's Hottest Charity," 52.

10. From Avon grant-application materials, which were circulated by the National Association of Breast Cancer Organizations (NABCO) in an outreach letter dated April 26, 1996.

11. Quoted in Hwang, "Linking Products to Breast Cancer Fight Helps Firms Bond with Their Customers."

12. Belkin, "How Breast Cancer Became This Year's Hottest Charity," 52.

13. Quoted in Hwang, "Linking Products to Breast Cancer Fight Helps Firms Bond with Their Customers."

14. Fernandez, "Mamm's Guide to Breast Cancer Corporate Bucks," 45.

15. Ibid., 39.

16. Ibid., 34.

17. See Altman, *Waking Up, Fighting Back,* 314.

18. Quoted in Belkin, "How Breast Cancer Became This Year's Hottest Charity," 42. For a slightly different version of this story, see J. Davidson, "Cancer Sells," *Working Woman,* May 1997, 36–39.

19. Susan Claymon, interview by author, January 21, 1998.

20. Illinois (1981) and North Carolina (1982) were the first two states to pass legislation mandating reimbursement for mammographies, followed by Texas, Hawaii, and Massachusetts in 1987. In 1988 these states were joined by six more, including California. Between 1989 and 1992 twenty-four additional states passed mammographic screening reimbursement legislation, and Illinois and North Carolina revised their codes. See Centers for Disease Control and Prevention, "State Laws Relating to Breast Cancer."

21. Braun, "The History of Breast Cancer Advocacy."

22. Veronica Chater, "The Run of Their Lives," *Northern California Woman,* October 1997, 3–5.

23. *San Francisco Chronicle,* October 21, 1996.

24. See Richard W. Scott et al., *Institutional Change and Healthcare Organizations: From Professional Dominance to Managed Care* (Chicago: University of Chicago Press, 2000).

25. For an overview of baby boomers as a health care market, see Kevin Lumsdon, "Baby Boomers Grow Up," *Hospitals and Health Networks,* September 20, 1993, 23–34.

26. The "pill" in this context referred to tamoxifen (brand name Nolvadex), the most frequently prescribed breast cancer treatment drug in the world. See Michael W. DeGregorio and Valerie J. Wiebe, *Tamoxifen and Breast Cancer: What Everyone Should Know about the Treatment of Breast Cancer* (New Haven: Yale University Press, 1999).

27. According to even the most conservative estimates, mammograms (and the radiologists who interpret them) fail to diagnose breast cancers large enough to be visualized by this technology at least 15 percent of the time—even more often among premenopausal women. Most breast cancers do not appear on mammograms and cannot be "seen" by radiologists until they have been growing for about eight years. For a view of how these issues were being discussed during the mid-1990s, see especially Love and Lindsey, *Dr. Susan Love's Breast Book.*

28. Beverly Rhine, "A Faith Centered Model for Activism and Advocacy" (paper presented at the World Conference on Breast Cancer, Kingston, Ontario, Canada, July 13–17, 1997).

29. R. M. Henson, S. W. Wyatt, and N. C. Lee, "The National Breast and Cervical Cancer Early Detection Program: A Comprehensive Public Health Response to Two Major Health Issues for Women," *Journal of Public Health Management Practice* 2 (1996): 36–47.

30. The BCEDP and BCCCP were eventually merged (while maintaining separate

funding streams), renamed Every Woman Counts, and reorganized into ten (rather than fourteen) regional partnerships.

31. California Department of Health Services Cancer Detection Section, "Request for Applications, Breast Cancer Partnerships for Early Detection of Breast Cancer," (Sacramento: California Department of Health Services, 1996).

32. The BCEDP certainly did not invent the strategy of community mobilization or the focus on racial and ethnic minority communities. According to Patricia Kaufert, for example, the ACS's BCDA projects of the 1980s seemed to be "based on principles of community mobilization from the 1960s, shrewd marketing strategies, and elements of evangelical revivalism." But the size, scope, and systematicity of the California BCEDP's utilization of community mobilization make it a particularly important site of this strategy's implementation. Kaufert, "Women and the Debate over Mammography," 172.

33. California Department of Health Services Cancer Detection Section, "Request for Applications, Breast Cancer Partnerships for Early Detection of Breast Cancer."

34. Ibid.

35. Ibid.

36. Ibid.

37. Nelly Oudshoorn and Trevor Pinch, *How Users Matter: The Co-Construction of Users and Technologies* (Cambridge: MIT Press, 2003).

38. At the time I conducted my fieldwork, there was a popular debate regarding the breast cancer risk profile of lesbians. The notion that lesbianism was a risk factor for breast cancer can be traced to a 1993 study conducted by Suzanne Haynes in which she concluded, on the basis of data collected by the National Lesbian Health Care Survey, that lesbians were two to three times more likely to develop breast cancer than heterosexual women. This conclusion was based on data indicating that lesbians, on average, had higher body-mass indexes, fewer pregnancies, and more pregnancies at older ages (for example, over the age of thirty) and that they consumed more alcohol than heterosexual women—all of which were considered risk factors for breast cancer. This rather alarming conclusion was then taken up, misinterpreted, and recirculated in the mainstream and alternative (gay, lesbian, feminist) media. In response to this controversy, the Lyon Martin Women's Health Services (a San Francisco medical clinic serving the lesbian community), in collaboration with the University of California, San Francisco, and with funding from the California Breast Cancer Research Program, conducted a study measuring the risk factors of lesbians compared to those of heterosexual women. In their final report to the California BCRP, the principal investigators concluded that although "lesbians may have a higher risk profile for developing breast cancer . . . it is by no means two to three times higher than for heterosexual women." Suzanne Dibble and Stephanie Roberts, "Breast Cancer Risk Factors: Lesbian and Heterosexual Woman; Final Report," California Breast Cancer Research Program Research Portfolio; abstract of original proposal (1998) and final report (2002) are available at http://www.cbcrp.org/research/PageGrant.asp?grant_id=224. See Liz Galst, "Lesbians

and Cancer Risk," *Mamm: Women, Cancer, and Community,* December–January 1999, 46; Stephanie Roberts et al., "Differences in Risk Factors for Breast Cancer: Lesbian and Heterosexual Women," *Journal of Gay and Lesbian Medical Association* 2 (1998): 93–101. For an analysis of lesbian-gay-bisexual-transgendered activism oriented toward their inclusion in medical research, see Steven Epstein, "Sexualizing Governance and Medicalizing Identities: The Emergence of 'State-Centered' LGBT Health Politics in the United States," *Sexualities* 6 (2003): 131–71.

39. Viewers familiar with lesbian culture and communities in the United States know that golf and softball are often coded as lesbian sports. This is a public health version of what Anthony Cortese calls "lesbian image adverting" that, in the words of Karen Stabiner, "speak[s] to the homosexual consumer in a way that the straight consumer will not notice." Anthony J. Cortese, *Provocateur: Images of Women and Minorities in Advertising* (Rowman and Littlefield, 1997); Karen Stabiner, "Tapping the Homosexual Market," *New York Times Magazine,* May 2, 1982, 35–36, quotation on 35. For a thoughtful discussion of these techniques in the context of contemporary forms of American "orientalism," see Minjeong Kim and Angie Y. Chung, "Consuming Orientalism: Images of Asian/American Women in Multicultural Advertising," *Qualitative Sociology* 28 (Spring 2005): 67–91.

40. California Department of Health Services Cancer Detection Section, "Breast Cancer Early Detection Program Quality Indicator Report (Issue No. 2, December 11)" (Sacramento: California Department of Health Services, 1998).

41. California's Public Benefit Program was created in 1994, when the nonprofit health insurance company Blue Cross of California converted to a for-profit company.

42. In order to stretch the funding as far as possible, guidelines were adopted to ration services. These guidelines limited medical treatment to a maximum of eighteen months per recipient, excluded women who suffered metastases of their original breast cancers, and restricted reimbursement to medically necessary procedures. This meant, among other things, that treatment funds could not be used to pay for reconstructive surgery. The exclusion of low-income, uninsured, and underinsured women from reconstructive surgery constituted yet another bitter irony, given the centrality of normative femininity and the nearly ubiquitous images in breast cancer awareness campaigns, including BCEDP media, of breast cancer survivors with unmarred, unscarred bodies. California Breast Cancer Treatment Fund, "Questions and Answers about the California Breast Cancer Treatment Fund" (Fresno: California Health Collaborative Foundations, 1997).

43. Ruth Rosen, "Where Is the Governor's Compassion?" *Los Angeles Times,* October 7, 1998.

44. King, "An All-Consuming Cause." See also King, *Pink Ribbons, Inc.*

45. Fernandez, "Mamm's Guide to Breast Cancer Corporate Bucks," 32.

46. David H. Harris et al., "Stage of Breast Cancer Diagnosis among Medically Underserved Women in California Receiving Mammography through a State Screening Program," *Cancer Causes and Control* 15 (September 2004): 721–29.

## 6. PATIENT EMPOWERMENT AND FEMINIST
## TREATMENT ACTIVISM

1. In 1988 Winnow found another lump in the same breast where her cancer had been diagnosed three years earlier. Further tests revealed that her breast cancer had metastasized to her lungs and bones. She underwent an oophorectomy (removal of the ovaries) and in the summer of 1989 began radiation and chemotherapy to slow the spread of her cancer. She died on September 7, 1991. See Sandy Polishuk, "Jackie Winnow and the Women's Cancer Resource Center (an Interview)," *Bridges: A Journal for Jewish Feminists and Our Friends* 2 (Fall, 1991): 72.

2. Jackie Winnow, conference speech, as printed in "Lesbians Working on AIDS: Assessing the Impact on Health Care for Women," *Out/Look* 2 (Summer 1989): 10.

3. Ibid.

4. Ibid.

5. Ibid.

6. Ibid.

7. More recent analyses of AIDS activism have confirmed and expanded upon Winnow's analysis of AIDS exceptionalism. In his stunningly thorough and insightful investigation of the AIDS movement, for example, Steve Epstein argued that "the unique features of the clinical picture of AIDS" and its "distinctive social epidemiology" shaped the development of an activist response to AIDS and its character. See Epstein, *Impure Science,* 10. See also the excellent volume edited by Elizabeth Fee and Daniel M. Fox, *AIDS: Burdens of History* (Berkeley and Los Angeles: University of California Press, 1988).

8. Winnow, "Lesbians Working on AIDS," 10.

9. See especially Steven Epstein, "Democratic Science? AIDS Activism and the Contested Construction of Knowledge," *Socialist Review* 91 (1991): 35–64; Steven Epstein, "The Construction of Lay Expertise: AIDS Activism and the Forging of Credibility in the Reform of Clinical Trials," *Science, Technology, and Human Values* 20 (1995): 403–37; Epstein, *Impure Science;* Steven Epstein, "Activism, Drug Regulation, and the Politics of Therapeutic Evaluation in the AIDS Era: A Case Study of ddC and the 'Surrogate Markers' Debate," *Social Studies of Science* 27 (1997): 691–727; Steven Epstein, "Democracy, Expertise, and AIDS Treatment Activism," in *Science, Technology, and Democracy,* ed. Daniel Lee Kleinman, 15–32 (Albany: State University of New York Press, 2000).

10. The Komen Foundation was founded by Nancy Brinker in Dallas in 1982, and Y-ME was founded by Mimi Kaplan and Ann Marcou in Chicago in 1978 as a patient support organization. These organizations did not, however, develop a national network of local chapters until the early 1990s. A third breast cancer organization, the National Association of Breast Cancer Organizations, was founded by Rose Kushner, Nancy Brinker, Ruth Spear, and Diane Blum in 1986. NABCO, which was heavily funded by the pharmaceutical industry, did not develop in the activist direction that Kushner had hoped, however, and she left NABCO in 1988 to create Breastpac, a

political action committee. Breastpac dissolved upon Kushner's death. Although NABCO played a key role in the formation of the National Breast Cancer Coalition, as an organizational entity it primarily functioned as a resource for its member organizations, most of which were in the health care or pharmaceutical industries. NABCO closed its doors in 2004. One of the reasons it folded, according to a prominent leader in the breast cancer movement with whom I spoke, was that NABCO had lost its appeal to pharmaceutical corporations and health care providers, who had shifted their philanthropic activities and public relations machines to breast cancer organizations with greater public visibility and a broader base of popular support.

11. Lorde, *The Cancer Journals,* 16.

12. The DES controversy is an interesting case because it bridges between the politics of cancer and reproduction. DES (diethylstilbestrol) was prescribed to pregnant women in the United States from 1940 to 1971. As a result, between 500,000 and 3 million women—known as "DES daughters"—were exposed prenatally to this drug. These in utero exposures led to a variety of reproductive problems among DES daughters, including miscarriages, infertility, and vaginal and cervical cancer. In 1978 DES Action was founded by women's health activists to provide information and support for women exposed to DES. Because of its relationship to the women's health movement and the movement's focus on the politics of reproduction, DES was viewed through a lens of reproductive rather than cancer activism. See especially Susan Bell, "Becoming a Political Woman: The Reconstruction and Interpretation of Experience through Stories," in *Gender and Discourse: The Power of Talk,* ed. A. D. Todd and S. Fisher, 97–123 (Greenwich, Conn.: Ablex, 1988); Bell, "Narratives and Lives: Women's Health Politics and the Diagnosis of Cancer for DES Daughters," *Narrative Inquiry* 9 (1999): 347–89.

13. For a detailed account of the first decade of the women's health movement, see Ruzek, *The Women's Health Movement.* For an edited volume with a number of fascinating contributions, see Dreifus, *Seizing Our Bodies.* For analyses of the organizational development of the women's and women's health movements, see especially Ferree and Martin, *Feminist Organizations;* Morgan, *Into Our Own Hands;* Weisman, *Women's Health Care;* Ruth Rosen, *The World Split Open: How the Modern Women's Movement Changed America* (New York: Penguin, 2001); Myra Marx Ferree and Beth Hess, *Controversy and Coalition: The Feminist Movement across Three Decades of Change,* 3rd ed. (New York: Routledge, 2000).

14. Two important exceptions to this rule are the Boston Women's Health Book Collective and the National Women's Health Network. Neither of these organizations, however, prioritized breast cancer, although they did include breast cancer among their concerns and played a key role in politicizing the disease. For an analysis of the importance of the Boston Women's Health Book Collective, see especially Gordon and Thorne, "Women's Bodies and Feminist Subversion."

15. For a more recent history of the politics of the cancer research establishment, see Proctor, *Cancer Wars.*

16. See Jackie Winnow, "Lesbians Evolving Health Care: Cancer and AIDS," in

"Disability," *Sinister Wisdom* 39 (Winter 1989–1990): 2–13; Winnow, "Lesbians Evolving Health Care: Our Lives Depend On It," in *Cancer as a Women's Issue: Scratching the Surface*, ed. Midge Stocker, 23–36 (Chicago: Third Side Press, 1991); Winnow, "Lesbians Evolving Health Care: Cancer and AIDS," in *1 in 3: Women with Cancer Confront an Epidemic*, ed. Judith Brady, 233–44 (Pittsburgh, Pa.: Cleis Press, 1991); Winnow, "The Politics of Cancer," in *Confronting Cancer, Constructing Change: New Perspectives on Women and Cancer*, ed. Midge Stocker, 153–64 (Chicago: Third Side Press, 1993). For a more recent collection of essays that includes contributions by Jackie Winnow, see Victoria Brownworth, ed., *Coming Out of the Closet: Writings from the Lesbian Cancer Epidemic* (Emoryville, Calif.: Seal Press, 2000).

17. Bridging between "collective action frames"—what David Snow and his colleagues term "frame bridging"—is an "alignment process" that serves as an important strategy for many social movements. Frame bridging is the process of creating linkages between two collective action frames that are ideologically congruent but structurally unconnected. For discussions of "collective action frames" and "frame alignment processes" in the context of social movements, see especially David A. Snow et al., "Frame Alignment Processes, Micromobilization, and Movement Participation," *American Sociological Review* 51 (1986): 464–81; David A. Snow and Robert D. Benford, "Ideology, Frame Resonance, and Participant Mobilization," in *International Social Movement Research: From Structure to Action*, ed. Bert Klandermans, Hanspeter Kriesi, and Sidney Tarrow, 197–217 (Greenwich, Conn.: JAI Press, 1988); Robert D. Benford and David A. Snow, "Framing Processes and Social Movements: An Overview and Assessment," *Annual Review of Sociology* 26 (2000): 611–39.

18. The emotion culture supported by feminist cancer activists was, interestingly enough, the exact opposite of the dominant public emotions displayed by informed consent activists during the 1980s. Theresa Montini's research has shown that informed consent activists encouraged the public display of sadness and vulnerability but censored the public display of anger, though many activists acknowledged this emotion when they were no longer in public. Montini, "Gender and Emotion in the Advocacy of Breast Cancer Informed Consent Legislation." See also Montini, "Women's Activism for Breast Cancer Informed Consent Laws"; Montini, "Resist and Redirect."

19. *Center News*, Winter 1994, 2.

20. *The Women's Cancer Resource Center Newsletter*, Fall 2000, 2.

21. Historical information is based on WCRC newsletters, interviews with staff and volunteers who had been involved since the beginning, and the published speeches and interviews of Jackie Winnow, including Polishuk, "Jackie Winnow and the Women's Cancer Resource Center."

22. Susan Liroff, "Director's Farewell," *Women's Cancer Resource Center Update and News* 3 (Spring 1993): 10.

23. Claymon, interview.

24. Charlotte Maxwell Complementary Clinic was named in honor of a former patient of Savitz.

25. Complementary therapy refers to therapies that are used in conjunction with—as a complement to—mainstream therapies (surgery, radiation, chemotherapy, and hormone therapy). Complementary therapies, which include acupressure, acupuncture, massage, meditation, Chinese herbs, homeopathy, and special diets, are typically used to mitigate the side effects of mainstream treatments and to strengthen patients' immune systems.

26. These goals were stated in *Charlotte's Web*, the newsletter of CMCC.

27. Andrea Martin, interview by author, November 26, 1996.

28. Claymon, interview.

29. Joe Thornton, *Chlorine, Human Health, and the Environment: The Breast Cancer Warning; A Greenpeace Report* (Washington, D.C.: Greenpeace, 1993).

30. Breast Cancer Action, "Why Do We Say 'Cancer Sucks'?" *Breast Cancer Action Newsletter,* Summer 2003.

31. The signatory organizations were BCA, the Bay Area Black Women's Health Project, WCRC, Lyon Martin Women's Health Services, Bay Area Breast Cancer Network (in San Jose), Cancer Support Community, CMCC, and the Medical Effectiveness Research Center for Diverse Populations. A copy of this letter was obtained from BCA, courtesy of Barbara Brenner.

32. Data from "The Susan G. Komen Breast Cancer Foundation/San Francisco Chapter Grants Report" for 1995 and 1996. Data from 1995 and 1996 are no longer available from the Web site of what is now called the Komen San Francisco Bay Area Affiliate, but data from 1998 to 2006 are available at http://www.sfkomen.org/k_grants_awards.html.

33. The historical data for this background section is based on an interview (1997) with Abby Zimberg, who served as the key organizer of the Women and Cancer Walk during the years—1994, 1995, 1996—that I volunteered. It also draws on Carrie Spector, "Before the Battle of the Corporate Walkathons, There Was the Women and Cancer Walk," *Breast Cancer Action Newsletter,* November–December 2003.

34. Spector, "Before the Battle of the Corporate Walkathons, There Was the Women and Cancer Walk."

35. Abby Zimberg, interview by author, July 12, 1997.

36. The term "corporeal styles" is borrowed from Judith Butler, "Performative Acts and Gender Constitution: An Essay in Phenomenology and Feminist Theory," in *Performing Feminisms: Feminist Critical Theory and Theatre,* ed. Sue-Ellen Case, 270–82 (Baltimore: The Johns Hopkins University Press, 1990), 272.

37. For an excellent brief overview of Bay Area treatment activism focusing on clinical trials, including the episode of civil disobedience at Genentech, see R. Ruth Linden, "Re-inventing Treatment Activism," *Breast Cancer Action Newsletter,* December 1995, 3–4.

38. The term "universe of political discourse" is borrowed from Jenson, "Changing Discourse, Changing Agendas."

39. Although Elenore Pred (one of the cofounders and the first president of BCA),

for example, was a lesbian, that fact was not part of her public life or the public face of BCA. For thoughtful discussions of the role of lesbians in women's cancer activism, see Ulrike Boehmer, *The Personal Is Political: Women's Activism in Response to the Breast Cancer and AIDS Epidemics* (Albany: State University of New York Press, 2000). Also see Andrea Densham, "The Marginalized Uses of Power and Identity: Lesbians' Participation in Breast Cancer and AIDS Activism," in *Women Transforming Politics: An Alternative Reader,* ed. Cathy J. Cohen, Kathleen B. Jones, and Joan C. Tronto, 284–301 (New York: New York University Press, 1997).

40. For a full statement of BCA's policy on corporate contributions, go to http://www.bcaction.org/index.php?page=policy-on-corporate-contributions.

41. Andy Coghlan, *Art.Rage.Us: Art and Writing by Women with Breast Cancer* (San Francisco: Chronicle Books, 1998). The exhibit traveled to Los Angeles for twelve weeks, then to Hong Kong and elsewhere.

42. Claymon interview.

43. One of the most original and arresting artwork and activism projects that I encountered during my fieldwork in the Bay Area was called "Who Holds the Mirror? Breast Cancer, Women's Lives, and the Environment: A Traveling Mural." Beth Sauerhaft, the project's inspired organizer, oversaw the creation of a mural made up of numerous panels, each of which depicted a different aspect of breast cancer and its relationship to a wide range of social issues, including environmental justice, immigrant rights, body image and self-esteem, access to health care, and the politics of research. Sauerhaft used the mural as an aid in her efforts at community outreach, education, and activism. Additional information is available at http://whoholdsthemirror.com.

For an interesting new literature that examines the relationship between artwork and breast cancer activism from a scholarly perspective, see especially Alan Radley and Susan Bell, "Artworks, Collective Experience, and Claims for Social Justice: The Case of Women Living with Breast Cancer," *Sociology of Health and Illness* 29, no. 3 (2007): 366–90. Also see Susan Bell, "Living with Breast Cancer in Text and Image: Making Art to Make Sense," *Qualitative Research in Psychology* 3 (2006): 31–44.

44. Irving Saraf and Allie Light's 1991 documentary, *In the Shadow of the Stars,* won an Oscar. Their 1994 documentary, *Dialogues with Mad Women,* won an Emmy. For additional information on these remarkable filmmakers and their films, see Light-Saraf Films, http://www.lightsaraffilms.com.

45. For correspondence between Rachel Carson and George Crile, the maverick activist-doctor with whom Carson consulted after her original doctor lied to her, see Leopold, *A Darker Ribbon.* For discussions of Carson's life and legacy, see Sandra Steingraber, "We All Live Downwind," in Brady, *1 in 3,* 36–48; Steingraber, "'If I Live to Be 90 Still Wanting to Say Something': My Search for Rachel Carson," in *Confronting Cancer, Constructing Change: New Perspectives on Women and Cancer,* ed. Midge Stocker, Women/Cancer/Fear/Power, 181–200 (Chicago: Third Side Press, 1993); Steingraber, *Living Downstream: An Ecologist Looks at Cancer and the Environment* (Reading, Mass.: Addison-Wesley, 1997).

46. The Jennifer Altman Foundation is connected to Commonweal, a nonprofit health and environmental research institute and a retreat center for people with cancer. Commonweal is located about an hour north of San Francisco, in Bolinas, California.

47. Nancy Evans, ed., *Rachel's Daughters: Searching for the Causes of Breast Cancer Community Action and Resource Guide* (San Francisco: Light-Saraf Films, n.d.), 2.

48. Susan Claymon died on January 18, 2000.

## 7. CANCER PREVENTION AND ENVIRONMENTAL RISK

1. In a speech that she gave at a community forum in 1996 entitled "The Politics of Breast Cancer," Nancy Evans, then president of BCA, quoted this passage, which she attributed to a speech delivered by Sandra Steingraber in Santa Fe, New Mexico, in 1994. I quote it here partly to illustrate the way discourses traveled within the culture of environmental cancer activism.

2. I began doing participant observation of the TLC in October 1994, shortly after its formation. Most of the information on the history of the TLC comes from my notes on those meetings and from my participation in early events, including the 1994 demonstration at Race for the Cure. The information about the first two meetings of the TLC is based on interviews with cancer activist Judy Brady and on the public recounting of this history at various events. I conducted participant observation research with the TLC from 1994 to 1999.

3. Quotation taken from AstraZeneca International, "Community and Company Projects: US Breast Cancer Awareness Month," http://www.astrazeneca.com/communityproject/110.aspx.

4. Although NBCAM's genealogy can be traced to 1985, there was no "National Breast Cancer Awareness Month" that year. Rather, there was a week of activities designed around the promotion of breast cancer early detection. As part of this effort Imperial Chemical Industries created a public service announcement featuring Susan Ford Bales and her mother, Betty Ford. The public service message elicited such a positive response that it led to the program's expansion into National Breast Cancer Awareness Month. See Johns Hopkins Health Information, "How It All Began."

5. This already-impressive vertical integration was later extended when Zeneca purchased Salick Health Care, which consisted of eleven comprehensive outpatient cancer treatment centers, six comprehensive breast centers, and a number of for-profit medical practices specializing in cancer, including one down the block from WCRC. Elisabeth Rosenthal, "Maker of Cancer Drugs to Oversee Prescriptions at 11 Cancer Clinics," *New York Times,* April 15, 1997.

6. In 1999 NBCAM was second on the Project Censored list of the most censored news stories in 1998. For reviews of Project Censored's list, see Jim Doyle, review of *Censored 1999: The News That Didn't Make the News—The Year's Top 25 Censored Stories,* by Peter Phillips and Project Censored, *San Francisco Chronicle,* June 6, 1999, Book Review Section, 5. See also Gabriel Roth, "Not Fit to Print? Project Censored Uncovers the Stories That Didn't Make the News in 1998," *Guardian,* March 24, 1999.

7. The term "National Cancer Industry Awareness Month" was coined in 1993 by the late Jeannie Marshall, an activist with the Women's Community Cancer Project in Cambridge, Massachusetts. I am indebted to Barbara Brenner for this insight.

8. The image was actually a parody of *Time* magazine. The image, which was printed on posters and postcards and was widely circulated in feminist and environmental cancer networks, said, "Cancer has been linked to chlorine in the environment." At the bottom, the alarm clock is followed by the words "for Prevention" [time for prevention]. At the very bottom it reads: "In early 1992 *TIME* assured its readers that it would use non-chlorine bleached paper in the magazine 'as soon as it is practical to do so.' TIME HAS YET TO KEEP THAT PROMISE." Matuschka, *Time for Prevention* (1994).

9. Northern California Cancer Center, "Breast Cancer in the Greater Bay Area: Highest Incidence Rates in the World," *Greater Bay Area Cancer Registry Report* 5 (1994). The first page of this report contained a chart comparing breast cancer rates for women living in twenty different regions that included Japan, India, Colombia, Israel, France, Spain, Australia, Hawaii, and the San Francisco Bay Area. In visually striking terms the bar chart showed that white women in the Bay Area had the highest recorded rates of breast cancer in the world. The data on black women in the Bay Area, however, were in many ways even more shocking, though they received less attention. They showed that black women in the Bay Area had the fourth-highest breast cancer incidence rate of any group of women anywhere in the world. It was well known that black women had the highest mortality rate, but high incidence rates were perceived as a white issue. As this report made clear, however, black women in the Bay Area had a higher incidence rate than almost any other group of women in the world. Northern California Cancer Center, "Breast Cancer in the Greater Bay Area." Northern California Cancer Center, "Breast Cancer in the Greater Bay Area: Highest Incidence Rates in the World," *Greater Bay Area Cancer Registry Report* 5 (1994).

10. WEDO, which is based in New York City, was founded in 1990 by former U.S. Congresswoman and "cancer fighter" Bella Abzug, who led WEDO until her death in 1998.

11. Francine Levien died from breast cancer in 2001.

12. I was a participant-observer with MBCW for about three years, beginning in the fall of 1995, when the group first began meeting in Levien's living room. Interestingly enough, however, I learned of the formation of this new group at Race for the Cure, where GayLynn Richards, an oncology nurse at Marin Medical Center, was staffing the hospital's display booth—demonstrating, once again, the density of linkages between these three COAs and the relatively unrestrained flow of information within the Bay Area field of contention.

13. For a study of the Bayview–Hunters Point case, see Fishman, "Assessing Breast Cancer."

14. Clarence Johnson, "S.F. Summit to Address High Breast Cancer Rate," *San Francisco Chronicle,* October 30, 1996.

15. Andrea Martin, interview by author, November 11, 1996.

16. For an important study on the "emotion work" of social movements and the role of emotion cultures in AIDS activism, see Deborah B. Gould, "Life during Wartime: Emotions and the Development of ACT UP," *Mobilization: An International Journal* 7 (2002): 177–200.

17. Wingspread Conference on the Precautionary Principle, "Wingspread Statement on the Precautionary Principle," January 26, 1998, Science and Environmental Health Network, http://www.sehn.org/wing.html.

18. Anthony S. Robbins, Sonia Brescianini, and Jennifer L. Kelsey, "Regional Differences in Known Risk Factors and the Higher Incidence of Breast Cancer in San Francisco," *Journal of the National Cancer Institute* 89 (July 2, 1997): 960–65.

## 8. THE IMPACT OF DISEASE REGIMES AND SOCIAL MOVEMENTS ON ILLNESS EXPERIENCE

1. The names of the main characters in this narrative—"Clara Larson," her partner "Regina," and her partner "Susan"—are pseudonyms.

2. National Institutes of Health, "The Treatment of Primary Breast Cancer and Management of Local Disease." The first consensus development conference, which focused on mammographic screening, was held in 1977. See chapters 3 and 4 for discussions of the NIH consensus development conferences on breast cancer.

3. Centers for Disease Control and Prevention, "State Laws Relating to Breast Cancer."

4. Sandra Butler and Barbara Rosenblum, *Cancer in Two Voices* (San Francisco: Spinsters, 1991).

5. See Kathryn Hollenbach and Barry Meisenberg, "Outpatient Stem Cell Transplants for Breast Cancer," grant application, 1996, http://www.cbcrp.org/research/PageGrant.asp?grant_id=89.

6. See Michelle M. Mello and Troyen A. Brennan, "The Controversy over High-Dose Chemotherapy with Autologous Bone Marrow Transplant for Breast Cancer," *Health Affairs: The Policy Journal of the Health Sphere* 20 (September–October 2001): 101–17; Hope Rugo, "High-Dose Chemotherapy for Breast Cancer: The Controversy Continues!" *Carol Franc Buck Breast Cancer Center Newsletter*, Winter 1999.

7. Mello and Brennan, "The Controversy over High-Dose Chemotherapy with Autologous Bone Marrow Transplant for Breast Cancer," 5. In 2000 the results of a major clinical trial of high-dose chemotherapy with bone marrow transplant for the treatment of metastatic breast cancer were reported in the *New England Journal of Medicine*. This trial, conducted by Edward Stadtmauer and colleagues, which confirmed the results of four other randomized trials, showed no survival advantage for this procedure, relative to standard-dose chemotherapy. An accompanying editorial concluded that "to a reasonable degree of probability, this form of treatment for women with metastatic breast cancer has been proved to be ineffective and should be abandoned in favor of well-justified alternatives." Quoted in Mello and Brennan, "The Controversy over High-Dose Chemotherapy with Autologous Bone Marrow Transplant for Breast Cancer," 5.

8. For an institutional analysis of these transformations in the Bay Area, see especially Scott et al., *Institutional Change and Healthcare Organizations*.

9. See especially Ellen R. Schaffer, "Breast Cancer and the Evolving Health Care System: Why Health Care Reform Is a Breast Cancer Issue," in *Breast Cancer: Society Shapes an Epidemic*, ed. Anne S. Kasper and Susan J. Ferguson, 89–118 (New York: St. Martin's Press, 2000).

## 9. BREAST CANCER IN THE TWENTY-FIRST CENTURY

1. Michael Lerner, "The Age of Extinction and the Emerging Environmental Health Movement" (n.d. [accessed November 11, 2006]), http://www.commonweal.org/pubs/lerner/article_extinction.html.

2. Quoted in "International Summit on Breast Cancer and the Environment: Research Needs" (conference held in Santa Cruz, Calif., May 22–25, 2002), http://cfch.berkeley.edu/reports/BC%20and%20Environment%20Summit%20Final%20Report.pdf, 32.

3. The BCCPTA provided states with the option of using enhanced federal matching funds to extend Medicaid eligibility to women diagnosed with breast or cervical cancer through publicly funded screening programs. California activists, legislators, and policy makers worked with one eye on the national policy-making arena, altering and adjusting their proposals in anticipation of and in response to the progress of the federal legislation. For an analysis of the Breast and Cervical Cancer Prevention and Treatment Act of 2000, see Paula M. Lantz, Carol S. Weisman, and Zena Itani, "A Disease-Specific Medicaid Expansion for Women: The Breast and Cervical Cancer Prevention and Treatment Act of 2000," *Women's Health Issues* 13 (2003): 79–92.

4. The legislation was not a perfect solution, and it was the source of fairly rancorous debates. The chief complaint was that it established a two-tiered system that provided inadequate care for disenfranchised immigrants. Only citizens and legal residents were able to qualify for the full range of Medic-Cal (Medicaid) benefits. Women who did not meet the citizenship or legal residency requirements established by the federally subsidized program were authorized to receive treatment for breast and cervical cancer, but the state would not pay for other medical services, regardless of need.

5. This press statement, along with the images and educational materials used in the campaign, may be found at http://www.breastcancerfund.org/site/pp.asp?c=kwkXLdPaE&b=83016.

6. The BCF's Art-Reach program was launched in 1998 with Art.Rage.Us. "Obsessed with Breasts" was part of this larger campaign of art-based education and activism. See http://www.breastcancerfund.org/site/pp.asp?c=kwkXLdPaE&b=83002.

7. See Think before You Pink: A Project of Breast Cancer Action, http://www.thinkbeforeyoupink.org.

8. Cited in "Critical Questions to Ask," Think before You Pink: A Project of Breast Cancer Action, http://www.thinkbeforeyoupink.org/Pages/CriticalQuestions.html.

9. Nancy Evans, ed., *State of the Evidence: What Is the Connection between Chemicals*

*and Breast Cancer?* (San Francisco: Breast Cancer Fund and Breast Cancer Action, 2002), 20; also *State of the Evidence: What Is the Connection between the Environment and Breast Cancer?* 4th ed. (San Francisco: Breast Cancer Fund and Breast Cancer Action, 2006).

10. For information on this campaign, see http://www.safecosmetics.org.

11. The summit was funded through a grant to the UC–Berkeley Center for Family and Community Health.

12. "International Summit on Breast Cancer and the Environment: Research Needs," 39. I use the term "painstaking" because the planning and preparation activities that proceeded the summit were as thoroughly documented in the official report as any I have ever seen. Likewise, the report-writing and approval process was as democratic and participatory as any I have seen—to the point of including participants' comments in response to the report itself. The report was submitted to the CDC by Patricia Buffler, who served as the "principal investigator" for the CDC grant application, and other researchers at the University of California, Berkeley, School of Public Health. The report was submitted to the CDC and released to the public in March 2003.

13. In 2006 MBCW changed its name to Zero Breast Cancer. Executive Director Janice Barlow explained in the summer newsletter, "The name Marin Breast Cancer Watch has served us well for the past decade, but it no longer reflects what we are doing or what we are setting out to do in the future." Because MBCW's focus had grown to include a broader geographic region and issues that extended beyond Marin County, the organization decided to change its name to something that reflected this expanded focus. Janice Barlow, "Marin Breast Cancer Watch Celebrates 10th Anniversary with a New Name and Visual Identity," *Zero Breast Cancer,* Summer 2006.

14. "Community Outreach and Translation," Early Environmental Exposures: Breast Cancer and the Environment Research Centers, http://www.bcerc.org/cotc.htm.

15. Sara Shostak has written extensively about the shift toward genomics in the NIEHS and the environmental health sciences. See Sara Shostak, "Disciplinary Emergence in the Environmental Health Sciences, 1950–2000" (Ph.D. diss., University of California, San Francisco, 2003); Shostak, "Locating Gene–Environment Interaction: At the Intersections of Genetics and Public Health," *Social Science and Medicine* 56 (2003): 2327–42; Shostak, "Environmental Justice and Genomics: Acting on the Future of Environmental Health," *Science as Culture* 13 (2004): 539–62.

16. Early Environmental Exposures: Breast Cancer and the Environment Research Centers, http://www.bcerc.org. The passage appears to be authored by the NIEHS program director, Leslie Reinlib. I am assuming that the meaning of "outcomes," in this case, is "goals."

17. See, for example, the article written by BCA's executive director, Barbara Brenner, after she attended the first annual meeting of the BCERC in Princeton, New Jersey: "Breast Cancer and the Environment Research Centers: Promises and Pipe Dreams," *Breast Cancer Action Newsletter* (December 2004–January 2005).

18. For additional information on biomonitoring, see Commonweal Biomonitoring

Resource Center, http://www.commonweal.org/programs/brc. Also see Centers for Disease Control and Prevention, *Third National Report on Human Exposures to Environmental Chemicals* (Atlanta, Ga.: CDC, 2005), available at http://www.cdc.gov/exposurereport/report.htm.

19. The NIH established the Women's Health Initiative (WHI) in 1991 to address the most common causes of death, disability, and impaired quality of life for postmenopausal women—a group whose health, historically, had been undervalued and overlooked by biomedical researchers and funding agencies. The WHI focused on cardiovascular disease, cancer, and osteoporosis. The WHI was a fifteen-year, multimillion-dollar undertaking—one of the largest U.S. prevention studies of its kind. It included a community preventions study, an observational study, and three clinical trials, one of which consisted of two studies of hormone-replacement therapy. For information on the HRT studies, see http://www.nhlbi.nih.gov/whi/whi_faq.htm.

20. V. F. Semiglazov et al., "[Interim Results of a Prospective Randomized Study of Self-Examination for Early Detection of Breast Cancer (Russia/St. Petersburg/WHO)]," *Vopr Onkol* 45 (1999): 265–71; D. B. Thomas et al., "Randomized Trial of Breast Self-Examination in Shanghai: Final Results," *Journal of the National Cancer Institute* 94 (2002): 1445–57.

21. Gina Kolata, "Study Sets Off Debate over Mammograms' Value," *New York Times,* December 9, 2001.

22. Quoted in ibid.

23. Quoted in ibid.

24. Lisa M. Schwartz et al., "Enthusiasm for Cancer Screening in the United States," *Journal of the American Medical Association* 291 (January 7, 2004): 71–78.

25. Karsten Juhl Jørgensen and Peter C. Gøtzsche, "Presentation on Websites of Possible Benefits and Harms from Screening for Breast Cancer: Cross Sectional Study," *British Medical Journal* 328 (January 17, 2004): 148.

26. Donald A. Berry et al., "Effect of Screening and Adjuvant Therapy on Mortality from Breast Cancer," *New England Journal of Medicine* 353 (October 27, 2005): 1784–92.

27. "The Benefits of Mammography," editorial, *New York Times,* November 6, 2005. Also see Gina Kolata, "New Study Finds Mammograms Have Benefits in Fighting Cancer," *New York Times,* October 26, 2005.

28. Theresa Agovino, "Genetic Tests to Get Marketing Push," *Miami Herald,* June 6, 2002.

29. See Lesley Henderson and Jenny Kitzinger, "The Human Drama of Genetics: 'Hard' and 'Soft' Media Representations of Inherited Breast Cancer," *Sociology of Health and Illness* 21 (1991): 560–78; National Cancer Institute and National Action Plan on Breast Cancer, "Genetic Testing for Breast Cancer Risk: It's Your Choice," (Washington, D.C.: National Institutes of Health, 1997); Lerner, "Great Expectations"; Robertson, "Embodying Risk, Embodying Political Rationality." For a comparative study of the politics of genetic screening in the United States and the United Kingdom, see Parthasarathy, "Regulating Risk."

30. Mutations in BRCA genes are not exclusive to women. Men with an altered BRCA1 or BRCA2 gene (especially the latter) have an increased risk of breast cancer (approximately 6 percent) and possibly of prostate cancer. See especially http://www .cancer.gov/cancertopics/factsheet/Risk/BRCA.

31. For additional information on genetic testing for BRCA1 and BRCA2, see especially http://www.cancer.gov/cancertopics/factsheet/Risk/BRCA.

32. See http://www.cancer.gov/cancertopics/factsheet/Risk/BRCA. Interestingly enough, the risk of developing breast cancer before the age of fifty appears to be increasing for women with BRCA1 and BRCA2 mutations. A recent study conducted by Mary-Claire King shows that among mutation carriers born before 1940, the risk of developing breast cancer before the age of fifty was 24 percent. Among those born after 1940, however, the risk was 67 percent. This raises intriguing questions about the role of gene–environment interactions. See Mary-Claire King et al., "Breast and Ovarian Cancer Risks Due to Inherited Mutations in BRCA1 and BRCA2," *Science* 24 (October 2003): 643–46.

33. See Nina Hallowell, "Reconstructing the Body or Reconstructing the Woman? Problems of Prophylactic Mastectomy for Hereditary Breast Cancer Risk," in Potts, *Ideologies of Breast Cancer,* 153–80.

34. For a study of the Breast Cancer Prevention Trial and the promotion of tamoxifen to healthy, high-risk women, see Hogle, "Chemoprevention for Healthy Women"; Klawiter, "Risk, Prevention, and the Breast Cancer Continuum"; Wooddell, "Codes, Identities, and Pathologies in the Construction of Tamoxifen as a Chemoprophylactic for Breast Cancer Risk Reduction in Healthy Women at High Risk"; Klawiter, "Regulatory Shifts, Pharmaceutical Scripts, and the New Consumption Junction." For a study of the STAR trial (Study of Tamoxifen and Raloxifene), see Jennifer Ruth Fosket, "Breast Cancer Risk and the Politics of Prevention: Analysis of a Clinical Trial" (Ph.D. diss., University of California, San Francisco, 2002); Fosket, "Constructing 'High-Risk Women.'"

35. IBIS-I and IBIS-II, which were funded by the United Kingdom, were conducted in Australia, New Zealand, Austria, France, Germany, Italy, and Switzerland.

36. Victor G. Vogel et al., "Effects of Tamoxifen vs. Raloxifene on the Risk of Developing Invasive Breast Cancer and Other Disease Outcomes," *Journal of the American Medical Association* 295 (June 21, 2006): 2727–41.

37. The literature on online support for women with breast cancer includes Barbara F. Sharf, "Communicating Breast Cancer On-Line: Support and Empowerment on the Internet," *Women and Health* 26 (1997): 65–84; Victoria Pitts, "Illness and Internet Empowerment: Writing and Reading Breast Cancer and Cyberspace," *Health: Interdisciplinary Journal of Health, Illness, and Medicine* 8 (2004): 33–59; Patricia Radin, "'To Me, It's My Life': Medical Communication, Trust, and Activism in Cyberspace," *Social Science and Medicine* 62 (2006): 591–601. For studies of "cyberactivism," see Martha McCaughey and Michael D. Ayers, eds., *Cyberactivism: Online Activism in Theory and Practice* (New York: Routledge, 2003).

38. All quotations from Franklin Hoke, "Struggle over Online Cancer Service Spurs Larger Medical Ethics Debate," *Scientist* 9 (April 3, 1995): 1.

39. Quoted in Gina Kolata, "Shift in Treating Breast Cancer Is under Debate," *New York Times,* May 12, 2006.

40. Personal communication, e-mail, March 23, 2005.

41. Personal communication, e-mail, February 12, 2005.

42. Kolata, "Shift in Treating Breast Cancer Is under Debate."

## CONCLUSION

1. Foucault, *History of Sexuality,* 1:89.

2. The expansion of clinical breast exam also incorporated a new group of voluntary subjects—primary care physicians—more fully into the regime of breast cancer. This, however, lies beyond the scope of my focus on involuntary subjects of the regime.

3. See for example Brady, *1 in 3;* Stocker, *Cancer as a Women's Issue;* Stocker, *Confronting Cancer, Constructing Change.*

4. Amy Blackstone has written extensively about activism among Komen volunteers in one local chapter. See especially Amy Blackstone, "Racing for the Cure and Taking Back the Night: Constructing Gender, Politics, and Public Participation in Women's Activist/Volunteer Work" (Ph.D. diss., University of Minnesota, 2003); Blackstone, "'It's Just about Being Fair.'"

5. Meyer and Whittier, "Social Movement Spillover."

6. The fact that AIDS was not simply coded as a men's disease (in the late 1980s and early 1990s) but as a *gay* men's disease—in other words, the disease of a stigmatized minority—was elided by breast cancer activists who sought, instead, to emphasize sex-based rather than sexuality-based inequalities, the latter of which would have cut against the largely (but not entirely, thanks to Susan Love) heterosexual public image of breast cancer activists. The influence of AIDS activism on breast/cancer activism (along with the influence of feminism, the environmental movement, and the lesbian community) is particularly strong in Winnow, "Lesbians Working on AIDS"; Winnow, "Lesbians Evolving Health Care: Cancer and AIDS."

7. These influences are easily visible, for example, in Stocker, *Cancer as a Women's Issue;* Stocker, *Confronting Cancer, Constructing Change.* For analyses of the organizational and cultural impact of the women's movement, the women's health movement, and lesbian feminism, broadly speaking, see especially Taylor and Whittier, "Collective Identity in Social Movement Communities"; Suzanne Staggenborg, Donna Eder, and Lori Sudderth, "Women's Culture and Social Change: Evidence from the National Women's Music Festival," *Berkeley Journal of Sociology* 38 (1993): 31–64; Ferree and Martin, *Feminist Organizations;* Weisman, *Women's Health Care;* Morgan, *Into Our Own Hands;* Rosen, *The World Split Open.*

8. The strength of these influences is particularly visible, for example, in Brady, *1 in 3;* Steingraber, *Living Downstream.*

9. Personal correspondence, August 11, 1998. Wanna Wright, "Alive/To Testify," 1997.

10. Wright, in turn, continued to be shaped by the Bay Area COAs. In the spring of 2005 Wright became one of twelve Californians "known for their integrity, wisdom, and commitment to community health and justice" who were invited by the Commonweal Biomonitoring Resource Center to participate in a study testing their bodies for the presence of chemical pollutants. She later commented, "My beloved friend, Andrea Martin, who founded the Breast Cancer Fund, was tested for the presence of chemicals in her body, and strongly believed that many of those chemical found were connected to the cancers she suffered from. Before then, I had focused on early detection as key, in terms of cancer activism, but when we lost Andrea to cancer [in 2003], I became more focused on prevention and wanted to be tested as a way to raise public awareness about the possible environmental connections to cancer." Quoted in Commonweal Biomonitoring Resource Center, "Taking It All In: Documenting Chemical Pollution in Californians through Biomonitoring" (2005), http://www .commonweal.org/programs/brc/Taking_It_All_In.html, 33. The report of this study and the publicity it generated helped secure the success of the California biomonitoring legislation in 2006. See Commonweal Biomonitoring Resource Center, "Taking It All In."

11. For thoughtful treatments of this point, see especially Bell, "Living with Breast Cancer in Text and Image," and Radley and Bell, "Artworks, Collective Experience, and Claims for Social Justice."

12. Brown et al., "Embodied Health Movements."

13. A number of journals have devoted special issues to social movements; for example, see *Sociology of Health and Illness* 26, no. 6 (2004), edited by Phil Brown and Steve Zavestoski; *Science as Culture* 13, no. 4 (2004), edited by David Hess; and *Social Science and Medicine* 62, no. 3 (2006), edited by Kyra Landzelius and Joe Dumit. Also see Frickel and Moore, *The New Political Sociology of Science;* Epstein, "Patient Groups and Health Movements."

14. Quoted in Matuschka, "Why I Did It," 163.

15. Ibid., 162.

16. Jon Carroll, "The Image of the Century," *San Francisco Chronicle,* December 31, 1999.

## APPENDIX

1. Michael Burawoy, Teaching Participant Observation," in *Ethnography Unbound: Power and Resistance in the Modern Metropolis,* ed. Michael Burawoy et al., 291–300 (Berkeley and Los Angeles: University of California Press, 1991), 291.

2. Millie Thayer, "Social Movements, Ethnography, and Power," *Political Sociology: States, Power, and Societies,* the newsletter of the Political Sociology section of the American Sociological Association, 11, no. 2 (2005): 1, 4–5, quotation on 4.

3. Michael Burawoy, "Reaching for the Global," introduction to *Global Ethnography: Forces, Connections, and Imaginations in a Postmodern World,* ed. Michael Burawoy et al., 1–40 (Berkeley and Los Angeles: University of California Press, 2000), 27.

4. I had never heard of "multisited" ethnography when I began my research in 1994, but it was an approach that many of the graduate students in Burawoy's Global Ethnographies Group seemed, more or less, to spontaneously pursue. Many years later I discovered that the anthropologist George Marcus had formally coined the term in 1998, juxtaposing it to traditional ethnography, where the parameters of the field are determined in advance. See especially Burawoy et al., *Global Ethnography;* George Marcus, *Ethnography through Thick and Thin* (Princeton: Princeton University Press, 1998).

5. The term "non-innocent" is borrowed from Donna Haraway, "Situated Knowledges: The Science Question in Feminism and the Privilege of Partial Perspective," in *Simians, Cyborgs, and Women,* 183–202.

6. See especially Burawoy, "The Extended Case Method," *Sociological Theory* 16, no. 1 (1998): 4–33; Burawoy, "Critical Sociology: A Dialogue between Two Sciences," *Contemporary Sociology* 27, no. 1 (1998): 12–20; Burawoy, "Revisits: An Outline of a Theory of Reflexive Ethnography," *American Sociological Review* 68 (2003): 645–79. Also see Burawoy et al., *Ethnography Unbound,* and Burawoy, "Reaching for the Global."

7. Burawoy, "Reaching for the Global," 28.

8. Ibid., 27.

9. Burawoy et al., *Ethnography Unbound,* 6.

10. Melucci, "The Symbolic Challenge of Contemporary Movements"; Melucci, "Getting Involved: Identity and Mobilization in Social Movements," *International Social Movements Research* 1 (1988): 329–48; Melucci, *Nomads of the Present: Social Movements and Individual Needs in Contemporary Society* (London: Hutchinson Radius, 1989).

11. Consciousness-raising groups, in turn, were fed by experiences in the civil rights and new left movements. See especially Sara Evans, *Personal Politics: The Roots of Women's Liberation in the Civil Rights Movement and the New Left* (New York: Vintage Books, 1980). Also see Ferree and Hess, *Controversy and Coalition.*

12. Verta Taylor is one of the few scholars who has studied women's self-help from a feminist, social movements perspective, and she has done so in exemplary fashion. See Taylor, *Rock-a-Bye Baby;* Taylor, "Gender and Social Movements: Gender Processes in Women's Self-Help Movements," *Gender and Society* 13, no. 1 (1999): 8–33; Taylor, "Emotions and Identity in Women's Self-Help Movements," in *Self, Identity, and Social Movements,* ed. Sheldon Stryker, Timothy J. Owens, and Robert W. White, 271–99 (Minneapolis: University of Minnesota Press, 2000); Taylor and Van Willigen, "Women's Self-Help and the Reconstruction of Gender."

# INDEX

Abbott, Dorothy, 76–77, 334n93
Abzug, Bella, 212–13, 356n10
access to medical treatment, unequal, 35,
103. *See also* medically marginalized
communities
access to resources: democratization of
access to information, 271–74; support groups and, 126
ACS. *See* American Cancer Society
activism: consensus, 134–35; Washington,
D.C., xx–xxii, 42, 284. *See also* cancer
prevention and environmental
activism, culture of; early detection
and screening activism, culture of;
patient empowerment and feminist
treatment activism, culture of
ACT UP, 172, 183, 184
ACT UP Golden Gate, 285
adjuvant chemotherapy, 113–17
adjuvant therapy, 232, 281; NIH consensus development conference on (1985),
114, 116; support groups reconceptualized as another form of, 125
advertising. *See* marketing
Advisory Council of California Breast
Cancer Research Program, 191

African American Task Force: of Bay
Area Partnership, 154; of Contra
Costa Breast Cancer Partnership, 286
African American women: in Bay Area,
153, 207, 213; Bay Area Partnership outreach and, 153–54, 157;
Bayview–Hunters Point community,
207, 214–16; BCDDP participation,
91; breast cancer incidence and
mortality rates among, 3, 155–56,
206–7, 356n9; DCIS incidence rate,
102; Essie Mormen, 204, 216–17. *See
also* race and ethnicity
"After Breast Surgery" *(Good Housekeeping)*, 78–79
Agnew, Hayes, 55, 56
*Agnew Clinic, The* (Eakins), 55–56
Agovino, Theresa, 360n28
AIDS activism, xvii–xviii, xxi, 311n5,
350n7, 350n9; comparing response
to breast cancer to, 164–68; influence
on breast/cancer activism, 172–73,
177–78, 190, 285, 362n6; mobilization of San Francisco lesbian and
gay communities, 164–66; women
and research on, 316n21

Breast Cancer Detection Awareness
(BCDA) project, 96–98
Breast Cancer Detection Demonstration
Project (BCDDP), 7, 88–95, 97; consent form, 93, 94; controversy over,
93–95; Data Management Advisory
Group (DMAG), 90; demographic
distribution of, 91; legacy of, 95;
medical history of subjects, 91–92;
misdiagnoses, notification of, 94–95;
practical and ethical considerations,
94–95; radiation risks, 93, 94;
recruitment for, 90–91
Breast Cancer Early Detection Program
(BCEDP), California, 42, 43, 147–51,
154, 155, 158, 159, 160, 162, 248, 307–8,
328, 347n30; Advisory Board, 308;
community mobilization, 348n32;
promotional materials, 150–51, 152;
significance of, 162
Breast Cancer Fund (BCF), 43, 168, 170,
190, 191, 195, 197, 211, 253–54, 328n119;
Art-Reach program, 249–50, 358n6;
Bay Area Study Group, 222–24; brief
historical overview, 174; growth and
change during second half of 1990s,
191; mission of, 174; mission of,
redefined, 253; Obsessed with Breasts
Educational Campaign, 249–50, 251;
style and strategy, 221
"Breast Cancer in Greater Bay Area:
Highest Incidence Rates in World"
(Northern California Cancer
Center), 211
breast cancer movement, xx–xxii;
activist-insider accounts of, 311n7;
biosociality and, 38–40; California,
42–43; corporate involvement in,
135–46, 161; diversity of goals and
dynamism fed by internal differences,
249; emergence from most medicalized
group, 9; factors shaping development

of, xxiv–xxv; hubs of women's
breast/cancer activism, 42; incidence
and mortality rates and emergence
of, 5–6; new forms of biosociality
and, xxviii, 281; partiality and
incompleteness of standard account
of, xxii; participation by cancer-free
women in, 281; poststructuralist
approach to studying, xxv–xxx;
regime of biomedicalization and, 281;
success in changing culture of breast
cancer, 293–94; support groups and,
121–27; viewed through lens of political process theory, xxv
breast/cancer movement: spillover from
AIDS movement to, 285; use of term,
328n117; visible pole of, 306–9;
women's cancer support groups as
invisible pole of, 301–6
"Breast Cancer Policymaking" (Weisman), 13–14
Breast Cancer Prevention Trial (BCPT),
263, 267, 361n34
Breast Cancer Quilt, 144
Breast Cancer Research Program
(BCRP), California, 42, 43, 328,
348n38
breast cancer survivor: activists, xx–xxii;
identity, 143–45, 209, 210; as new collective identity, xxi, xxix; as privileged
identity, 45; promotion of identity
of, 170; in Race for the Cure, 142–43
breasted existence, 344n57
breast health promotion: biopolitics of,
257–61; blurring boundaries between
anatomo-politics of breast cancer
and, 261–68; health-promoting
behaviors, 257
Breastpac, 350n10
breasts, cultural meaning/significance of
women's, xx, 118
breast self-examination (BSE), 78,

of deviance, 24–25, 322n75; feminist
critiques of medicine and, 323n76;
levels of, 29, 325n93; main forces
driving, 25–26; medical profession
involvement in, 29–30; negotiation
of process of, 25; as ongoing process,
30; politicization and, 305; of risk,
335n4; shifting engines of, 325n92;
shift toward theorizing gender and,
323nn77–78; social movements and,
20; theorizing (bio)medicalization,
24–32; use of term, 312n12; of
women's psyches and bodies, 25
medicalization, regime of, xxvii, 36–37,
39, 51–84; changes in, 85; danger
signals and dangerous/endangered
women, 52, 53, 65–75, 82, 83; diagnosis and treatment in, 75–80, 82–83;
era of therapeutic pluralism prior to,
36, 51, 53–59, 82; illness experience
and, 230, 231–37, 244–46; inventing
a curable disease, 63–65, 82; norms
of nondisclosure, 80–84, 279; shift
to, 59–63; summary of characteristics,
278–79; surgeons and, 52; temporary
sick role and the architecture of
closet, 53, 75–80, 82–84
medically marginalized communities:
expansion of state into and mobilization of, 146–61; mammographic
screening for, 133–34, 135, 136, 139, 140,
159, 162; practical support services
for, 190; Race for the Cure and,
145–46; treatment for, 147, 173–74;
treatment for, funding for, 159–60,
349n42
medical management of disease, 34;
changes in management of breast cancer, 268–74; medicalization of breast
cancer and, 36. See also anatomo-
politics of individual bodies/treatment
medical oncology, development of, 114

medical professions: sexism, paternalism, and patriarchalism of, 8. See also
physicians; surgeon(s)
Medicare, 100
medicine in America, history of, 55–59
Meisenberg, Barry, 357n5
Mello, Michelle M., 240, 357nn6–7
Melucci, Alberto, 10, 18–19, 20, 302,
320nn47–48, 364n10
Memorial Sloan-Kettering Cancer
Center, 315n15
Mendoza, Jenny, 195
mercury, 220
metastatic breast cancer: Herceptin for,
268; high-dose chemotherapy with
bone marrow transplant for, 357n7;
illness experience, 237; race and, 4;
support groups and, 124, 172; tamoxifen for, 116; "Walkers of Courage"
with, 183
Metropolitan Life Insurance Company,
67
Meyer, David S., 319n46, 326n101, 362n5
middle-class movements, 17
Mikkelsen, Edwin J., 326n101
Miller, Barry A., 336n6
mobile mammography van, 140
mobilization: community (see community
mobilization); of medically marginalized communities, 146–61
modified radical mastectomy, 107
Monro, Alexander, 54
Montague, Eleanor D., 334n95
Montini, Theresa, 108–9, 110, 111,
332n58, 341n13, 341n15, 342n17,
352n18
Moore, Kathryn Glovier, 339n69
Moore, Kelly, 327n103, 363n13
moral imperative, mammograms for
medically marginalized women as,
139, 151
Morantz-Sanchez, Regina, 317n21, 329n18

**Maren Klawiter** holds a Ph.D. in sociology from the University of California, Berkeley. She was a postdoctoral fellow in the Robert Wood Johnson Foundation Scholars in Health Policy Research Program at the University of Michigan, and an assistant professor in science, medicine, and technology studies at the Georgia Institute of Technology. She is currently pursuing a law degree at Yale University.